THE ART OF FITNESS

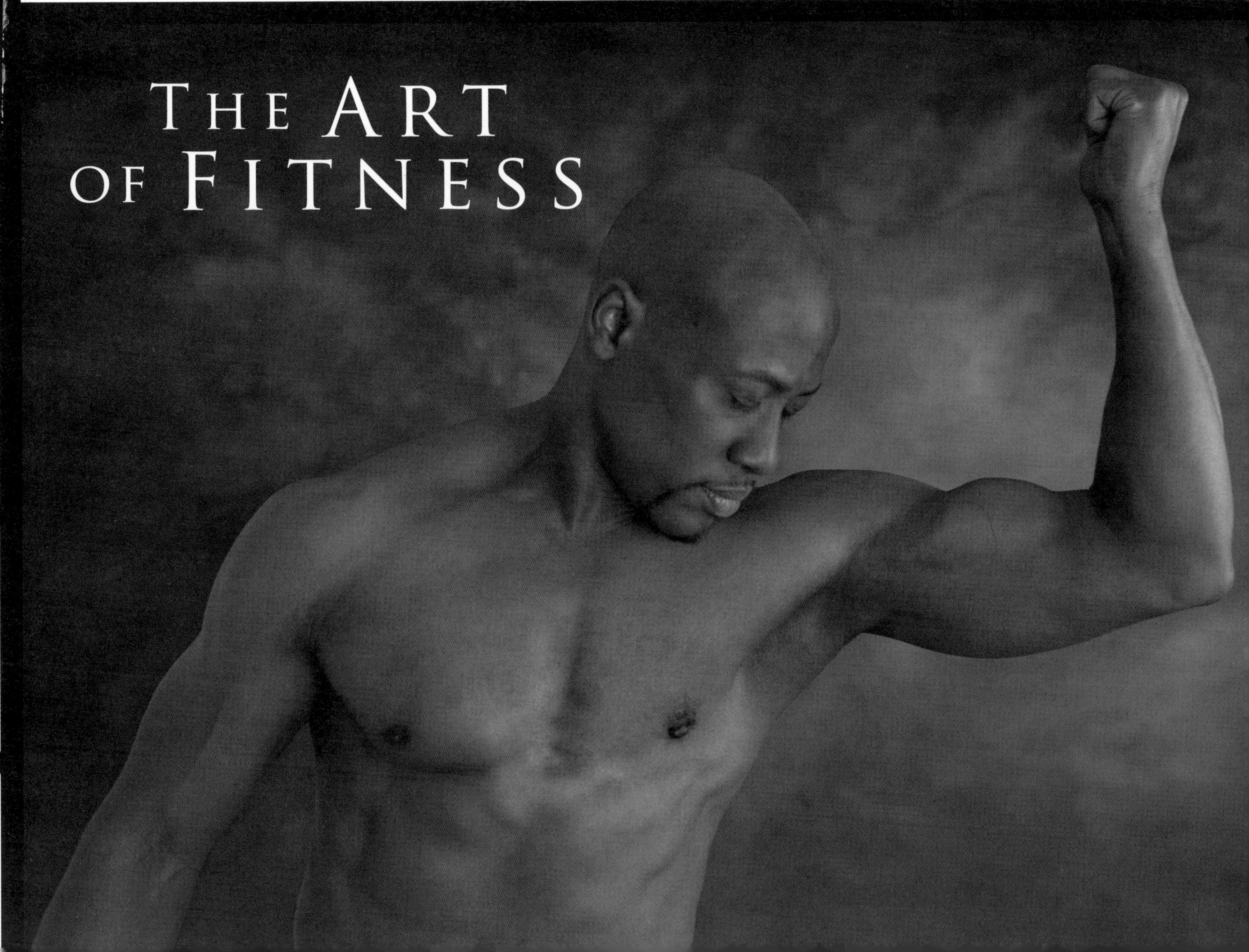

The Art of Fitness

by

D. Levi Harrison, MD

High Wisdom Publishing

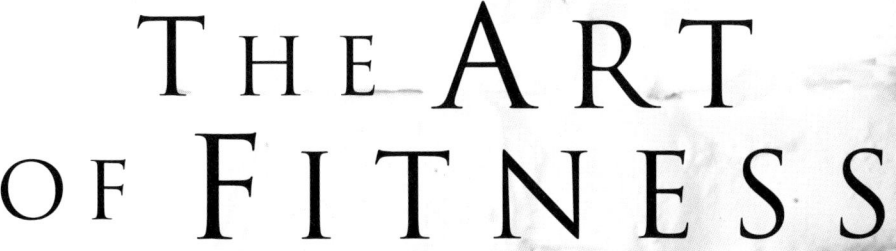

Copyright © 2016 by D. Levi Harrison, MD

All rights reserved. No part of this publication may be reproduced, distributed, or transmitted in any form or by any means, including photocopying, recording, or other electronic or mechanical methods, without the prior written permission of the publisher, except in the case of brief quotations embodied in critical reviews and certain other noncommercial uses permitted by copyright law. For permission requests, write to the publisher, addressed "Attention: Permissions Coordinator," at the address below.

High Wisdom Publishing, Inc.
3940 Laurel Canyon Blvd., #998
Studio City, CA 91604
www.highwisdompublishing.com

The Art of Fitness is a registered trademark of the Art of Fitness, Inc., Los Angeles, California.

Quantity sales. Special discounts are available on quantity purchases by corporations, associations, and others. For details, contact the "Special Sales Department" at the address above.

Orders by US trade bookstores and wholesalers. Please contact BCH: (800) 431-1579 or visit www.bookch.com for details.

Printed in the United States of America

ISBN: 978-1-943776-11-5

Second Edition

20 19 18 17 16   10 9 8 7 6 5 4 3 2 1

All rights reserved. No part of this document may be reproduced or transmitted in any form, by any means (electronic, photocopying, recording, or otherwise) without the prior permission of the authors.

Photographs by Antonio Busiello
Design by Michael Dean

Disclaimer:
The diet, exercise and lifestyle changes in this book are not intended as a substitute for any exercise or diet plan that may be prescribed by your doctor. It is recommended that you get your doctor's approval before starting any exercise or diet plan so that you can be cleared to safely and effectively begin your specific program. The information contained in this book is to enhance and supplement but not to replace proper exercise training programs. Any form of exercise can present an inherent risk of injury. Before performing the exercises in this book be sure that your equipment is well maintained and it is imperative to not take risks extending beyond your level of fitness, strength, flexibility, aptitude, endurance or training. The author of this book advises readers to take complete responsibility for their safety and to be aware of their strength and endurance limits.

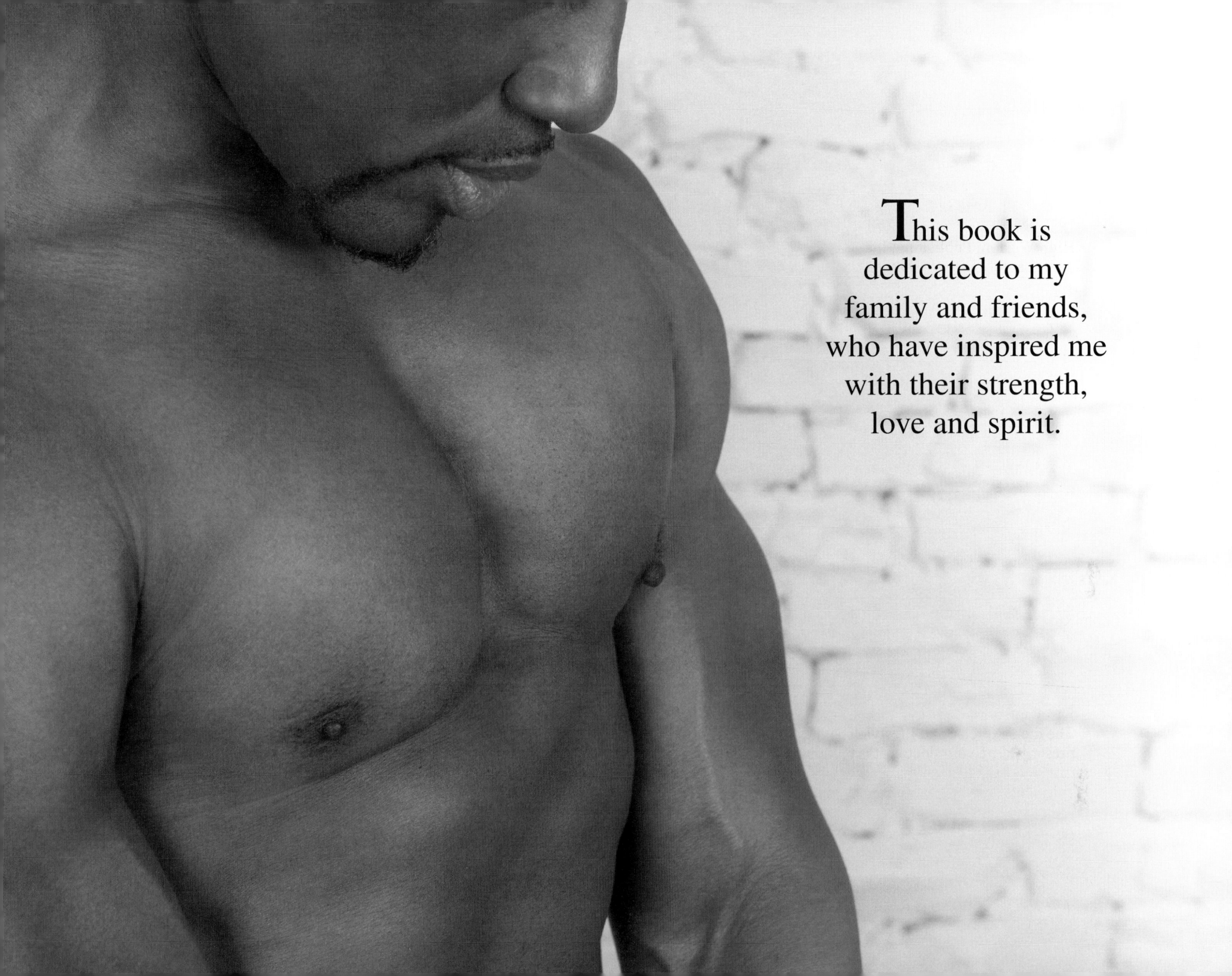

This book is dedicated to my family and friends, who have inspired me with their strength, love and spirit.

TABLE OF CONTENTS

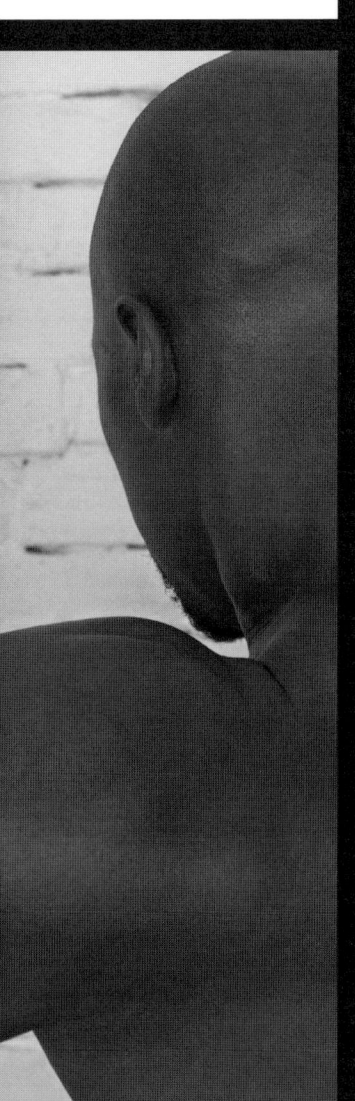

Foreword ix

Mission Statement x

Acknowledgments xi

Introduction xii

Chapter 1 • Commitment 1

Chapter 2 • Consistency 11

Chapter 3 • Exercise 15

    Section 1: Stretching and Warm Up 27

    Section 2: Arms 51

    Section 3: Legs and Gluteals 85

    Section 4: Chest and Back 99

    Section 5: Abs and Core Strengthening 113

Chapter 4 • Diet 193

Chapter 5 • Rest and Recovery 201

Chapter 6 • Conclusions 205

Gym Basics 209

Master Exercise Guide • Part 1 210

Master Exercise Guide • Part 2 216

Index 218

FOREWORD

BY REV. DR. MICHAEL BERNARD BECKWITH
AUTHOR OF "SPIRITUAL LIBERATION: FULFILLING YOUR SOUL'S POTENTIAL"

Many years ago, I coined the term *blissipline* to describe the practice of devoting oneself to a worthwhile endeavor with passion and commitment. Oftentimes, it goes against the grain to think of discipline as a blissful practice. Instead, we usually think of it as forcing ourselves to do something that may be good for us, but that we'd really rather not have to do. This, however, is an erroneous definition. To be disciplined means to be a disciple of something. In the consecration of our time, energy and resources to a noble endeavor, we carve a pathway to a greater way of being in the world.

In *The Art of Fitness*, Dr. Levi Harrison skillfully draws us into a level of deep blissipline, encouraging us to become disciples of the beauty, symmetry, integrity, endurance and flexibility that is the human body at its best. He asks us to tap into the highest potential of this magnificent instrument, which we may live as full expressions of vitality and wholeness. The exercises that he shares also have the wonderful side effect of causing the endorphin and serotonin levels to rise, creating an organic cheerfulness.

As you embrace the teachings in *The Art of Fitness*, you'll find that you're no longer living circumstantially—you're living pro-actively. These teachings can assist you in using the body temple as a living metaphor that invites health, well-being and excellence to permeate the rest of your life.

Excellence in any area of life doesn't just happen. It happens justly. In other words, there's a direct correspondence between our preparation, our practice and our outcome. The exercises in this book encourage us to live in a way that enables our daily practice to become a life-long habit. Ultimately, our habits yield an automatic competency, where we no longer have to think about striving for physical excellence. It's just how we live our life.

Unfortunately, too many individuals take better care of their car than they do of their body temple. They are under the misguided notion that the body will just continue to heal itself and duplicate cells at a healthy pace, regardless of this lack of consideration and attention. However, when one sees the body temple as an instrument that has to be finely tuned through proper nutrition, rest, recovery and exercise, then taking care of it becomes a deeply ingrained way of living. You keep your instrument tuned up.

The maintenance of good physical health is one of the developmental lines that we, as spiritual beings, have come here to practice. Some people are very developed spiritually but have allowed their body temples to deteriorate. Others advance themselves using universal principles to acquire great sums of wealth but have very little integrity, are out of sorts emotionally, or are physically depleted. The truth is that over-enhancement of any one of these developmental lines can leave the whole being out of balance.

It is also possible to use the development of one area to improve the others. For example, one can use the same qualities that helped to create a healthy, revitalized body temple (discipline, commitment, consistency, etc.) to stabilize the mental body, emotional body, the body of one's relationships or the body of one's affairs (which includes success, finances and living your vision). It simply requires a commitment to being better than you've ever been before.

The physical body is a divine work of art. Each individual is here to reflect that divine creativity by being an artist in his or her own way. It is through our joyful commitment that we take each task at hand and turn it into an art form. With this book, Dr. Harrison invites you to become conscious of yourself as an artist, sculpting your body temple. And here is more good news: The same energy of commitment and consistency that support the regeneration of your body will also contribute to your sculpting a life that celebrates all aspects of your walk on our magnificent planet.

– Rev. Dr. Michael Bernard Beckwith

Mission Statement

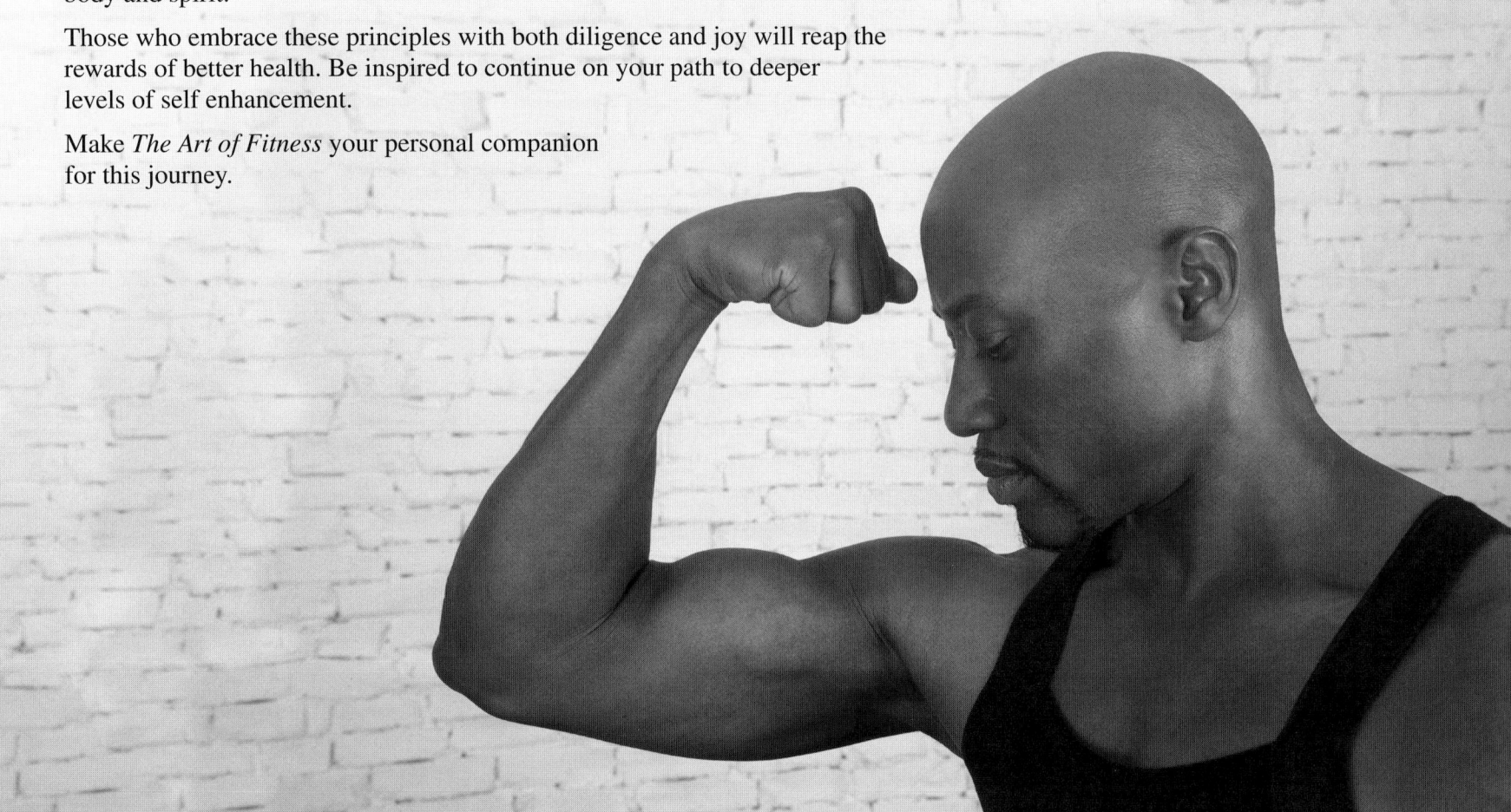

The Art of Fitness is a way of living. It was conceived to provide you with insightful and invigorating life-style changes. It has been created to enhance and improve your life by empowering you with the means to achieve a more fulfilling, healthy life. The core principles of Commitment, Consistency, Diet, Exercise, and Rest and Recovery will assist you on your journey with the hope of improving the quality and vitality of your mind, body and spirit.

Those who embrace these principles with both diligence and joy will reap the rewards of better health. Be inspired to continue on your path to deeper levels of self enhancement.

Make *The Art of Fitness* your personal companion for this journey.

ACKNOWLEDGMENTS

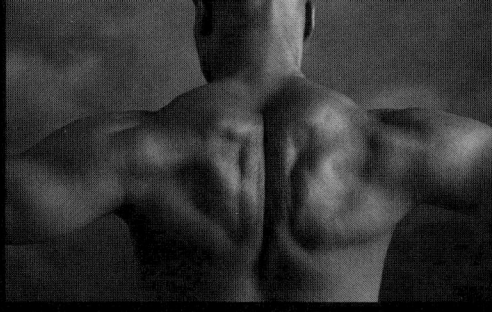

I want to thank God for giving me the strength, insight and intellect to write this book, *The Art of Fitness*, with a great team of good people. I believe it will encourage people to live healthy, fit, well-balanced and grateful lives. To everyone who makes this investment in themselves with *The Art of Fitness*, I hope it brings you joy, peace and health. God bless you.

A special and profound thanks to Rev. Dr. Michael Bernard Beckwith for his emotional and spiritual guidance. You are an extraordinary gift, epitomizing integrity, service, gratitude and love. Awesome Rev. Dr. Beckwith saw the book with clarity before I did during a conversation at The Bodhi Tree. You are my aspirational avatar. Thank you.

Antonio Busiello, the photographer, is a genius behind the lens. I am so grateful for his extraordinary ability to find inspiration, truth and strength in every image.

Michael Dean, the graphic designer, is a mastermind of artistic layouts. His insights empowered *The Art of Fitness* team to see the beauty in unstructured formats.

Timothy R. Cline, PhD., MCC, the scientific editor and consultant, epitomizes effortless, creative brilliance. I am grateful for your constructive insights.

Cynthia Ochoa, the stylist, was able to bring her timeless beauty and grace to *The Art of Fitness*. I was blessed by her perfectionism and professionalism.

I am also grateful to my office staff, Yesika Cazares and Xenia Barrios. They have been wonderful in assisting me on this journey. I thank God for them.

Thank you to my wonderful family, Williana Harrison, Dana Harrison, Alma Smith, Marie Herpin, Elvira Muse, Nathaniel Harrison, Jr., Jalene Mack, Tandra Ribet, Jacqueline Stewart, Michel Lecomte and my great friends, Joan McNamara, Todd Clark, Glenda Lomack, Elgin Charles, Jackée Harry, Justin Miller, Damone Roberts, Denise Thackston, Novella Williams, Jeffrey Joseph, Bill Stutz, The Kelly Family (Edmond, Millie, Alana and Aidan), Lynn Peters, Marina Sterner, Don Jones, Carlton R. West, Michael Harris, Joel Crandall, Judy Scheer, Melanie Braude, Mr. Jesse Reid, Danny Garcia, Garth Redwood, Margaret Cox, Lisa Nichols, Jack Canfield, Ms. Miriam Thomas, Martin Biallas, Rita Valente, Nava Ben-Isaac, Cynthia Norman-Bey, Bernadette Gilds-Pinel, Carolin Devine, Sandra Bross, Suzette Rivera, Adele Hodge and Sandra Hodge for all of their love and support. My colleagues at The Glendale Outpatient Surgery Center, U.S. Healthworks Medical Group, Verdugo Hills Medical Center, Glendale Adventist Medical Center, The University of Notre Dame, Howard University, UCLA, UC Davis, St. Augustine High School in New Orleans and USC were also great blessings. I am also grateful for Dianne Moore, Belen Conde, Mimi Dreckmann, Yelena Polonskaya, Roxanne Chacon and Ivan Ivanov.

I would like to thank the great women and men of the armed services. You are my heroes.

I would also like to thank my great teachers: Dr. Nancy Adin, Dr. Kay F. Brooks, Mr. Andrew Davis, Dr. Carlos Garrett, Dr. A. P. Johnson, Dr. William Kleinman, Sister Roland LaGarde, Dr. Melanie Lenington, Dr. James Luck, Dr. Alexander Mih, Dr. Theodore Miller, Fr. Robert Pavlak, Dr. Mark Sakakura, Dr. Don Sanders, Rev. Thomas Streit, Dr. Jeffrey Tanji, Dr. Alesia Wagner, Dr. Eleby Washington, Dr. Denise Williamson, Dr. Clarence Woods, and Dr. Colby Young. I am grateful.

I'd also like to thank Dr. Mehmet Oz for his making a difference in the medical communtiy and inspiring me as a surgeon.

Introduction

Today, you begin to reach your goal of living a life of fitness and well-being. As you begin this journey, you will enjoy the benefits of achieving your fitness goals. You can do it! We will take this journey together as you achieve and celebrate your goals. Remember that every day is a celebration. Every day is a gift. This is for everyone, no matter what your weight or size. It is important to know that where you are right now is perfect. You will continue to sculpt and enhance all that is you. So, as we go through the chapters of this book, remember to take one day at a time and to release any feelings of doubt or unworthiness.

You are worthy and beautiful as you are.

The Art of Fitness will enhance your ability to bring about greater health and self-acceptance. Take one day at a time and do not compare yourself to others. Your goals and your journey are unique. Enjoy being you. *This book does your body good!*

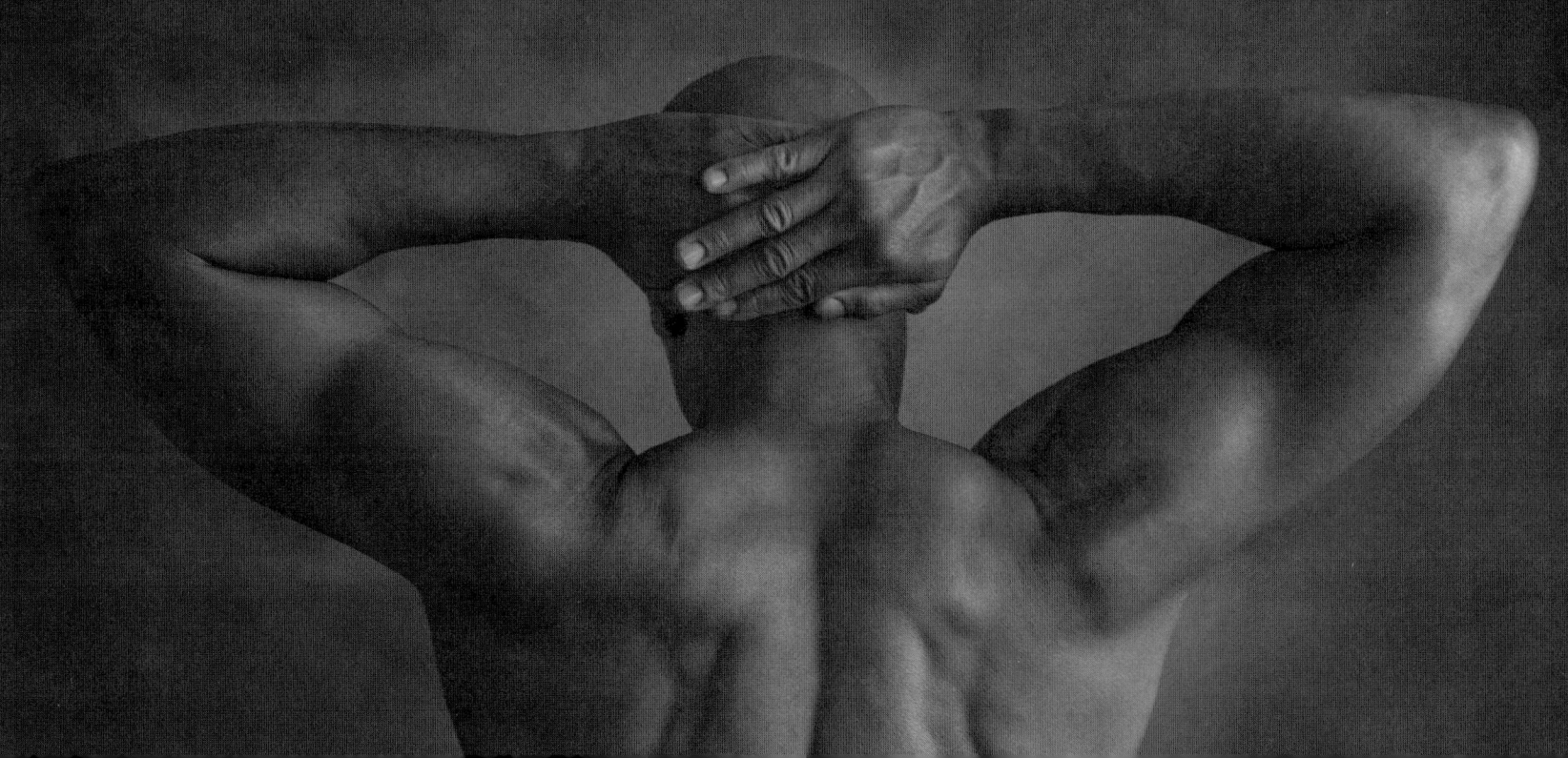

Chapter 1 • Commitment

"Commitment is the first step on the journey to realizing your fitness goals. You are on your way. Congratulations!"

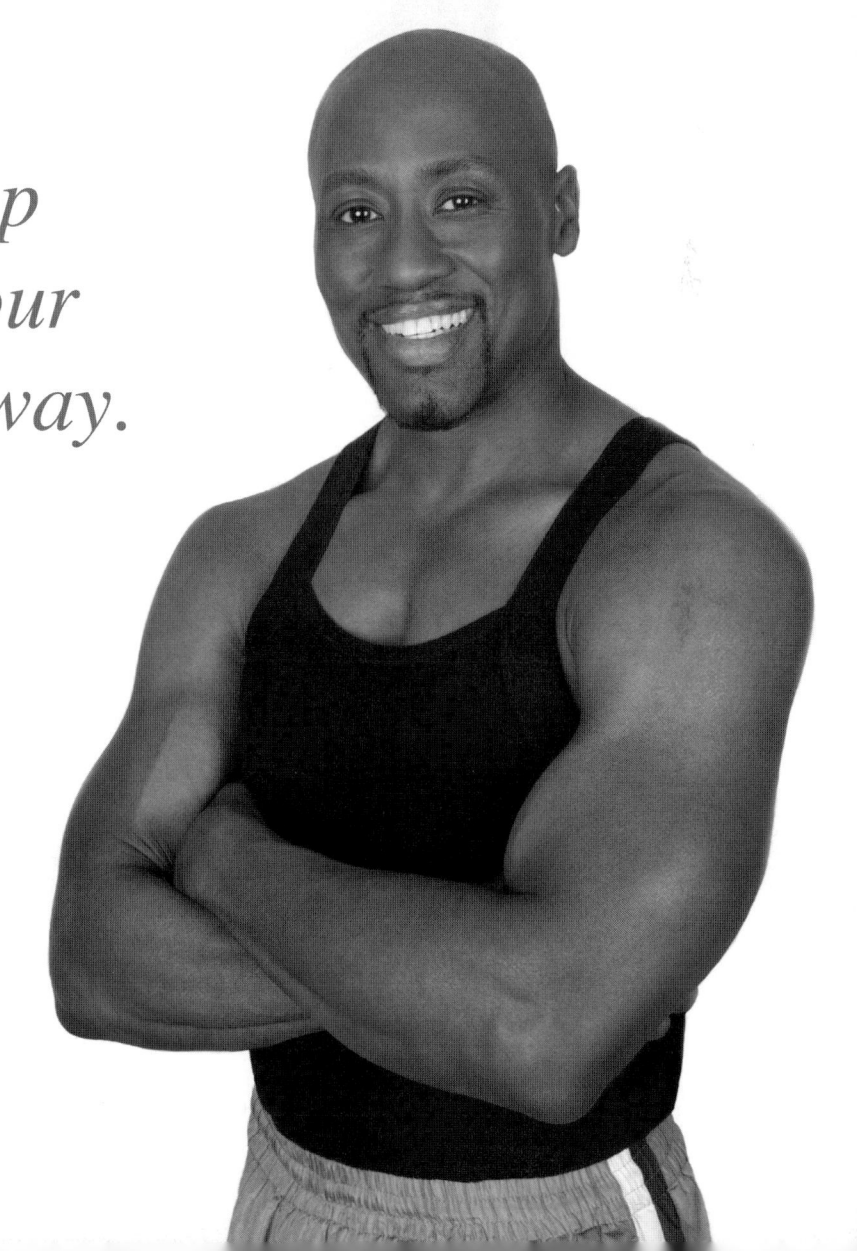

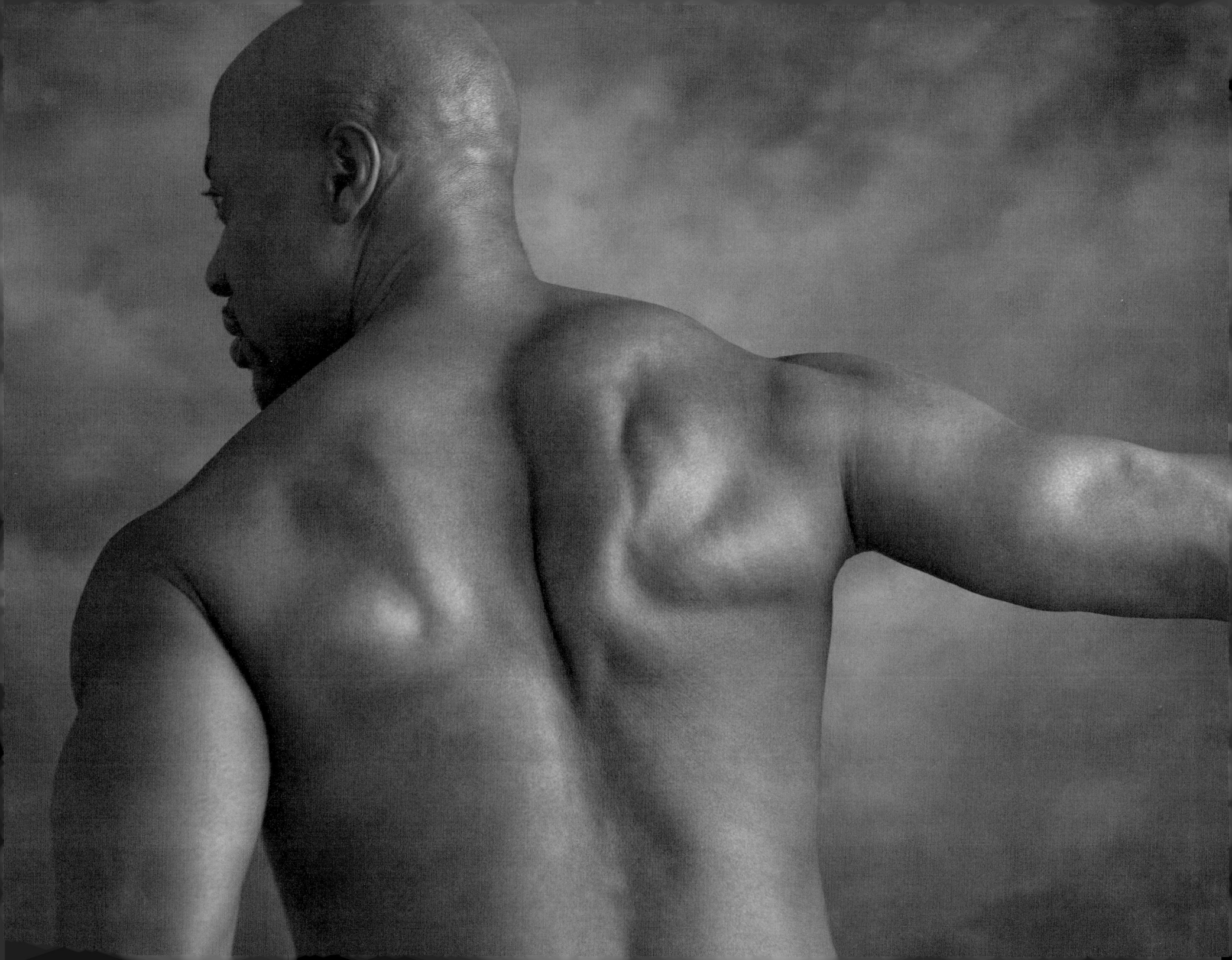

Commitment

Begin your journey by making an appointment with your primary care doctor. It is important to see your doctor before you begin any exercise program. He or she can advise you on the optimal program for your current physical condition.

I recommend a complete physical, including bloodwork, to establish baseline levels for your glucose, triglycerides, cholesterol, your blood pressure and your weight. This is important. Whatever state your body is in now, you will be taking steps to enhance your health and your life with this program.

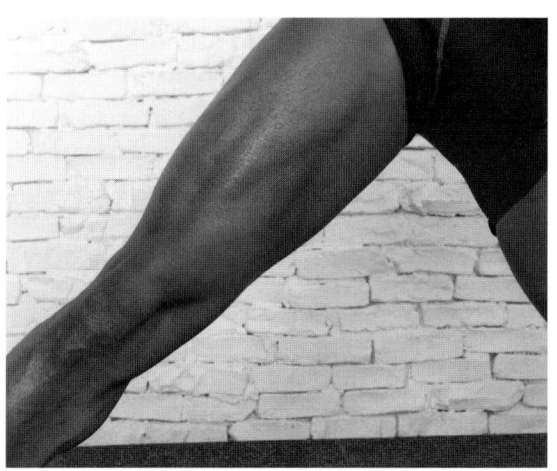

After your physical, recruit people that are supportive. This can be a spouse, a good friend, a co-worker, a neighbor, or one of your children. Support comes in different forms. It's up to you to look at your surroundings, and decide who could be of assistance to you. A workout partner will encourage regular exercise and increase the chance that you will stick to your goals.

Consider an online fitness group, a chat group, where everyone talks about what has been effective. These are great ways to achieve your goals. Start your own blog about enriching your life and enhancing your body. Your blog may motivate someone to get off the couch, start walking, join a gym, or simply go to a doctor for a physical exam. People wait years to get an examination and often have developed issues that need extensive medical care or pharmaceutical therapy.

Write down your goals. This is a great way to stay on track—to see where you've been and most importantly, where you're going. Post them in your bedroom, on the bathroom mirror, in your car or on the door of the refrigerator. Keep them on a card in your wallet. Before lunch, take them out and remind yourself why you will make healthier food choices.

Keep a journal. A journal is vitally important to achieving goals. On the first page, list your goals. The next page can be used for tracking your weight and how you plan to measure your progress on a weekly basis. Set up a separate page to record your gains in strength, distance and time, for example walking a mile in 30 minutes instead of 35. These things will help you feel good about your achievements. Write down how you feel about your challenges and how you rose to the occasion to achieve your goal. Write about the times you missed your mark and what got in your way. You can use this to help you plan for future success. Writing about what you don't achieve can provide that little push to get back on track.

Have no guilt, shame or grief about anything. Your goal is to be encouraged, to keep your journal personal, and take one day at a time, one step at a time, as you achieve your goals.

Change your routine. When you start your exercise program, walk, run, and consider a swimming program, an aerobic fitness program, or a water aerobics program. You want to do aerobic training not only to lose weight, but also to increase endurance, cardiovascular health, flexibility, and strength. You do this by creating a balanced, dynamic workout program.

To add greater versatility to your exercise program, you can change the order and type of exercises, as well as the places where you exercise. You can also consider changing the time of day you exercise. Instead of only doing strength training in the morning, try swimming or walking at that time. Variety doesn't have to mean major changes. Small changes can be enough to keep you motivated and on track.

Educate yourself about the basic food groups and how to read food labels including the amount of salt, saturated and trans-saturated fats and sugar. You will want to know what these terms mean: whole grain, salt-free, sugar-free, low-sodium, all-natural, and zero calories. The language of food should not be a pitfall for you. You want your program to be one that is super successful, that makes you feel good everyday when you wake up, and allows you to know that your commitment to this new life is not for temporary gain.

It's important that you reward yourself as you take these steps to greater fitness, and I want to reiterate these are small steps. The journey to fitness and better health is not made in leaps, but in a series of small steps over time. Start right now. With your commitment to yourself, you'll soon be in a better place. Your body will be stronger, your mind will be less stressed, and you will feel better. You will have more energy and your life will unfold with greater goodness.

The choice that you have made to become fit comes with an investment. That investment is not simply reading this book, going to your physician, buying a scale, or telling your spouse that you're going to do this. The investment is *you*. Consider this commitment you've made to exercise as essential as taking a breath. Infuse your lifestyle with fitness everyday. Even if you don't do any planned exercise on a given day, your commitment still carries over to your diet, dealing with your stress level and how you're feeling about work. Investment in wellness is not simply getting a gym membership, personal trainer, or fitness clothes, it is more than that. It's about your approach to every aspect of your life.

The things we enjoy, we do more often. The fun keeps us coming back. You may not enjoy tennis, golf or basketball. That's okay. Do not focus on what you don't like. Focus on a personal reason to exercise, like lower blood pressure, greater resilience to stress or feeling more energized. It's important that you have fun. If you enjoy walking, walk. Try to keep the best pace for your level of ability. Write in your journal how much 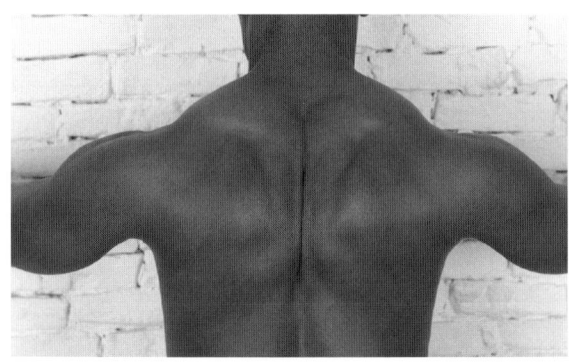 you're walking, where you're walking, with whom you're walking, and what was most fun. The fun can really be intensified as you continue exercising. You will discover new things that you like and are able to perform. Try a new sport to see if you like it. You will be exercising and that's what you want to do.

My goal is to get you moving. Movement burns calories and builds strength. Do it safely, effectively, and daily, but with enjoyment. Exercise with your kids and your spouse. Encourage them to adopt fitness as a lifestyle. Have fun!

Commitment Challenges

Many people intend to start exercising, but few of them actually follow through. In order to gain a deeper understanding of the major obstacles to maintaining a committed, physically active lifestyle, I conducted an informal survey of over four hundred individuals. My patients, their family members and other healthcare providers were included in the survey. It is clear that many people understand the benefits of enhancing mind and body through exercise and healthy diet. But it's clear that a lifestyle of exercise and healthy eating can be challenging. Listed are the top 10 responses people gave (I added number 11 as a bonus!) to the following question: "Why do people have difficulty committing to a focused exercise program?"

1. Lack of time
2. Lack of money
3. Pain caused by exercising
4. Family commitments
5. Illness
6. Stress
7. Distance to the gym
8. Laziness
9. Depression
10. Don't like exercising
11. Would rather watch TV

If you identify with any one of the above, the goal is to overcome that specific challenge and to get you moving. Here are some tips to get you started.

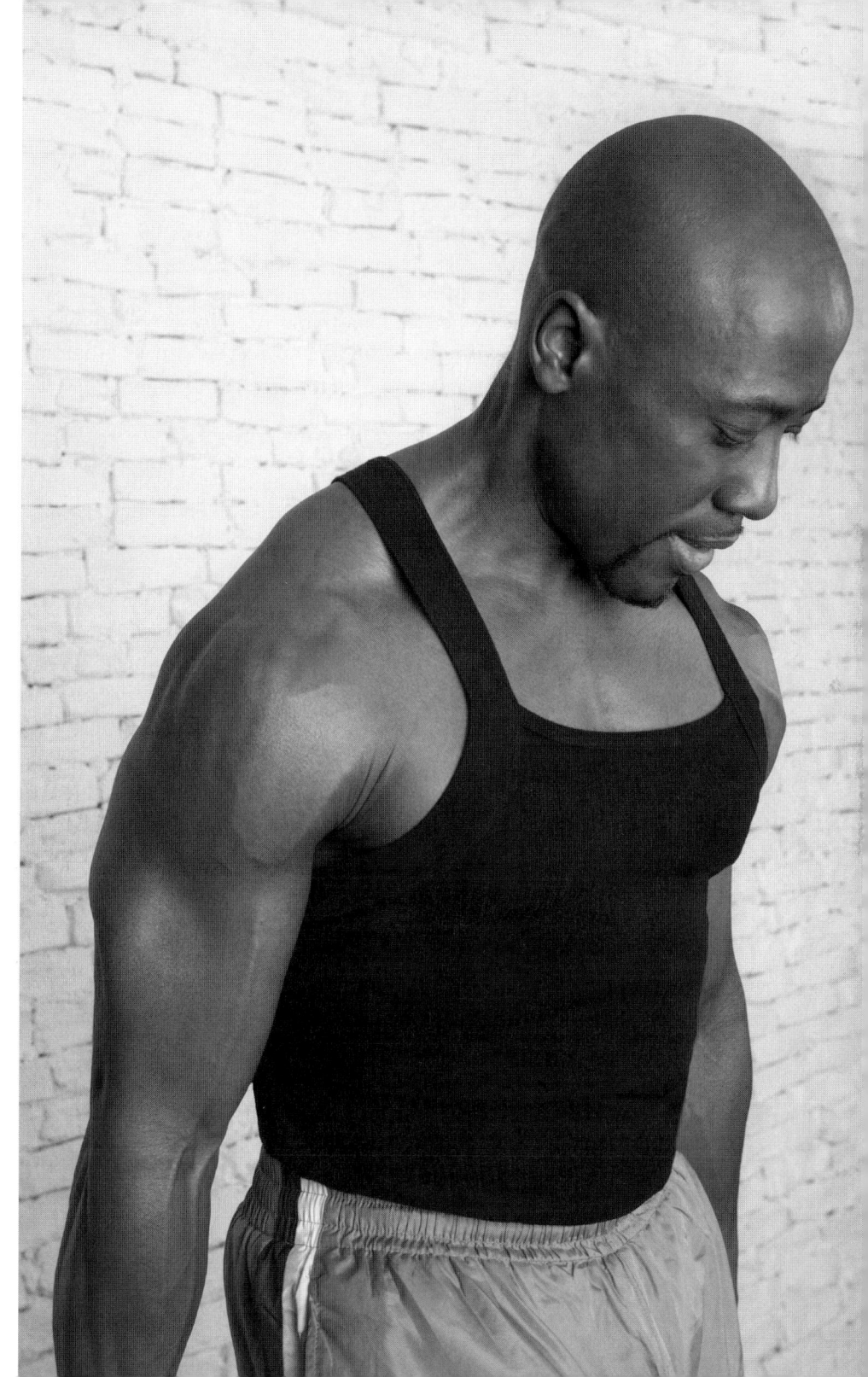

LACK OF TIME

Time is a problem for most people. Look at exercise as having the same intrinsic value as taking a breath. Prioritizing your schedule is essential.

Here are several ideas to assist with better time management.

- Get up earlier and go to the gym before work.

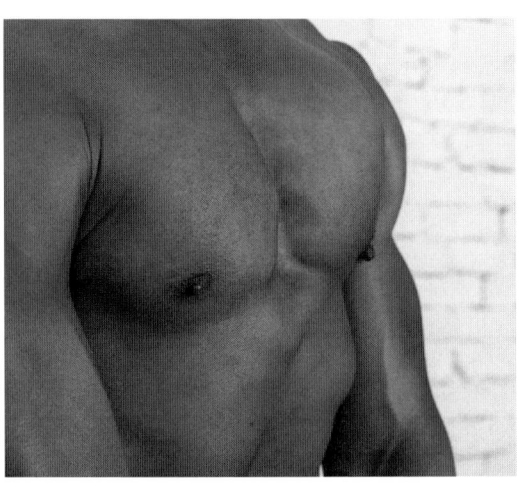

- If you are working out at home, get up and do half of your workout in the morning and the other half at night when you come home. Complete your workout at least two hours prior to bedtime so you can relax your body and calm your mind.

- Have a daily schedule that you stick to and someone that makes you accountable. The person who can help with accountability can be a workout partner. You can help them and they can help you. When you are tired or don't feel like going to the gym, knowing that your workout partner is waiting for you can be motivating.

- Consider working out with your spouse. This is not just a workout buddy or person; this is your spouse. You can work out together in the morning or later in the afternoon. Exercising with your spouse can cause you to grow closer as you both achieve your goals.

- Have your workout schedule mapped out for two weeks. By the end of the first week, you begin plotting the next two weeks. You're always two weeks ahead, which can help you to reduce stress when unexpected events occur.

LACK OF MONEY

Many of the responders said they don't belong to a gym because of money. Working out and exercising does not necessarily mean you have a gym membership. The gym is an asset and not a necessity.

You can get up in the morning and walk, jog, or swim. You can do push-ups, your sit-ups, and your leg lifts in the comfort of your home.

You can even do many exercises while sitting in a chair! Take the stairs at work instead of the elevator. The gym is not needed with any of these activities. Walk to the store in your neighborhood instead of taking the car. These alternatives remind you that you don't need a gym membership.

The good thing about a gym membership is having access to the equipment, fitness professionals and other motivated people.

If your budget doesn't allow for a gym membership, don't be dismayed. You can do very well with a few simple and inexpensive pieces of equipment. Most of the exercises demonstrated in *The Art of Fitness* can be done with a basic set of hand-held weights and rubber band pulleys.

A comfortable, sturdy pair of walking or running shoes and fitness gloves will round out your basic gear. You may want to consider purchasing a pedometer to track the number of steps you take on a daily basis. Tracking your steps regularly can increase your ability to sustain weight loss and fitness gains. Go to the website www.theartoffitnessbook.com for tips on creating a basic home gym.

Pain Caused by Exercising

Pain is the reason many people do not commit to exercise. Exercising may be uncomfortable; however, you need to understand that it should not be painful.

The human body is a very complex and dynamic system. Altering your eating and activity levels will result in many changes throughout your body. Some of those changes may cause discomfort, like muscle soreness and tightness, as your body adjusts to healthier routines. The human body was designed for movement. There truly is great joy in exercising, and pain should not be a part of the program, but discomfort may be. The job is to get you moving. That's what this book is about.

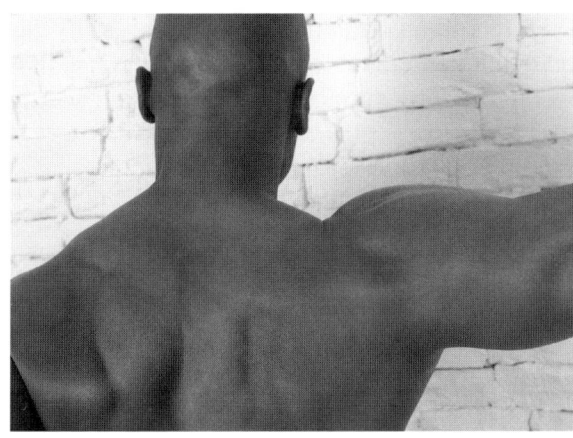

As you begin moving, there will be days when it will be slightly uncomfortable and you may feel achy. Pain is not the same as discomfort. Pain occurs when you try to do too much, too soon. Begin taking small steps to greater fitness. Start off slowly but very focused on one step at a time and one day at a time. Again, expect to feel some discomfort but not pain. The old adage of "no pain, no gain," should be "no pain, no gain, that's insane."

This book is a tool to help you reach and maintain the level of fitness you desire.

Family Commitments

Many of the responders said that they don't work out because exercise is not part of their family's routine. It's truly important to get the family involved. Getting fit together will necessitate commitment from everyone in the household. Mom and Dad are exercising and they're encouraging their children to exercise by taking long walks and hiking. Get the family involved in different types of activities such as competing in different sports. The whole family can join in a 5-k or 10-k walk for a charitable cause.

Reducing screen time, including computerized games and texting is a good start. Add activities that involve the whole family. I encourage you to look at family exercise as a healthy, wonderful and fun time. This gives time for greater bonding, deeper sharing, true empathy and fewer misunderstandings. Families that exercise together create healthy habits that can last a lifetime.

Illness

Many people said that they don't exercise because they have chronic health conditions, such as, diabetes, fibromyalgia, heart disease, or thyroid problems. If you have a medical condition or concern, it is very important to consult with a healthcare professional before you make changes to your exercise routine. A healthcare professional can help you design a program that will safely improve your health and well-being. Having an illness doesn't prevent you from exercising, but it may alter the way you exercise. It may simply mean taking a different path to achieving your personal best state of fitness and good health.

Stress

Stress was 6th in the top 10 list of why people don't exercise. Stress is not so much about what happens to us as it is about how we respond to life's challenges. We have to hone our coping skills.

- Take one day at a time.
- Do only what you can do.
- Do not feel guilty about how you're handling things—just do your best.

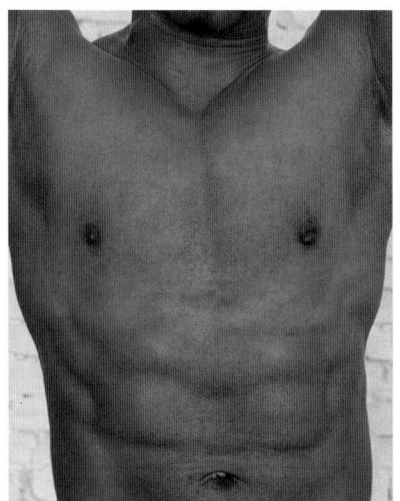

- Request help from family and friends and discuss the things that overwhelm you.
- Seek a healthcare professional about stress when you feel overwhelmed.

Stress is associated with many illnesses. These illnesses are often made worse by stress. Stress does overwhelm at times. Remember that you can't control everything. Despite your many roles and responsibilities, the only thing you can truly control is your own behavior. Practice being responsible for you. Embrace who you truly are.

Distance to the Gym

Many of the respondents indicated that they don't go to a gym, even after they've joined, because it's too far away. *This is an easy one!* Join a gym that's closer to your home, school, or work place. Make it convenient to work out and plan your schedule accordingly.

Laziness

I am grateful for the honesty of many respondents who said that they don't commit to exercising because they are lazy. Do not let laziness stop you from enriching your life.

Consider the implications of your health for your spouse or partner, your family, and those for whom you care. You may want to be able to enjoy being active with your grandkids, to share in their activities, and to be a good role model. Family can be a great motivator to overcome the obstacles to inactivity.

Think about how you appreciate your body and allow good thoughts to motivate you. *The desire for good health and longevity is self-motivating.*

Depression

Depression was also on the top 10 list. Depression has many faces. If you have been diagnosed with depression or think you have depression, get help. Many people silently struggle with depression because of its stigma. It affects many areas of their lives. There are many effective treatment options to consider for depression. Some are research based and proven, and some are not.

- Speak to your own healthcare professional so that they can advise you on medical treatments that may best meet your needs. Medication may provide significant relief.
- Consider seeing a therapist for talk therapy. Cognitive-behavioral therapy is one form of talk therapy that is especially good for the treatment of depression.
- Many people report that alternative treatments and activities such as yoga, T'ai Chi, and Chi Kung / Qi Gong can be helpful.
- *Get moving!* Recent studies show that a simple but regular program of brisk walking can be very effective in reducing the symptoms of depression.

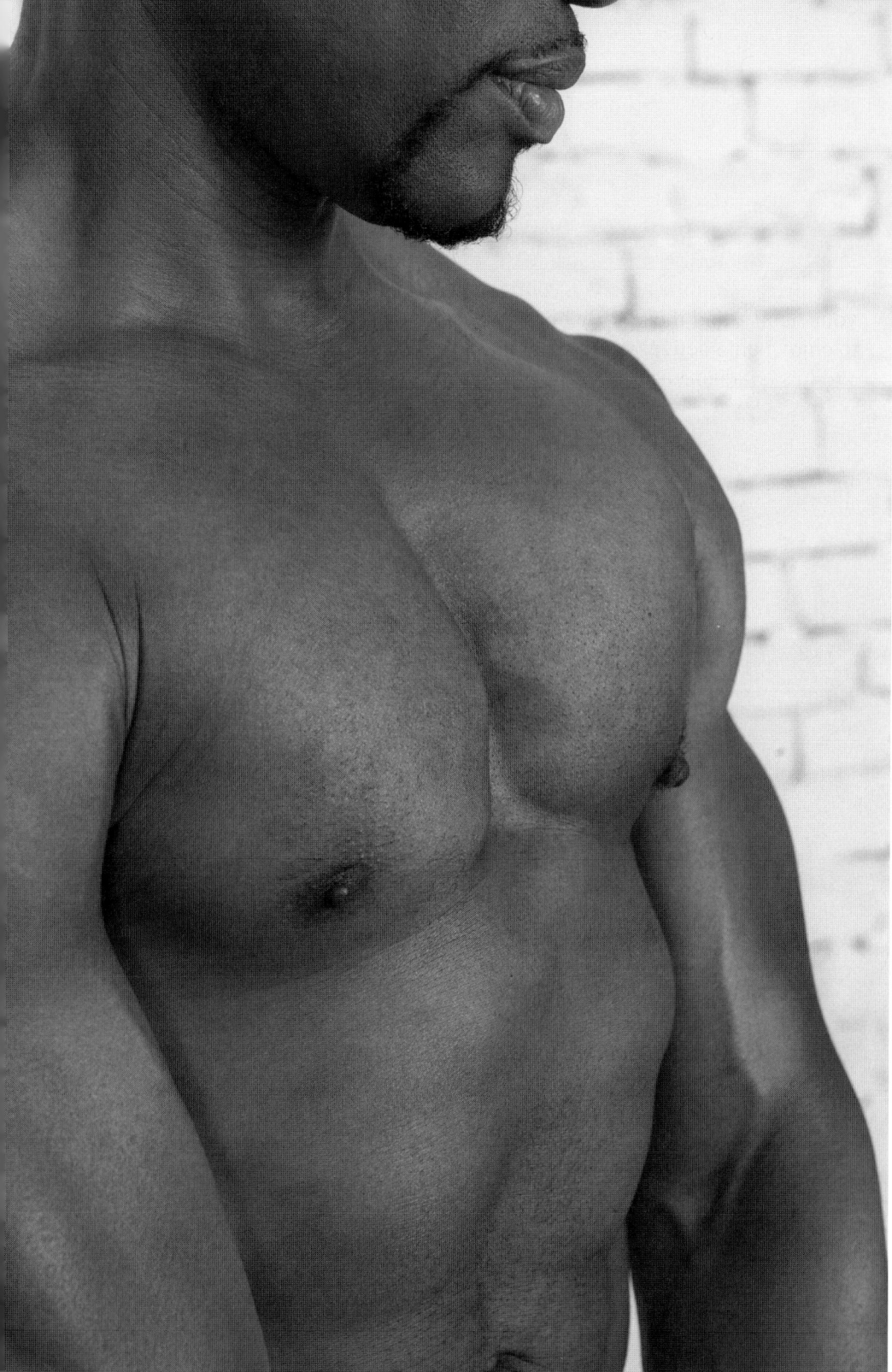

Seek professional assistance, be encouraged, and know that the healthcare communities, both eastern and western, are available to you.

Don't Like Exercising

Disliking exercise was the last response in the top 10 list. People honestly responded, "Hey, I don't do it because I just simply don't like it." Not liking exercise is not a reason to be inactive. The key is to find things you love!

Think of activities that you really like to do. Write them down and build them into a fitness plan. Create blocks of 30 to 60 minutes in your daily schedule to do the things you like.

As a kid I never really liked vegetables. However, my mom was very clear in letting me know, "That's okay, you don't have to like them; you just have to eat them." And I did eat them. And in time, I learned to love my vegetables. Not liking to exercise is okay, but don't let that stop you from staying active!

Watching TV

"Television addiction" was the 11th most popular reason people gave for why they don't commit to exercise. Even though it wasn't in the top 10, it was so high on the list and so pronounced in society that it should be discussed.

There is a high rate of "couch potatoism." Couch potatoism is resolved with one word…*activity*. Turn off the TV to simply take a walk. Your life is much more important than any television program that you might watch. As a family, turn off the television and exercise together. Get moving by walking, swimming, running, or jogging. Movement brings us to a greater place of fitness, health, and well-being. *Get out of the house, take a walk!*

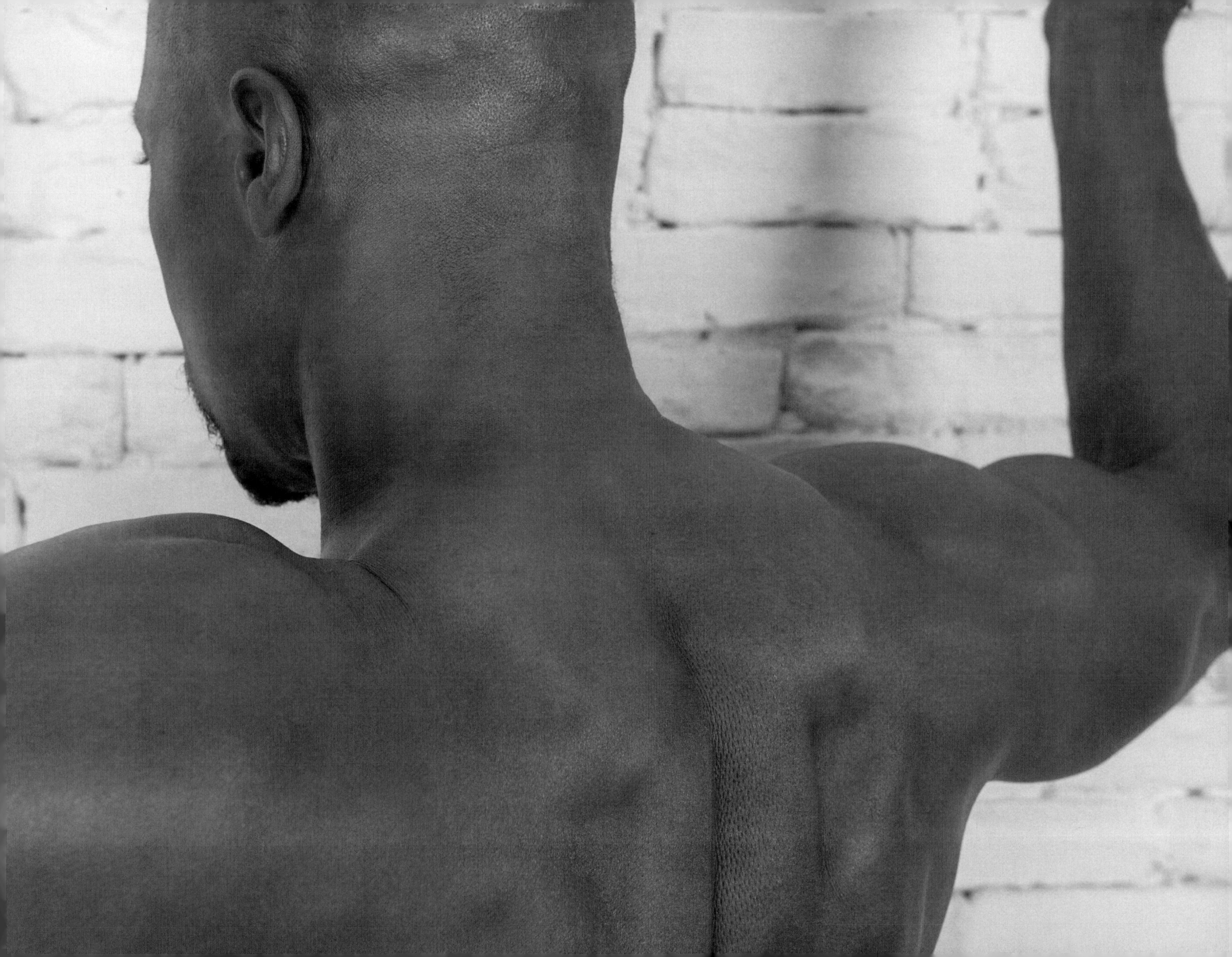

Chapter 2 • Consistency

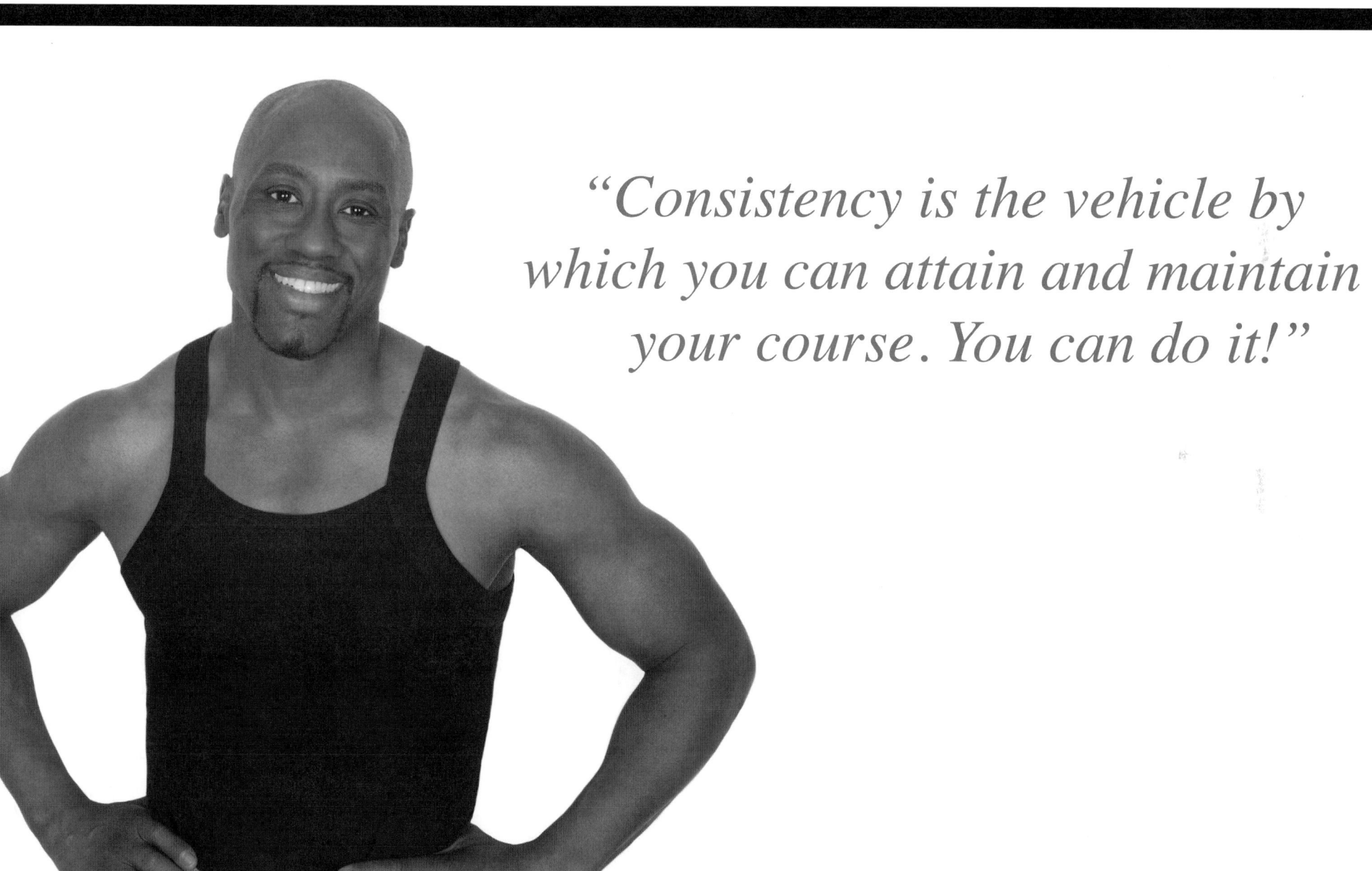

"Consistency is the vehicle by which you can attain and maintain your course. You can do it!"

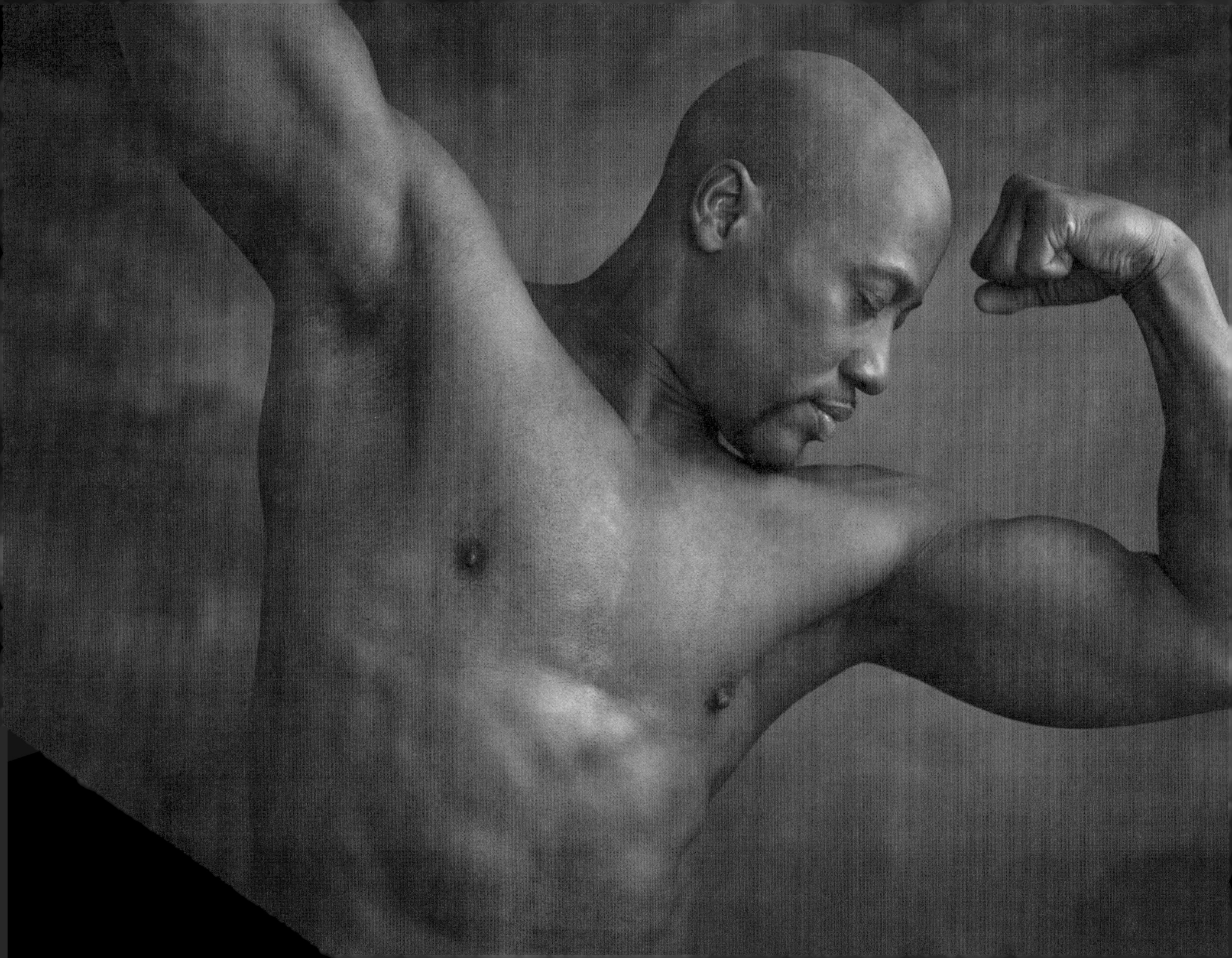

Consistency

Consistency is paramount to the achievement of health and a feeling of well-being. It is important to understand that practicing the techniques of *The Art of Fitness*, will have greater value when done on a regular basis. *Exercising creates a healthy lifestyle*. The goal is to follow your program every day. *Movement is the key*. Exercise every day. Be active every day. Small increases over time will provide big rewards.

Exercise can also decrease our stress levels. Chronic stress is unhealthy. Exercise is a known stress reducer. As we exercise we decrease our stress, thereby increasing the strength of our immune system.

With consistency, you will be able to maintain your level of exercise ability, as well as continue to reach and attain greater heights of fitness. By following a regular regimen of exercise, you will reach the goals of desired health. Exercising once a week is not a bad place to start; however, it is not the best. Grasp the idea of movement.

Recruit a workout partner. Just as it is good to have a workout partner with commitment; it is the same with consistency. Invite a family member, friend, co-worker, or a member of your spiritual community to work out with you. There is great intrinsic power in working out with someone. If you don't feel like exercising that day, the goal is for your partner to encourage you. Meet them at the gym or your home, or at their home, to exercise. If they do not feel like working out, then you can encourage them that day. The workout partner is also great if you want to take a class. Just taking a class with someone can increase the feeling that you are achieving your goals together. You will know that you are supported and that someone appreciates you.

Consistency can also be improved with Dynamic Core Cross-training. You won't get bored, the *b-factor*. This is a way to consistently maintain and elevate your fitness levels. Cross-training involves mixing different types of activities, such as: hiking, biking, walking, aerobic classes, swimming, kick boxing, mixed martial arts, yoga and Pilates. It is easy to become bored or tired doing the same exercises, day in and day out. Mix it up to avoid the b-factor.

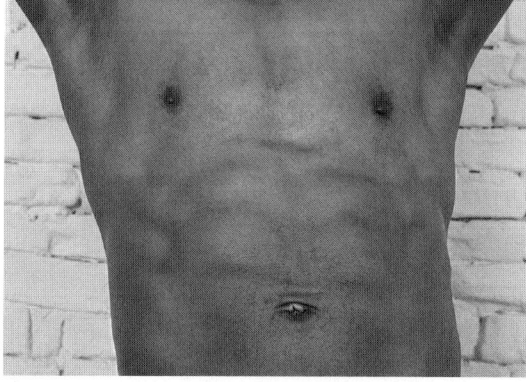

Time is a critical factor that keeps people from exercising consistently. Similar to commitment, one of the biggest challenges to maintaining a consistent workout schedule is the perception that there just isn't enough time. We addressed time management in the last chapter, but this is another area where a partner can really help.

I recommend that you always plan your fitness schedule two weeks in advance. Start out scheduling more than what you are doing now. Gradually build up to 45 minutes to an hour of some form of movement, five days or more per week. After you have carved out that period of time every day, if you have a workout partner, sit down and plan your schedules together.

Consistency will allow for improvement and maintenance of your level of physical abilities. You will see yourself reach greater heights of health. It is my hope that you are inspired to use the techniques suggested in this book. Your goal should be to work up to 5 or more days per week of physical activity. That said, truly embrace the *notion of motion*.

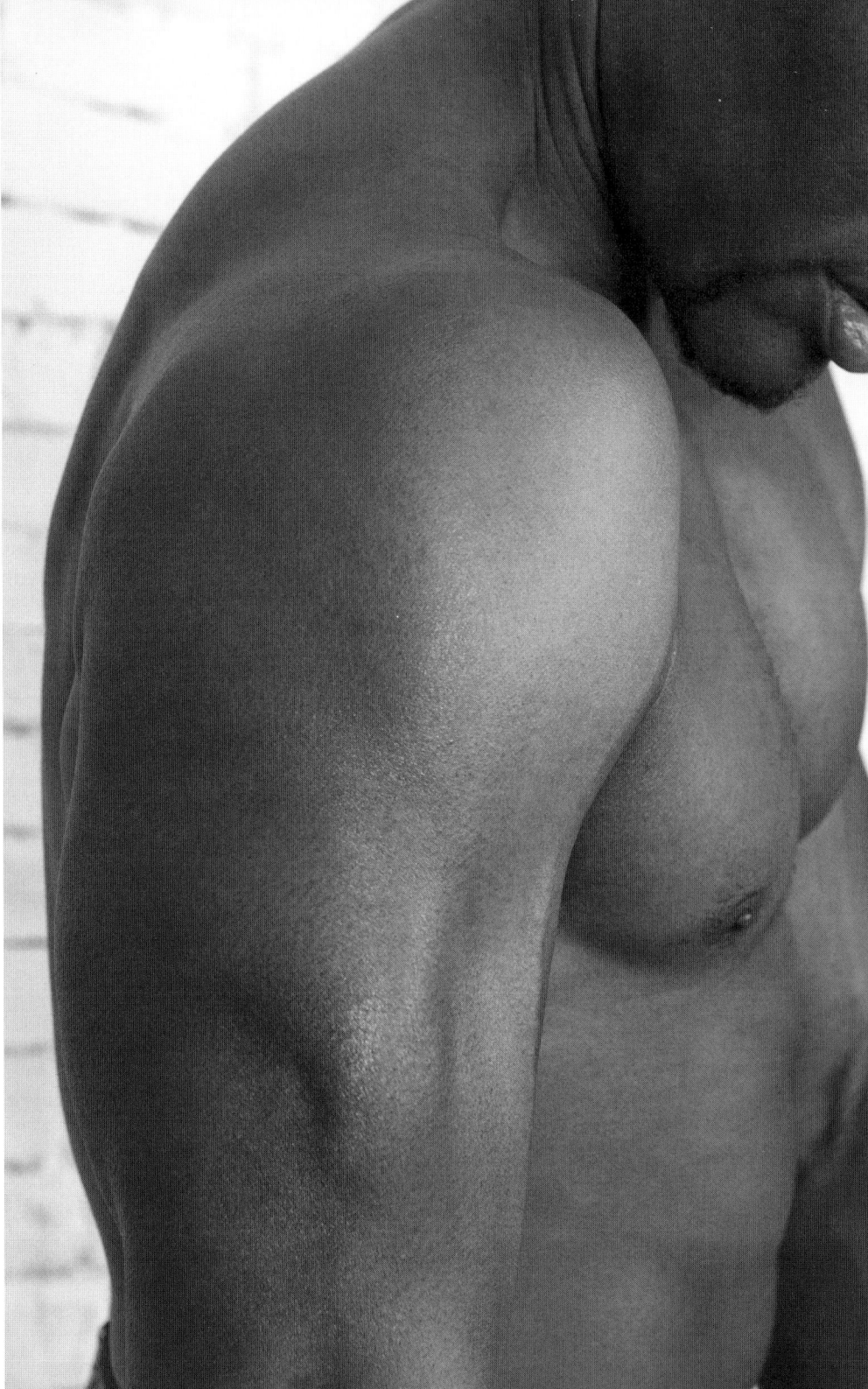

Chapter 3 • Exercise

"Exercise is essential for health and well-being. Enjoy its effects in your life."

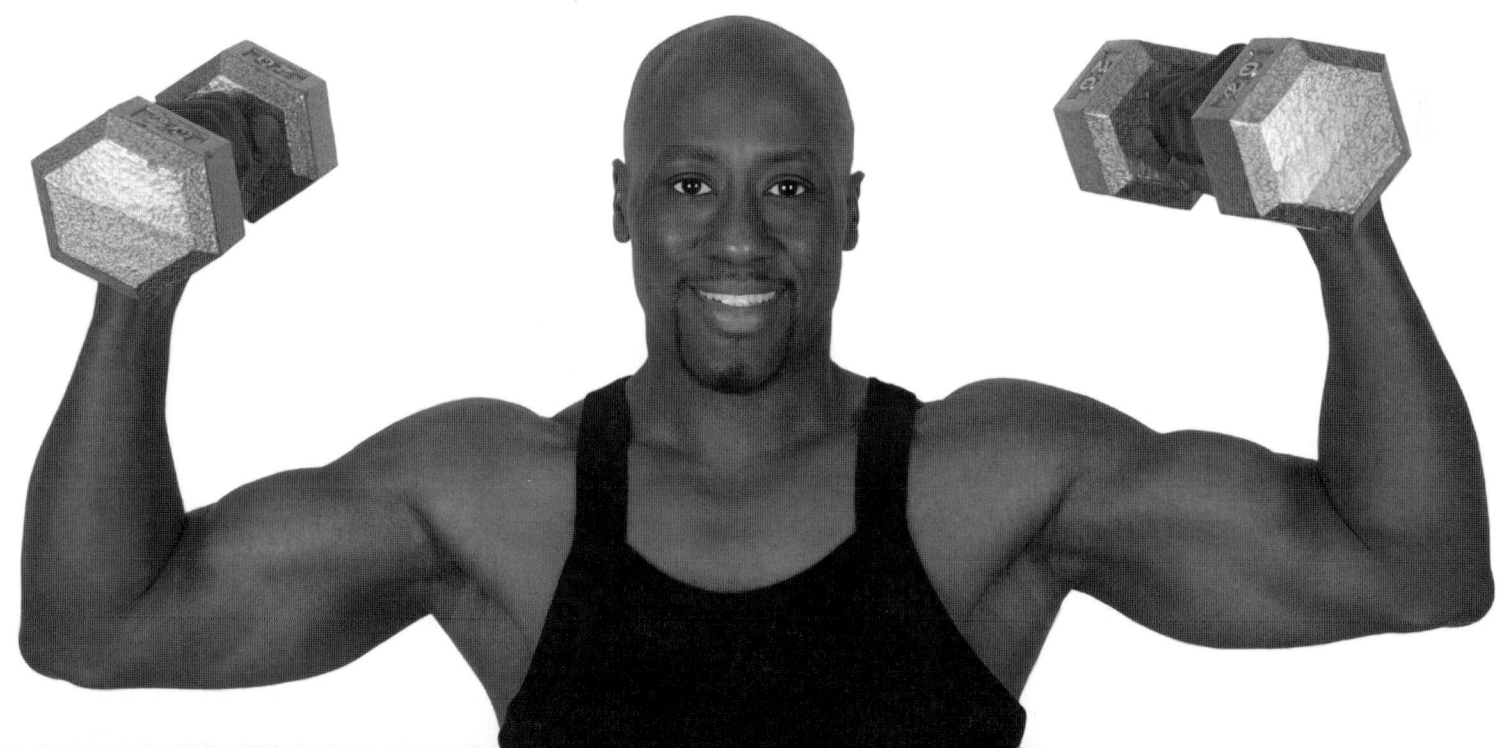

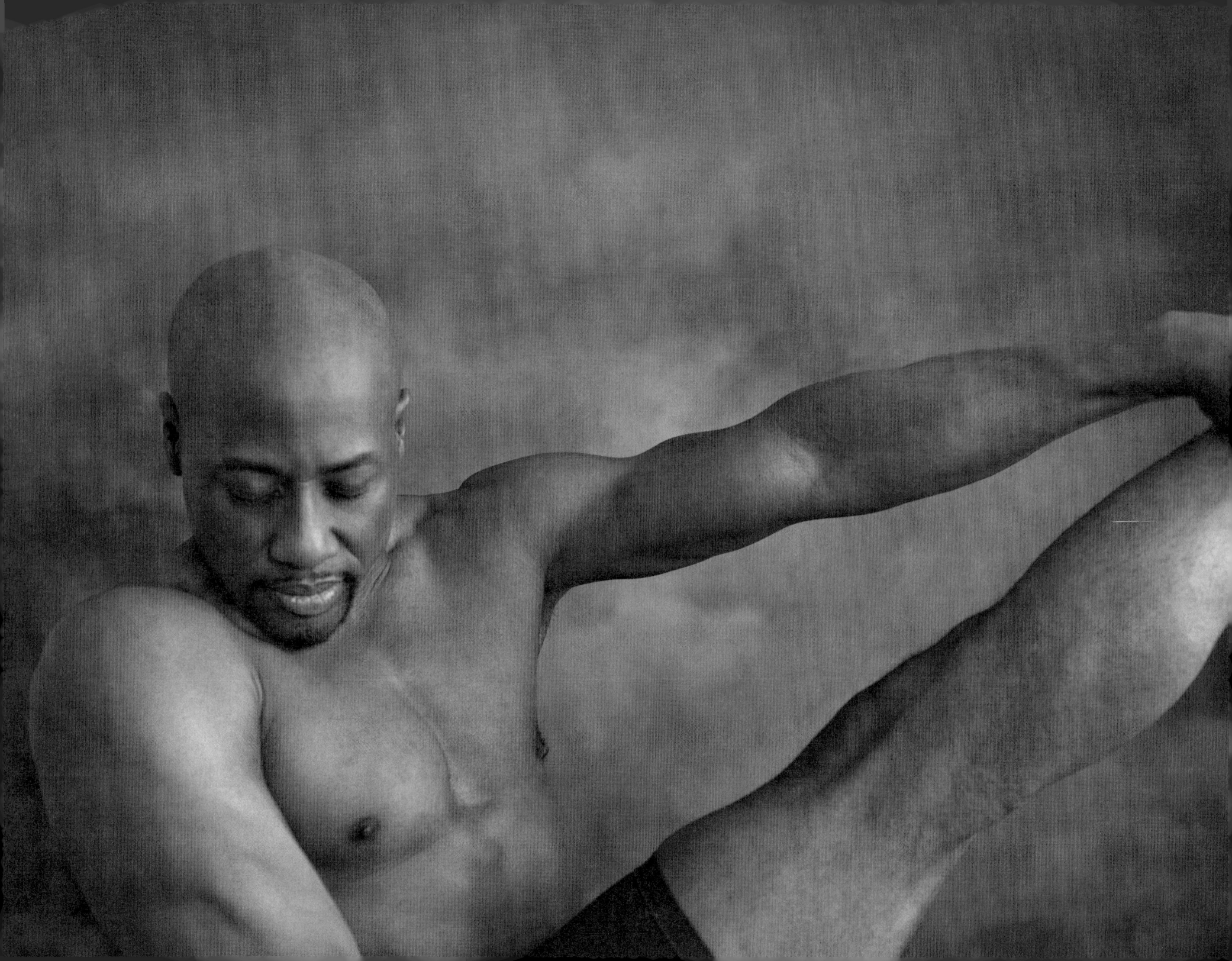

EXERCISE

Exercise is any activity that helps to improve or maintain physical fitness. For the purposes of this book we will look at three basic types of exercise: aerobics, strength training, and stretching.

The word "aerobic" literally means, "living in air." Aerobic exercise includes activities that require an increased supply of oxygen for prolonged periods of time. In turn, aerobic activities increase the body's ability to take in and to transport oxygen more efficiently throughout the body. Aerobic exercise includes activities such as brisk walking, cycling, swimming, jumping rope, hiking, and running. Aerobic exercise is good for your heart, lungs, and circulatory system. It can also support maintaining a healthy weight. When done at a moderately intense pace for ten minutes or longer at a time and on a regular basis, aerobic exercise can improve your cardiovascular endurance. This means that the more you do and the more often you do it, the more aerobic activity you will be able to do without feeling winded or getting fatigued.

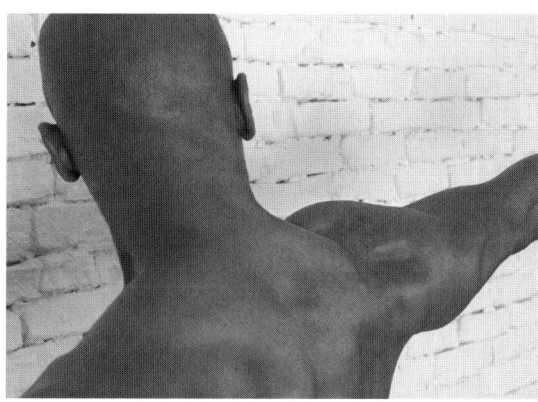

Strength training includes exercises that use your muscles to overcome resistance to movement. Resistance can be applied using only the weight of your body (such as push-ups, pull-ups, and squats) or with the aid of resistance equipment (such as free weights, exercise machines, pulleys and resistance bands). Strength training is necessary for increasing your muscular strength and endurance; the ability of your body to do work. Strength training can also increase the size of your muscles and help sculpt your physique. Many of the exercises illustrated in *The Art of Fitness* are strength training exercises.

Stretching is the third basic type of exercise, and is designed to improve range of motion to help prevent injury to your muscles, joints, and supportive tissues. Stretching increases your flexibility. There are two basic forms of stretching, static and kinetics. Static stretches involve stretching a muscle or group of muscles to the desired point and then holding that position for a given period of time. Holding still in a Yoga posture is a good example of a static stretch. Static stretches can be passive, meaning that you don't use muscular force to do the stretch. Imagine bending forward from a standing position, finger tips pointed toward your toes, and then simply relaxing to allow the weight of your upper body to stretch the muscles in the back of your legs and lower back. The seated hamstring stretch, illustrated on page 50 in *The Art of Fitness*, is another good example of a static-passive stretch. Static stretches can also be active. Static-active stretching involves using the force of some muscles to assist in stretching other muscles as they relax. Imagine doing the same stretch described above but grasping the backs of your legs with your hands and gently pulling your chest towards your legs to deepen the stretch. A great example of a static-active stretch is the Super Hamstring Stretch illustrated on page 47 in *The Art of Fitness*.

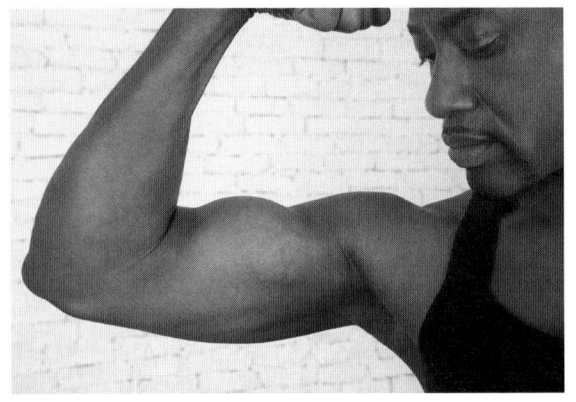

Kinetic stretching involves more than holding a stretch in a static position. Kinetic stretching involves adding various types of movement to a given stretch. This can be done many ways. If done correctly, kinetic stretching can add greatly to your flexibility. But when executed incorrectly, such as the "bouncing" method often observed in commercial gyms, kinetic stretching can significantly increase the odds of injury. To avoid such setbacks, only static stretches are illustrated in *The Art of Fitness*.

Don't hold your breath while stretching. Breathe through each stretch and imagine that you are releasing tension from the muscle being stretched with each exhalation. Finally, when doing any form of stretching, it's important to stretch to the point of slight discomfort, but not to the point of pain. Flexibility, like your overall fitness, will improve by taking small incremental steps, with commitment and consistency, towards your goals.

Basic Physical Activity Recommendations

The American College of Sports Medicine recommends doing 30 minutes of moderate intensity physical activity 5 days per week (150 minutes per week) as a baseline for all healthy adults. If achieving or maintaining weight loss is among your fitness goals, studies show that building up to 175 minutes or more of moderate intensity physical activity per week is better. And don't forget the "or more" part of this recommendation. When it comes to weight management, the more you do, the more you will benefit.

Your daily minutes of exercise do not have to be completed in a single session. Studies show that three 10-minute bouts of moderate intensity physical activity can provide similar health benefits as one 30-minute session. Break up your daily goal into smaller chunks of time to take advantage of shorter breaks in your schedule. While any amount of exercise is good, bouts lasting ten minutes or more will provide added health benefits.

Any activities that reach the threshold of moderate intensity, as defined above, for ten minutes or longer count towards your exercise minutes. That includes common activities such as raking the lawn or washing the car, to planned exercise bouts such as brisk walking, taking an aerobics class or lifting weights. For maximum benefit, a basic 150 minutes per week exercise regimen should include both aerobic and strength training activities. Remember to allow additional time for stretching. Finally, proper hydration is critically important to the overall success of your fitness program. Get in the habit of carrying a water bottle with you when you exercise and drinking frequently during and after your workout. Fill your clean water bottle before going to the gym to avoid possible contamination from contact between your water bottle and public drinking fountains.

Dynamic Core Cross-Training

Through *The Art of Fitness*, I would like to introduce you to a system of training that I believe will help you maximize the benefits of your personal investment in good health. It's called Dynamic Core Cross-training.

The benefits of Dynamic Core Cross-training include:

- A safeguard against injury
- Increased cardiovascular endurance
- Increased strength
- Improved flexibility
- Better balance and posture
- Support for achieving and maintaining a healthy body weight
- A highly efficient and effective workout

Your "core" includes muscles of the abdomen, mid and lower back, and pelvis. These muscles stabilize and align your pelvis, spine, ribs, and thorax. Your posture is determined by the strength of your core muscles. A strong core provides balance, stability and strength; and is important for everything from normal everyday activities to competing in sports.

Cross-training involves exercising each muscle group in a variety of ways to improve overall fitness and performance. Dynamic Core Cross-training combines core training and cross-training to give you the benefits of both while minimizing the demands on your time and energy.

Whether a novice or advanced exerciser, one of the first questions my patients ask during a fitness consultation is, "Where do I begin?". The answer depends on your starting point. I have included sample Dynamic Core Cross-training routines at each of four fitness levels to help you choose a good place to start. Since variety is one of the keys that sets Dynamic Core Cross-training apart from other exercise programs, I have included two different sample routines for each level of fitness.

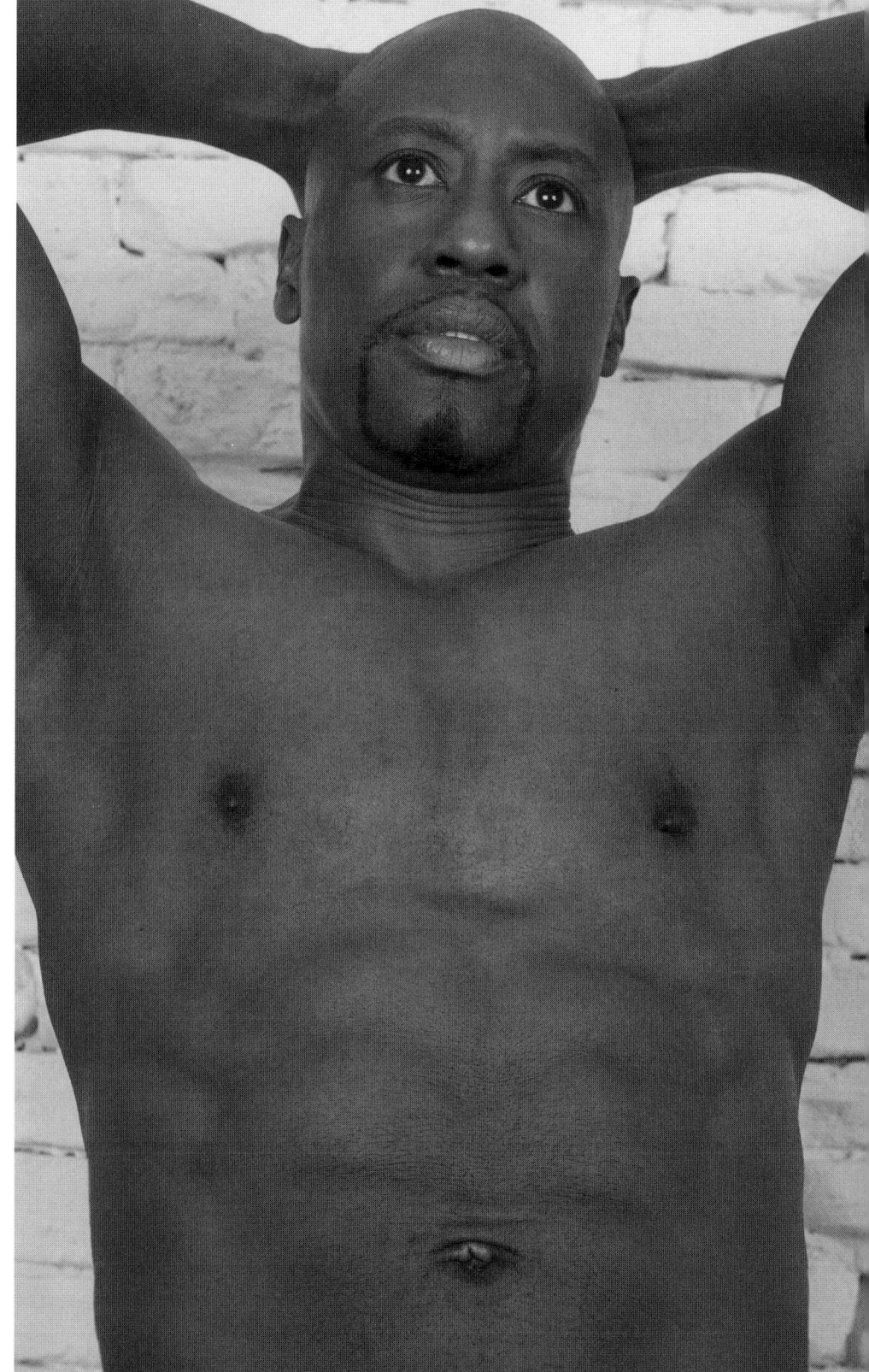

Fitness Levels

Level 1 routines are designed for the beginner. If you have never exercised on a regular basis, the first thing I want to say is, "Congratulations!" It takes courage and fortitude to venture into the unknown. Know that the rewards of shifting from a sedentary lifestyle to a physically active one are greater than those at any other exercise level. Your new commitment to self enhancement brings with it great potential to realize your fitness goals. As a Level 1 exerciser, it is essential to proceed slowly and safely. Celebrate the small successes along the way. You may not be able to start with a full routine and may need to begin with fewer exercises or fewer sets per exercise. Listen to your body as you build up to a complete Level 1 routine. Muscle tightness and discomfort are normal, especially for the beginner. Pain, however, is a sign that you are doing too much, too fast. Do more stretching between exercise sessions to relieve normal muscle tension and soreness. Your outlook on life will improve as you begin to foster a respect and love for the life-enhancing power of exercise.

Level 2 routines are for the individual who has adjusted well to Level 1 routines and is maintaining a consistent workout schedule. It is also a good starting place for those who have a working knowledge of aerobics, strength training and stretching; however, they have not been able to commit to a regular program with well-defined goals. As a Level 2 exerciser, you can expect to see and feel faster improvements as your body adjusts to a consistent and focused exercise plan that is both fun and diverse.

Level 3 routines are for those who are working out on a consistent basis (3 to 5 times per week) and are already meeting the American College of Sports Medicine guidelines discussed earlier. At this level, you are ready to step beyond basic fitness and venture into the realm of high-performance fitness. Level 3 exercise routines can be tailored to improve performance in specific sports or interests, such as tennis, downhill or cross-country skiing, and soccer, to name a few.

Level 4 routines are for individuals that far exceed the stated exercise guidelines for general health and well-being. These individuals are likely to be referred to as "elite" athletes. Level 4 exercisers are committed to their fitness and performance goals. Their commitment is evidenced by years of consistent, vigorous physical training.

The goal is to maximize the investments of time and energy to reach the highest levels of fitness and athletic achievement.

Now that I have defined the four exercise levels, I present two sample routines that are appropriate for each:

Level 1

Routine A

Aerobics: 10 minutes of brisk walking

Stretch: 3-5 repetitions each:
- Lateral neck side bends
- Neck and torso stretch
- Shoulder shrugs
- Right and left side bends
- Calf stretch
- Hamstring stretch

Legs: 2 sets of 5 repetitions each:
- Bench squat without weights

Chest: 2 sets of 5 repetitions each:

- Standard bench press
- Incline bench press

Core: 2 sets of 10 repetitions:
- Regular abdominal crunches

Stretch: 3-5 repetitions each:
- Lateral neck side bends
- Neck and torso stretch
- Shoulder shrugs
- Right and left side bends
- Calf stretch
- Hamstring stretch

Routine B

Aerobics: 15 minutes of brisk walking

Stretch: 2 sets of 3-5 repetitions each:
- Shoulder shrugs
- Right and left side bends
- Shoulder and back stretch
- Combined quadriceps, hamstrings and back stretch

Legs: 2 sets of 5 repetitions:
- Bench squats with hand weights

Back: 2 sets of 10 repetitions each:
- Rhomboid rows
- Lateral rhomboid raises

Core: 2 sets of 5 repetitions each:
- Short medicine ball twists
- Elevated leg crunches

Stretch: 2 sets of 3-5 repetitions each:
- Anterior and posterior shoulder rolls
- Right and left side bends
- Torso and oblique stretch

LEVEL 2

Routine A

Aerobics: 20 minutes of brisk walking, jogging, running, cycling or swimming

Stretch: 2 sets of 3-5 repetitions:
- Lateral neck stretch
- Shoulder and arm overhead stretch
- Right and left side bends
- Calf stretch
- Hamstring stretch

Legs: 2 sets of 5-10 repetitions:
- Wide squats with hand weights

Chest: 2 sets of five repetitions:
- Triangle push-ups

Arms: 5-10 repetitions:
- Biceps curls
- Triceps kickbacks
- Rotator cuff stabilizing side raises

Core: 2 sets of 5-10 repetitions:

- Medicine ball side twists
- Regular abdominal crunches

Shadow box: A set of 10 repetitions each:

- The jab, the cross, the hook and the upper cut

Stretch: 2 sets of 3-5 repetitions:

- Seated hamstring and calf stretch
- Shoulder shrugs
- Triceps stretch
- Torso stretch

Routine B

Aerobics: 25 minutes of brisk walking, jogging, running, cycling or swimming

Stretch: 2 sets of 3-5 repetitions:

- Lateral neck side bends
- Shoulder shrugs
- Deep lateral side bends and torso stretch
- Trapezium and neck stretch
- Seated hamstring and calf stretch

Legs: 2 sets of 5-10 repetitions:

- Combined upright rows and squats
- Bench squats with hand weights

Chest: 2 sets of 5-10 repetitions:

- Triangle push-ups
- Standard BOSU ball plank and push-up

Back: 2 sets of 5-10 repetitions:

- Lateral rhomboid raises

Arms: 2 sets of 5-10 repetitions:

- Rotator cuff stabilizing side raises
- Combination biceps curls and shoulder press
- Triceps kickbacks

Core: 2 sets of 5-10 repetitions:

- Knee raises
- Regular abdominal crunches
- Extended leg crunches

Stretch: 2 sets of 3-5 repetitions:

- Lateral neck side bends
- Shoulder shrugs
- Deep lateral side bends and torso stretch
- Trapezium and neck stretch
- Seated hamstring and calf stretch
- Quadriceps stretch
- Hamstring stretch

LEVEL 3

Routine A

Aerobics: 30 minutes of jogging, running, cycling, swimming, or jumping rope

Stretch: 2 sets of 3-5 repetitions:

- Deep lateral side bends and torso stretch
- Lateral neck side bends

- Combined quadriceps, hamstring and calf stretch

Legs: 2-3 sets of 10 repetitions:
- Leg extensions
- Hamstring curls
- Bench squats with weights

Chest: 2 sets of 5-10 repetitions
- Spider push-up
- BOSU ball plank and push-ups

Back: 2 sets of 5-10 repetitions:
- Roman chair back extensions
- Posterior deltoid rows
- Combined rhomboid rows and triceps kickbacks

Arms: 2-3 sets of 10 repetitions:
- Combined biceps curls and shoulder press
- Triceps kickbacks
- Rotator cuff stabilizing side raises
- Anterior and posterior wrist curls

Core: 2 sets of 10 repetitions:
- Balance plank
- Elevated leg crunches
- Extended leg crunches

Stretch: 2 sets of 3-5 repetitions:
- Quadriceps, hamstring & calf stretch combined
- Triceps stretch and torso stretch

Routine B

Aerobics: 30 minutes of jogging, running, swimming, cycling or jumping rope

Stretch: 2 sets of 3-5 repetitions:
- Back stretch
- Seated hamstring and calf stretch
- Right and left side bends
- Lateral neck stretches

Legs: 3 sets of 10 repetitions:
- Combined upright rows and squats
- Hamstring curls
- Leg extensions
- Forward standing calf raises

Back: 2 sets of 5-10 repetitions:
- Front one-arm dumbbell lat rows
- Lateral one-arm dumbbell lat rows
- Combined rhomboid rows and triceps kickbacks

Arms: 2-3 sets of 10-15 repetitions:
- Seated biceps hammer curls
- Inner biceps curls
- Chair triceps dips
- Anterior deltoid raises
- Posterior deltoid raises
- Rotator cuff stabilizing side raises

Core: 3-5 sets of 10 repetitions:
- Mountain climbers
- Triceps triangle push-ups
- Same-side plank and knee lifts
- Extended leg crunches
- Seated leg lifts

Stretch: 2 sets of 3-5 repetitions

- Shoulder and arm overhead stretch
- Shoulder and back stretch
- Triceps and torso stretch
- Quadriceps stretch
- Hamstring stretch

Level 4

Routine A

Aerobics: 30 minutes of running, jumping rope, power cycling, swimming, stair climbing or other intense cardio training of your choice

Stretch: 3 sets of 3-5 repetitions:

- Right and left side bends
- Trapezium and neck cervical stretch
- Super hamstring stretch and balance
- Quadriceps stretch

Legs: 3 sets of 10-15 repetitions:

- Leg extensions
- Hamstring curls
- Combined upright rolls and squats
- Bench assisted lunge

Back: 3 sets of 10 repetitions:

- Combined rhomboid rows and triceps kickbacks
- Front one-arm dumbbell lat rows
- Lateral one-arm dumbbell lat rows

Arms: 3-5 sets of 10-15 repetitions:

- Seated biceps hammer curls
- Combined biceps curl and shoulder press
- Triceps kick backs
- Overhead triceps extensions
- Rotator cuff stabilizing side raises
- Posterior and anterior wrist curls

Core: 3 sets of 5-10 repetitions:

- Exchange medicine ball push-ups
- Same-side plank and knee lifts
- BOSU ball plank
- Combined V-ups and leg lifts

Stretch: 3 sets of 3-5 repetitions:

- Right and left side bends
- Trapezium and neck cervical stretch
- Super hamstring stretch and balance
- Quadriceps stretch

Routine B

Aerobics: 30 minutes of running, jumping rope, power cycling, swimming, stair climbing or other intense cardio training of your choice

Stretch: 2 sets of 3-5 repetitions:

- Shoulder shrugs
- Quadriceps stretch
- Hamstring stretch
- Quadriceps, hamstring & calf stretch combined

Shadow box: A set of 10 repetitions each:

- The jab, the cross, the hook and the upper cut

Legs: 3 sets of 10-15 repetitions:
- Wide squats with weights
- Leg extensions
- Hamstring curls

Chest: 3 sets of 10 repetitions:
- Decline bench press
- Incline bench press

Arms: 3-5 sets of 10 repetitions:
- Combination of biceps curl and shoulder press
- Seated inner leg biceps curls
- Overhead triceps extensions
- Combined front deltoid rows and lateral triceps extensions

Core: 2 sets of 10 repetitions:
- Medicine ball side twists
- BOSU ball flying push-ups
- Overhead leg lifts
- Captain's Chair knee lift & leg extensions

Stretch: 3 sets of 3-5 repetitions:
- Super hamstring stretch
- Lateral super hamstring stretch
- Back stretch
- Seated hamstring and calf stretch
- Triceps and torso stretch

Building Your Own Dynamic Core Cross-Training Program

As you can see from the sample routines, there is a repeating pattern, or sequence of segments, to each Dynamic Core Cross-training session. I have witnessed the best results in myself and in my patients when adhering to this regimen. Remember, start slowly and build up.

Aerobics: Start with an aerobic activity that you like such as brisk walking, hiking, running, or swimming; however, switch to a different form of activity every 2 to 3 weeks. I prefer doing 2 or 3 different types of aerobic activities each week so that I don't get bored. In addition to providing cardiovascular conditioning, beginning with aerobics increases the circulation of blood and oxygen supply to your muscles, warming them up for the activities to follow.

Stretch: The initial stretches serve as a cool down from the aerobics as well as continuing to prepare muscles for the more intense strength training exercises.

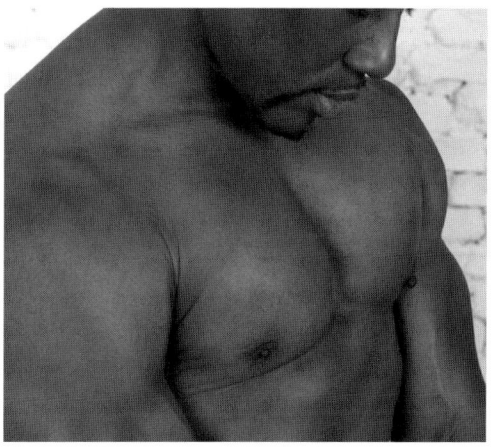

Strength Training: Choose 2 basic strength training exercises for each selected muscle group. Do 2-3 sets of each exercise, with 8-12 repetitions per set. The muscle groups include legs (quadriceps, hamstrings, and calves), chest, back, arms (deltoids, biceps, and triceps), and core (abdominals, mid and lower back, and pelvic muscles). Please note the following tips for strength training:

- Always work larger muscle groups (legs, chest, and back) before doing the smaller ones (arms).
- Save core exercises for the end of your strength training segment.
- Never hold your breath while training. Inhale as you contract

your muscles and exhale as you return to the starting position.

- Rest no more than 1 minute between sets when using lighter resistance and no more than 2-3 minutes when using maximum resistance.
- Start with lower resistance than you think you need and work up gradually. Add weight (resistance) when you can complete at least 10 repetitions of an exercise while maintaining perfect form and posture. Log in your journal all completed exercises as well as the number of sets, reps, and the weight/resistance used. By logging your progress, you can monitor the increase in strength gains.

Stretch: The final stretches serve to open circulation to the muscle groups just worked. This aids muscle recovery and helps prevent injuries from excessive tightness. The final stretches also serve as a cool-down from your workout session and a transition to the next part of your day. Choose 2 or 3 stretches and perform them after the strength training. Include stretches for the muscle groups you worked that day. Hold each stretch for 15-30 seconds. Avoid bouncing during the stretches. Do them in a slow, controlled manner. Go at your own pace. Remember, you are doing this for you. Do not worry about comparing your flexibility to anyone else. You will reach your goal.

As a bonus, add in some extra stretches that you can do outside of your exercise routine. At work, choose some stretches you can do at your desk during breaks. While at home, stretch during commercials when treating yourself to your favorite TV program.

You can customize the sample routines presented earlier and tailor them to your interests, schedule and fitness goals. Simply trade out any exercises from the sample routines with level-appropriate ones from the extensive list of exercises illustrated in *The Art of Fitness*. This book provides you with the ability to add infinite variety and texture to your workout routines and to always keep them fresh.

Working different body parts on different days of the week is another way to add diversity, for example:

Mondays and Thursdays: Chest, shoulders, triceps and core.

Tuesdays and Fridays: Back, biceps, and core.

Wednesdays and Saturdays: All leg muscles and core.

Sunday: Simply have fun doing any activity during your exercise time.

There are also a wide variety of abdominal and core exercises to choose from in *The Art of Fitness*. Remember to be versatile and change your aerobic exercises every two or three weeks as well. Why not try jumping rope? Most of us did this when we were kids, so why not remember those fun times!

Finally, I recommend that you aim to build up to:

- **Thirty minutes of aerobic activity per day to provide a cardiovascular benefit and 30 minutes of core and strength training.** The 30 minutes of aerobic activity can be split into two 15 minute or three 10 minute intervals.
- **One hour of exercise on a daily basis.** This can be divided into two 30 minute intervals or one 30 minute plus two 15 minute intervals.

Exercise your way to greater fitness!

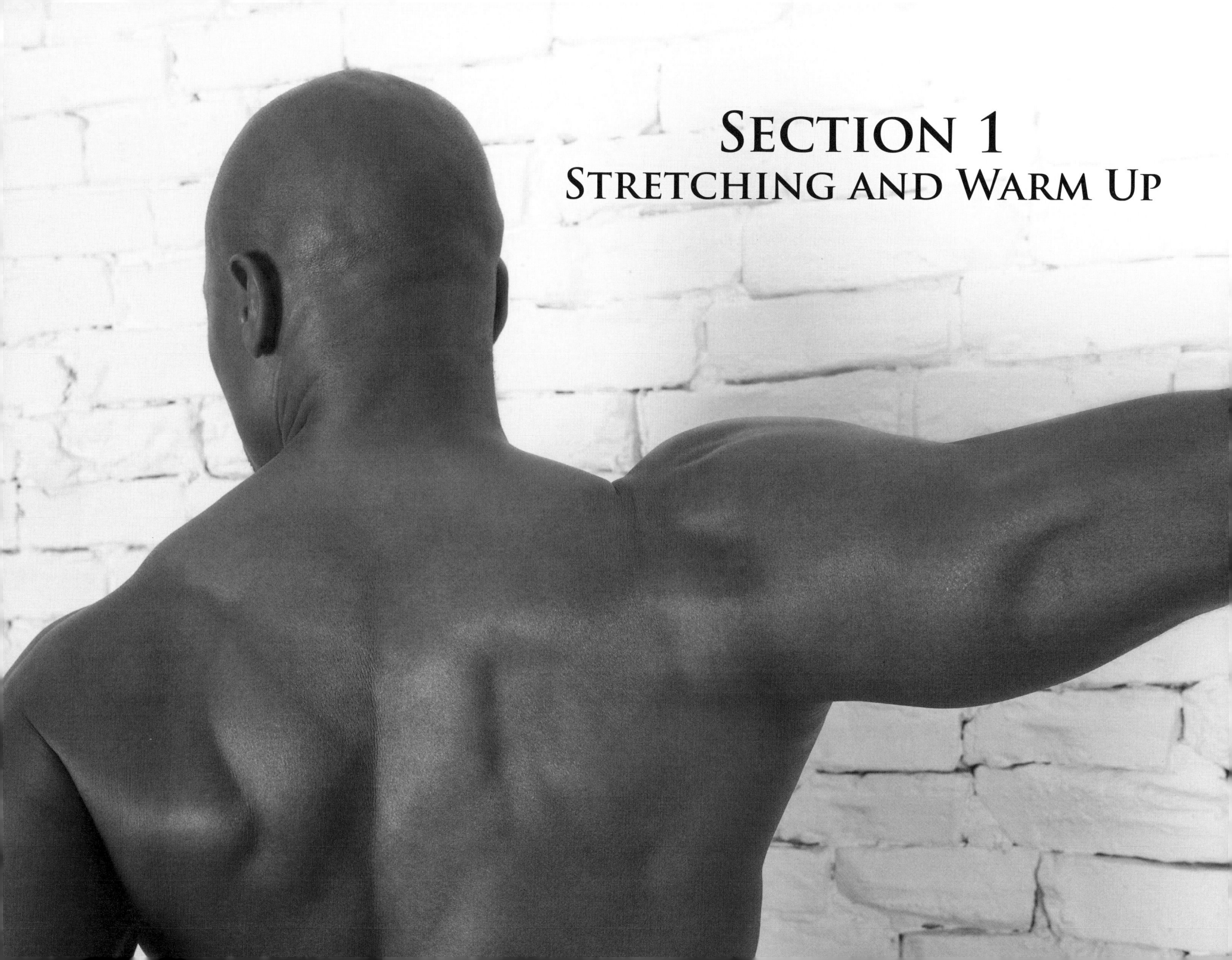

Section 1
Stretching and Warm Up

Lateral Neck Side Bends
Cervical Stretches

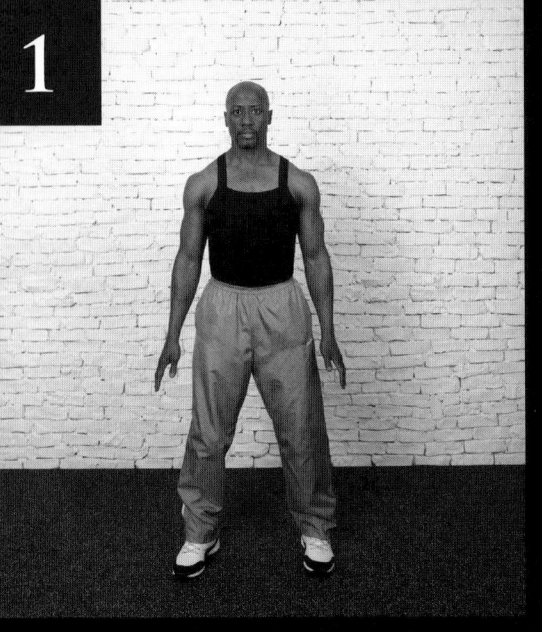

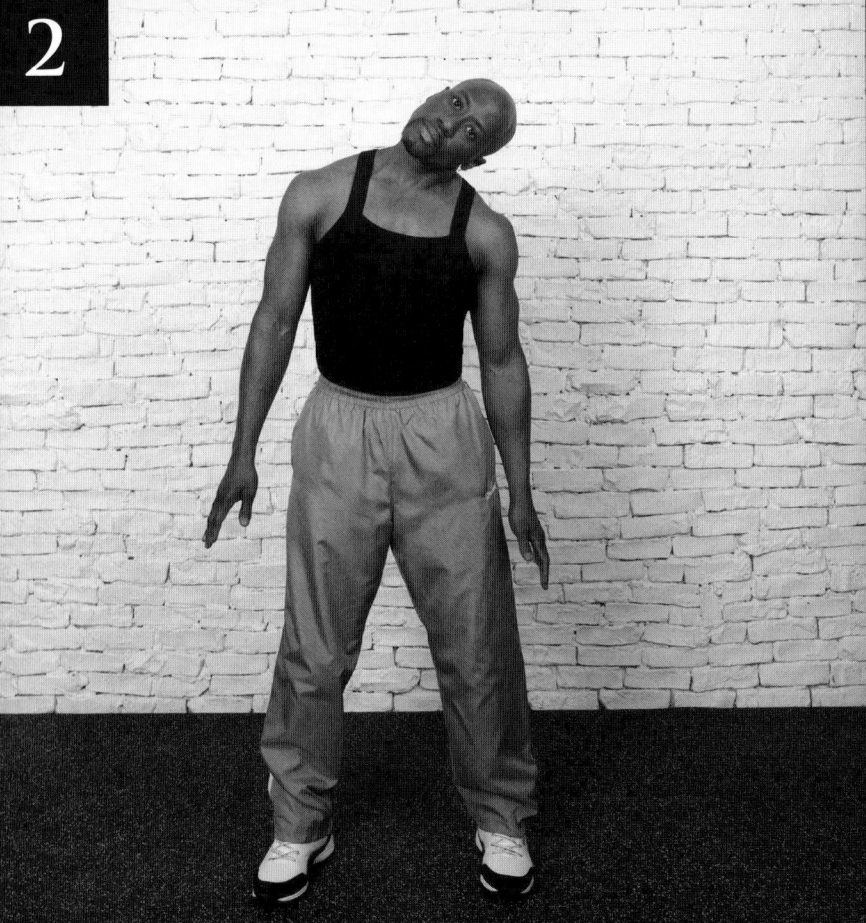

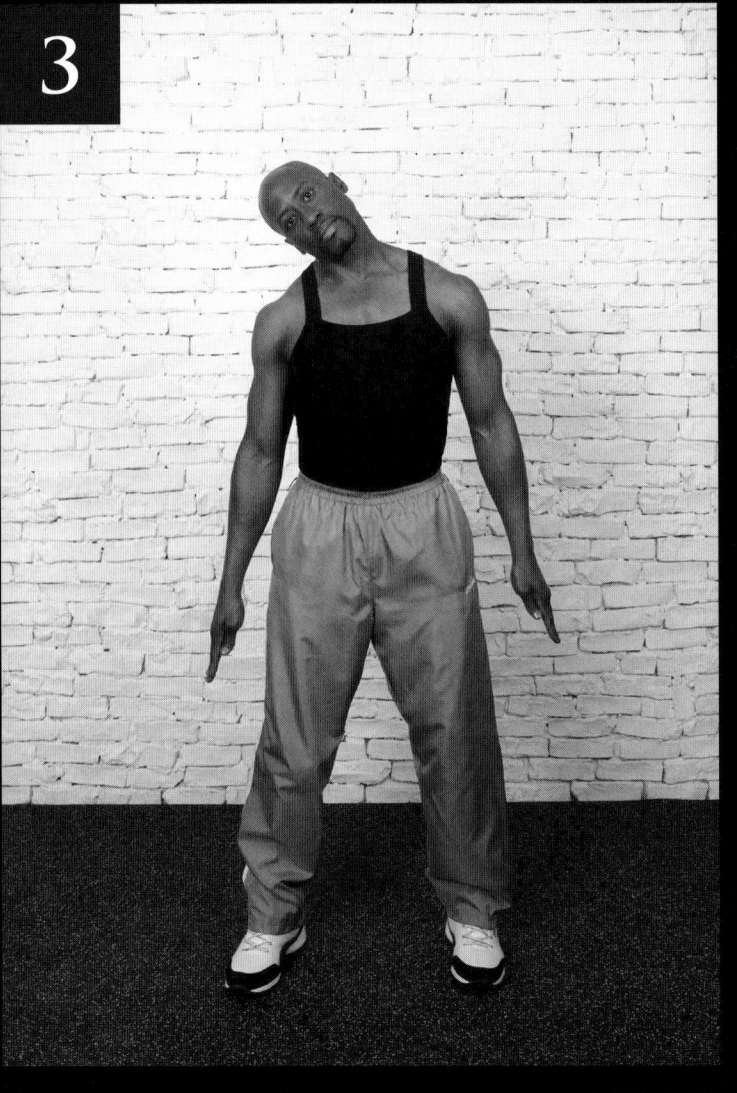

FIT TIP:
Keep your shoulders relaxed and focus your eyes on a point of attention during this exercise.

This exercise may be done sitting or standing.

Begin by standing with the feet slightly more than shoulder-width apart. Palms are open facing the thighs. Bend your head to the right and hold for 30 seconds and return to the upright position; then bend your neck gently to the opposite side and hold for 30 seconds before returning to neutral position.

Shoulder and Arm Overhead Stretch

The feet are wider than shoulder-width apart. The arms are at the sides. The arms are brought above the head and the palms of the hands are upward and pushed overhead. This position is held for 30 seconds.

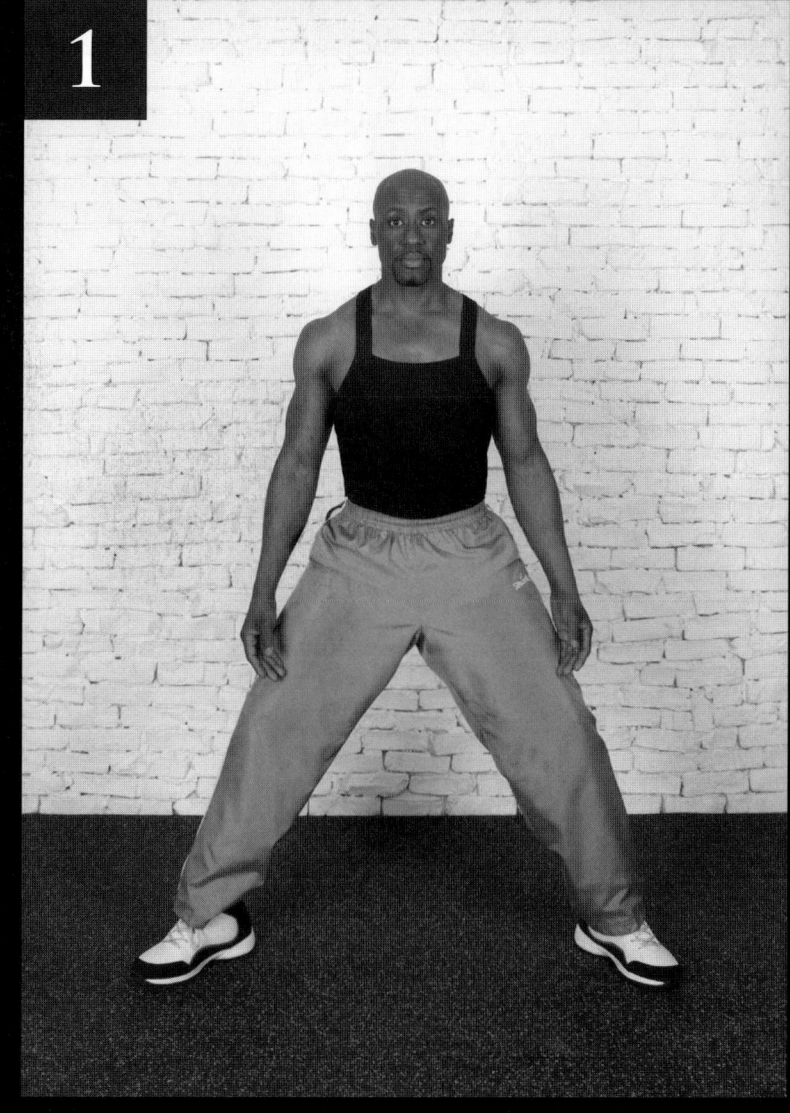

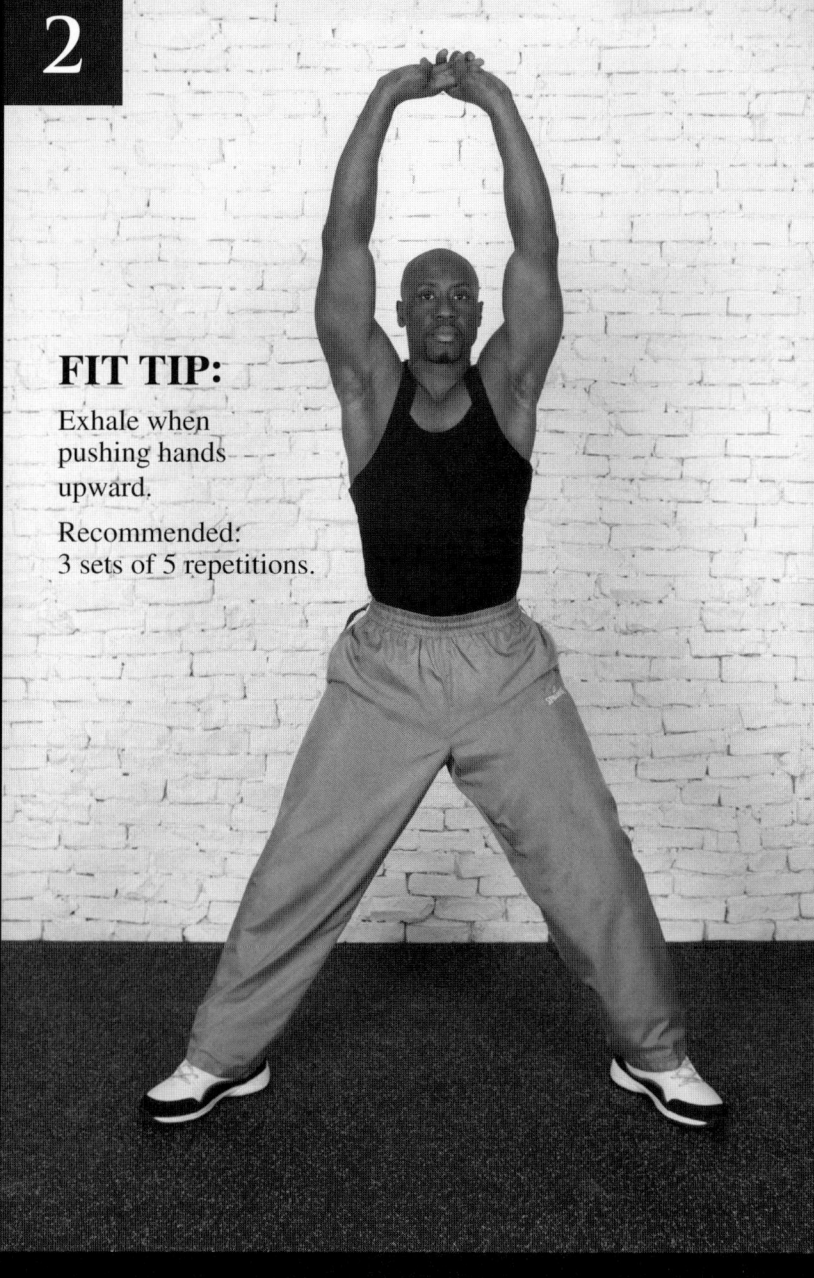

FIT TIP:
Exhale when pushing hands upward.

Recommended: 3 sets of 5 repetitions.

LATERAL NECK STRETCHES

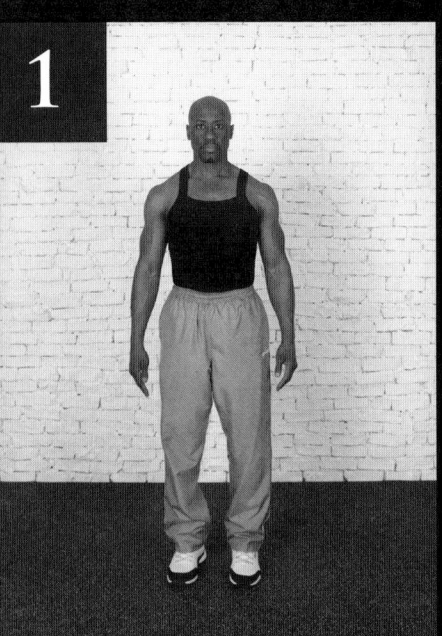

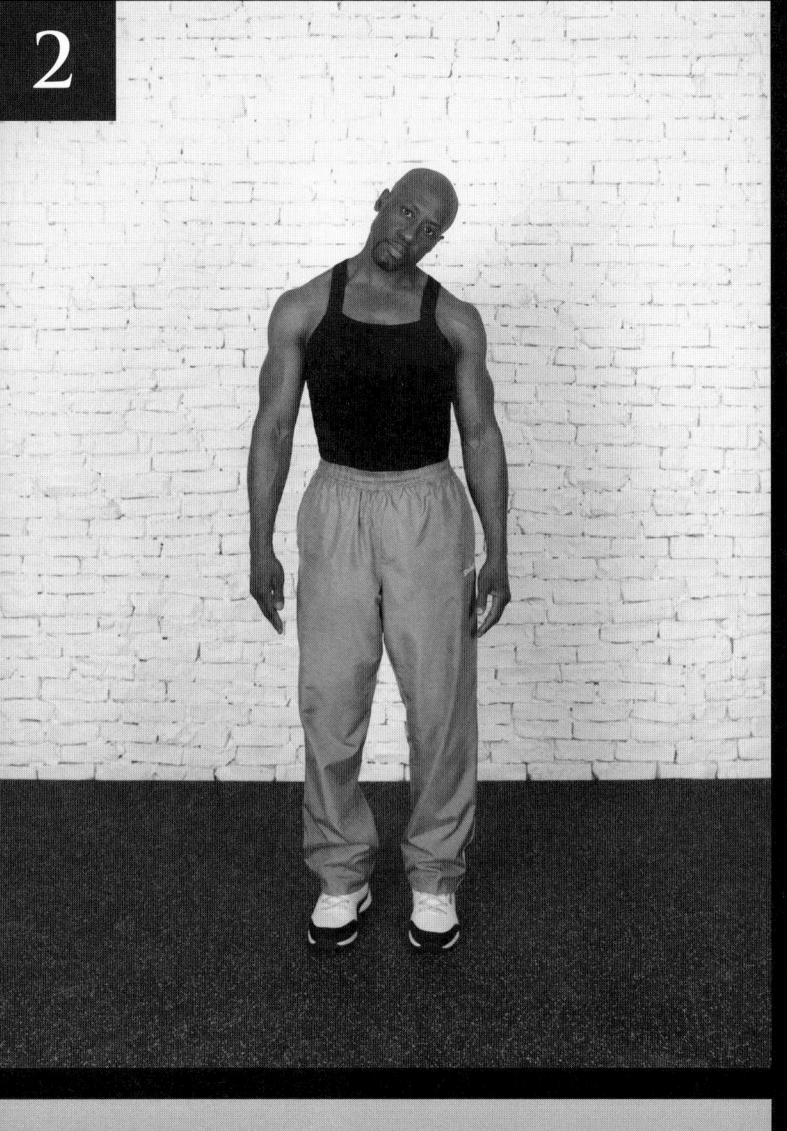

This is performed by starting in the neutral position, feet slightly more than shoulder-width apart. The head is tilted to one side and then the hand on that side gently stretches the neck to the side. This should be done with very gentle traction and held for 30 seconds. I recommend doing this while seated for most people.

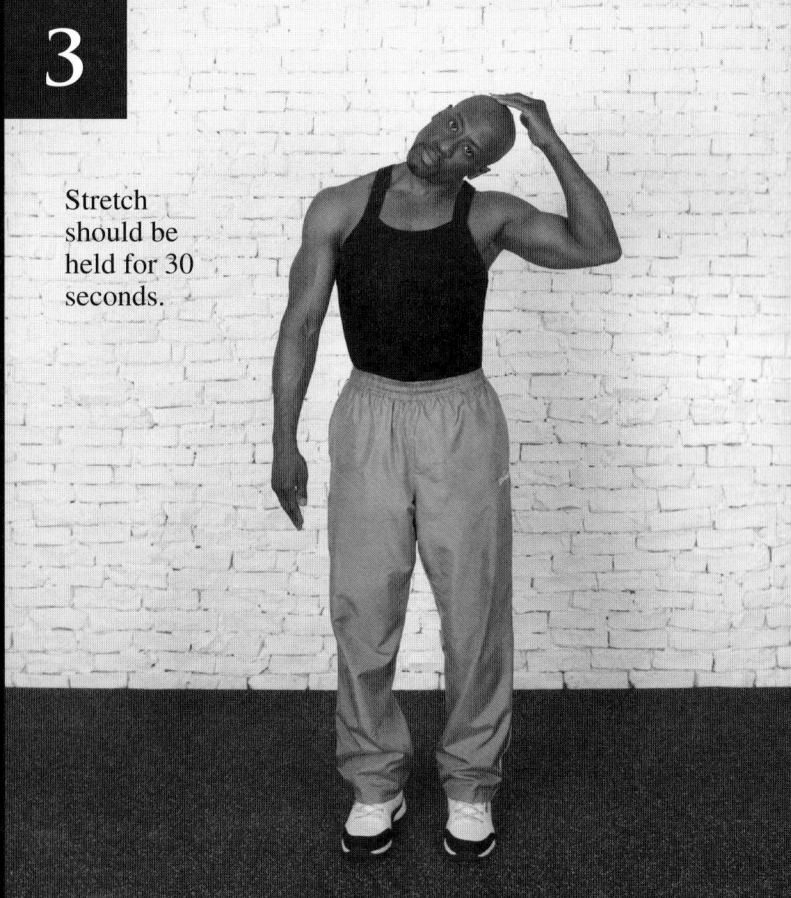

Stretch should be held for 30 seconds.

FIT TIP:

Inhale when stretching neck to each side. Breathe throughout the exercise.

Shoulder Shrugs

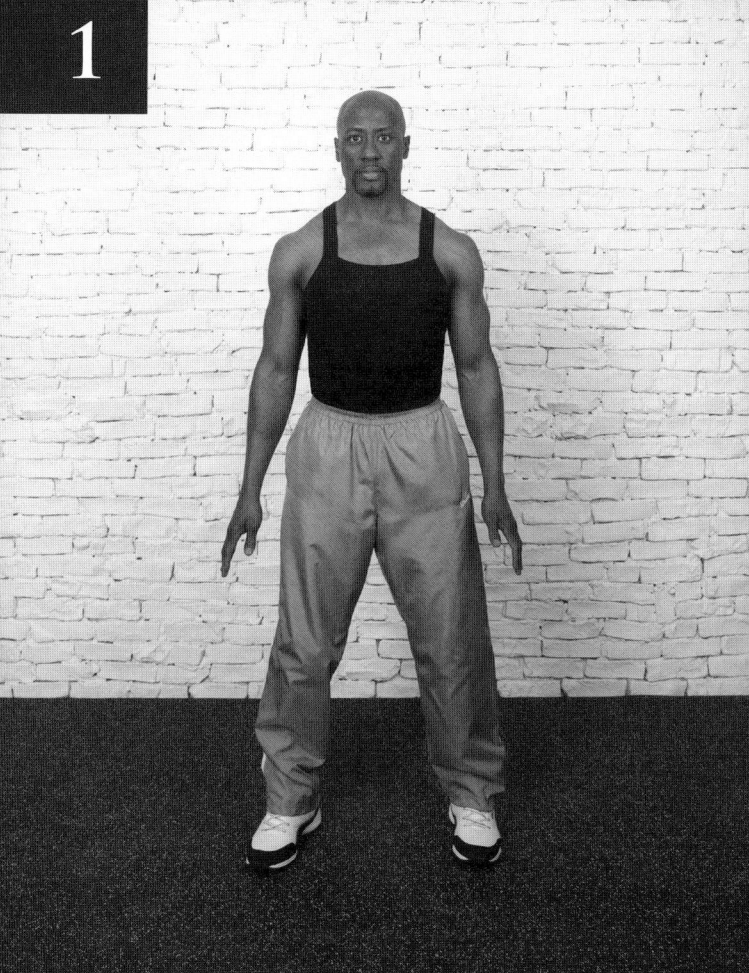

Recommended: 3 sets of 5 repetitions.

FIT TIP:
Inhale when bringing the shoulders up.

Stand with your feet shoulder-width apart, lift your shoulders up and gently bring your shoulders down. This is to be done for a sequence of five times

Posterior Shoulder Rolls

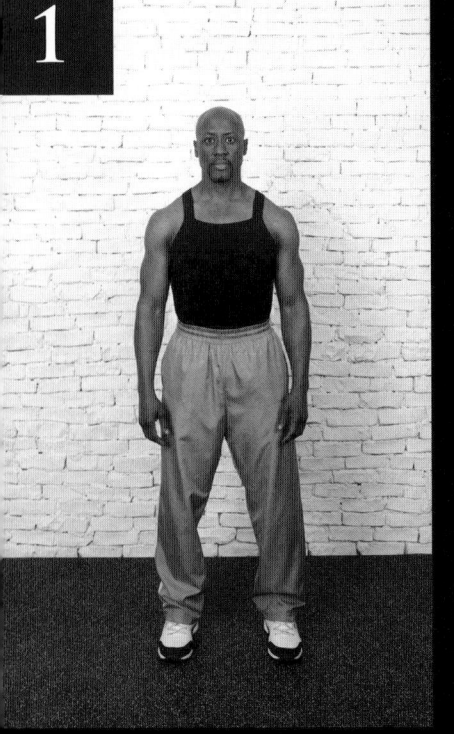

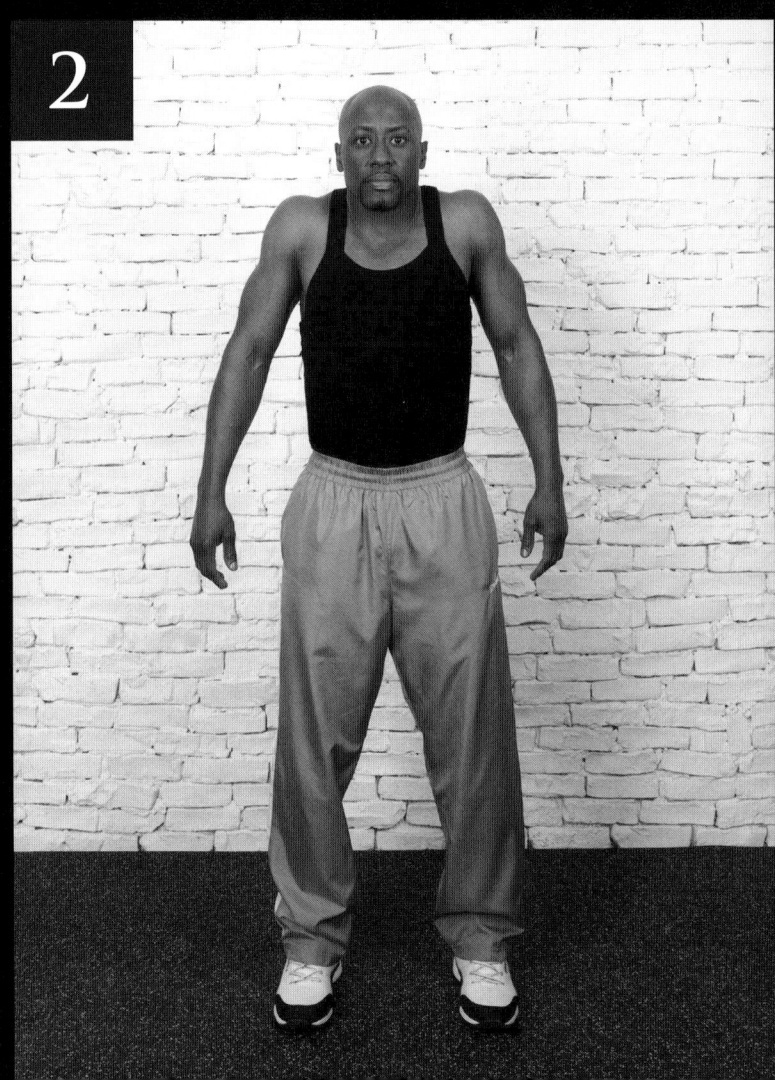

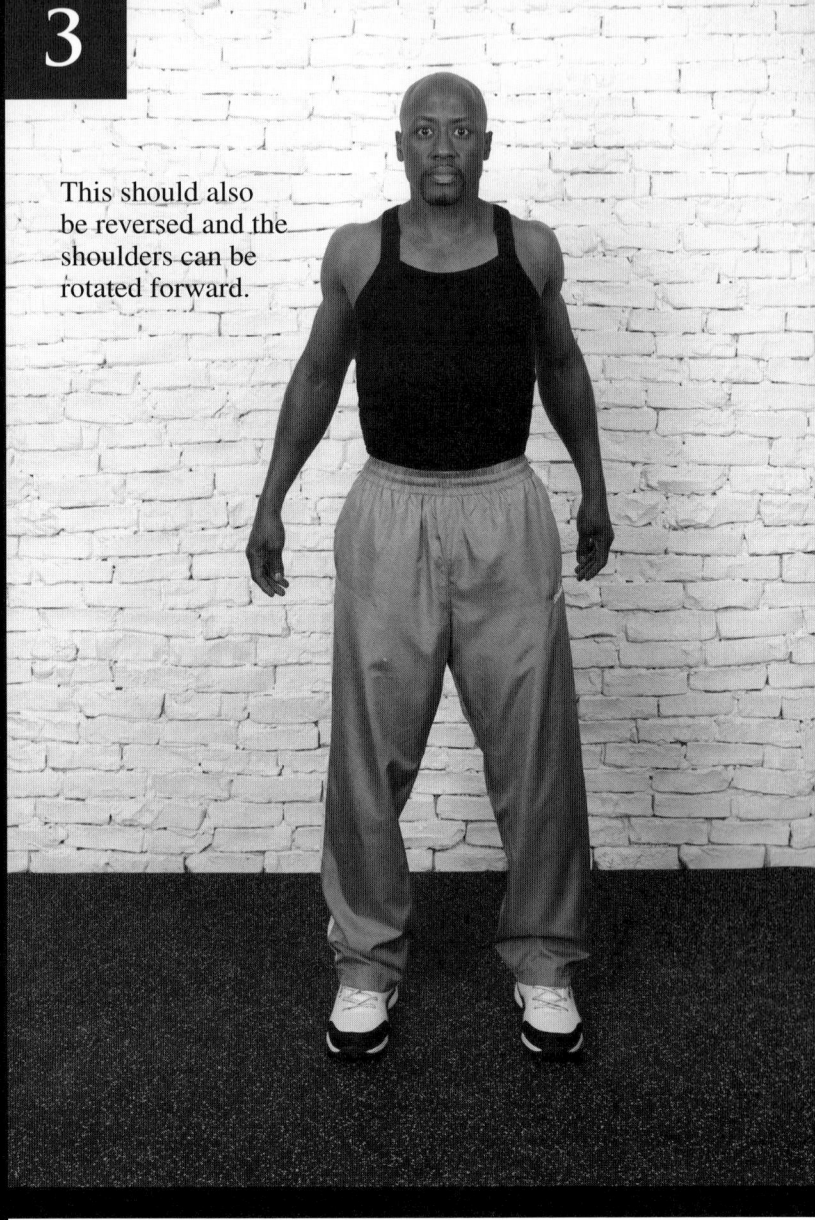

This should also be reversed and the shoulders can be rotated forward.

Stand with the feet shoulder-width apart in the neutral position. The shoulders should be shrugged and lifted upward toward your ears, then roll the shoulders backwards, and then roll the shoulders forward. This should be done slowly and gently five times.

Shoulder and Back Stretch

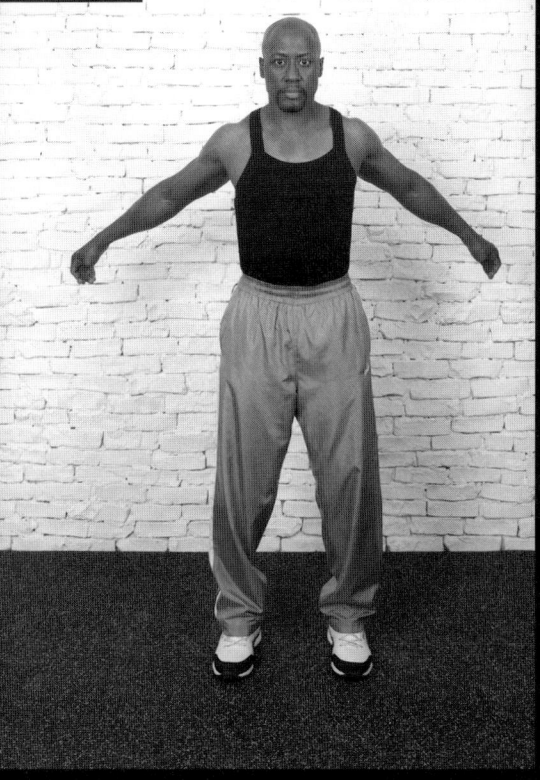

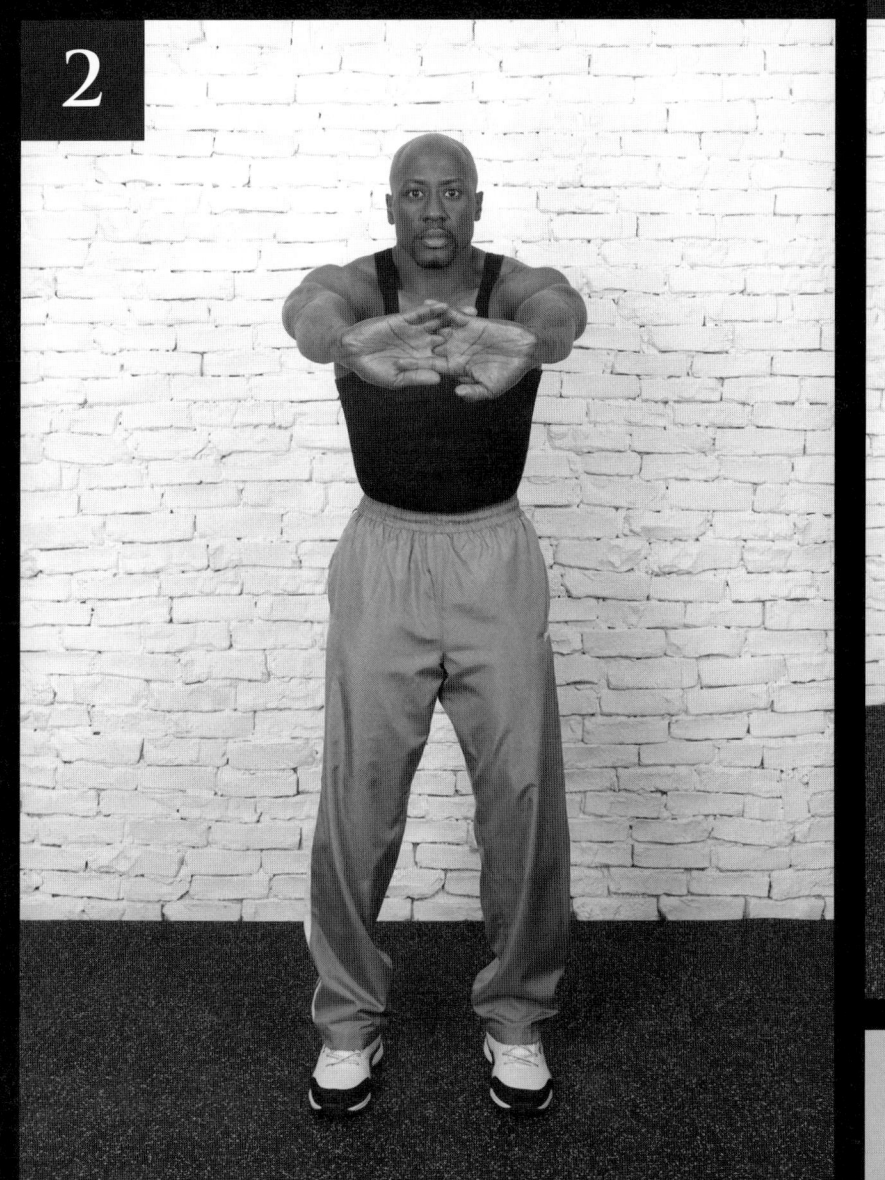

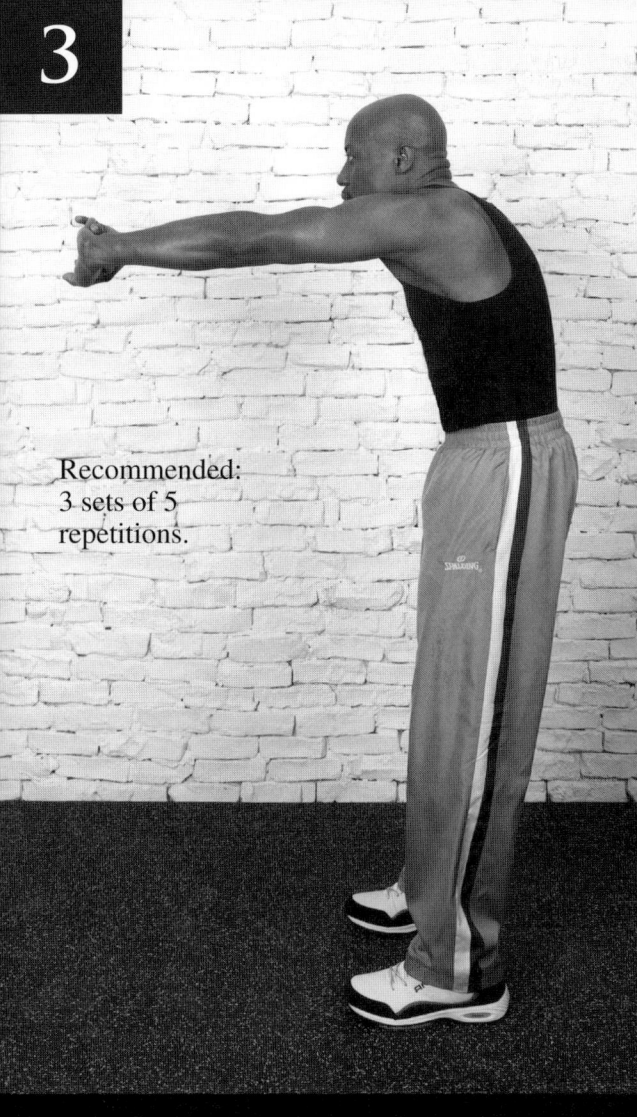

Recommended: 3 sets of 5 repetitions.

This exercise is done with the feet shoulder-width apart, the palms facing forward, roll the shoulders forward and roll the back gently forward.

Right and Left Side Bends

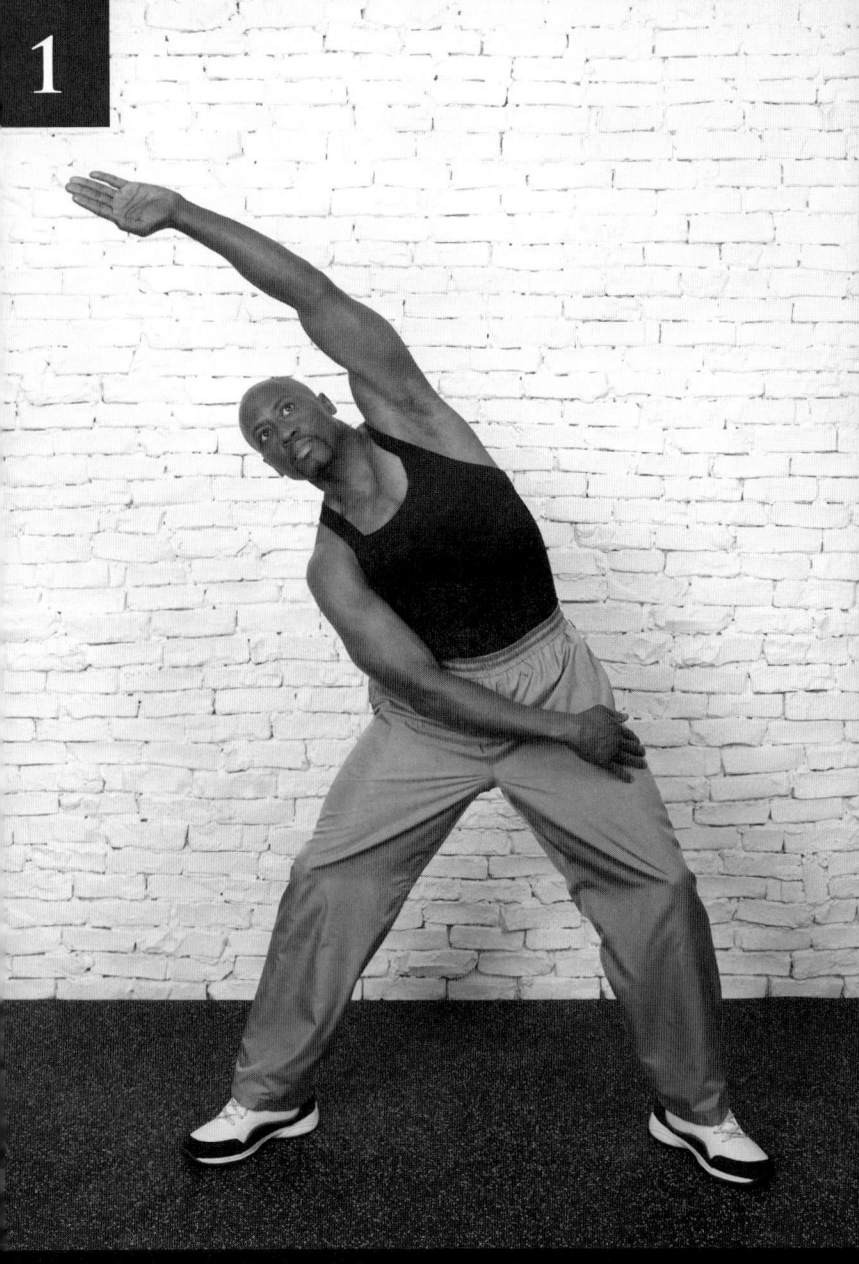

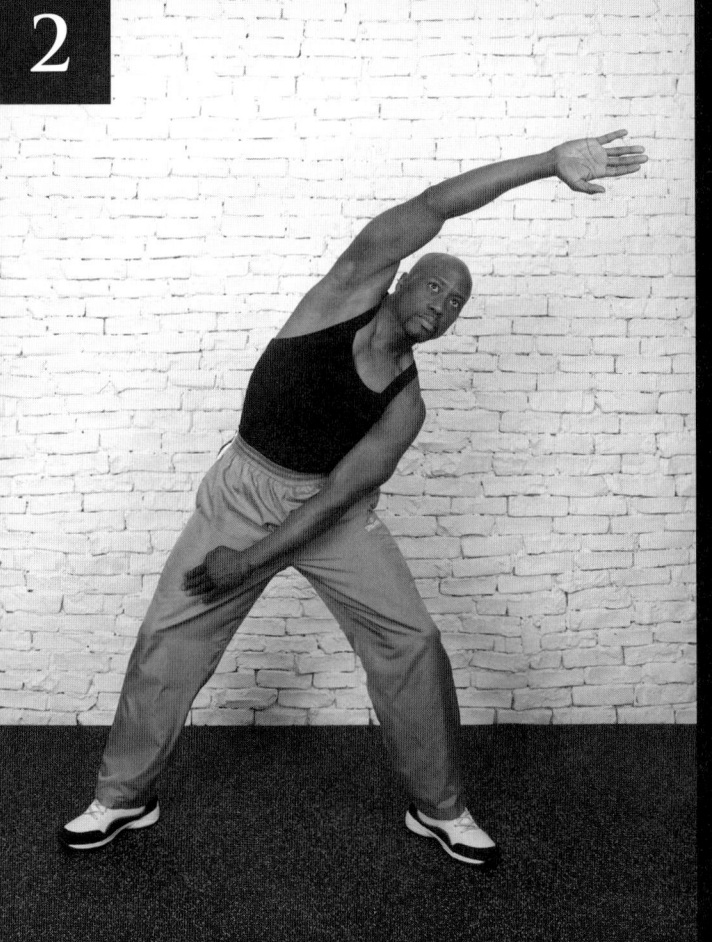

The feet are more than shoulder-width apart. The back is straight. One arm is across the abdomen and opposite thigh. The other arm is overhead. Knees are slightly bent. This position is to be held for 30 seconds. There should be no bouncing during this exercise. This is a static stretch.

FIT TIP:
Breathe throughout this exercise.

Triceps and Torso Stretch

FIT TIP:
The knees should be slightly bent during this exercise.

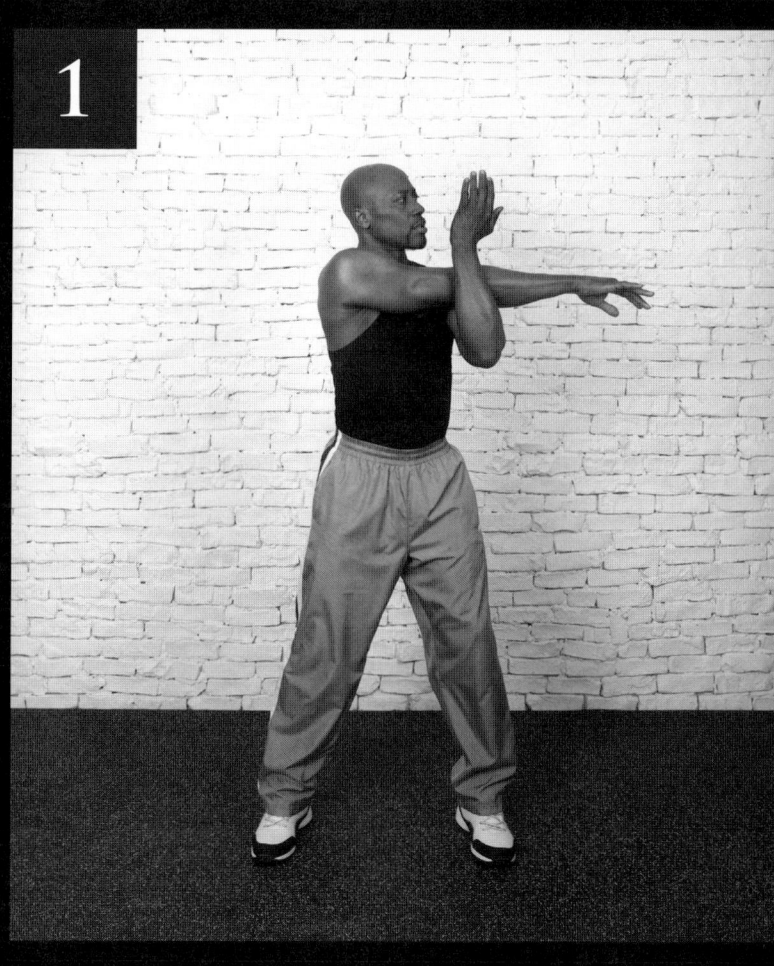

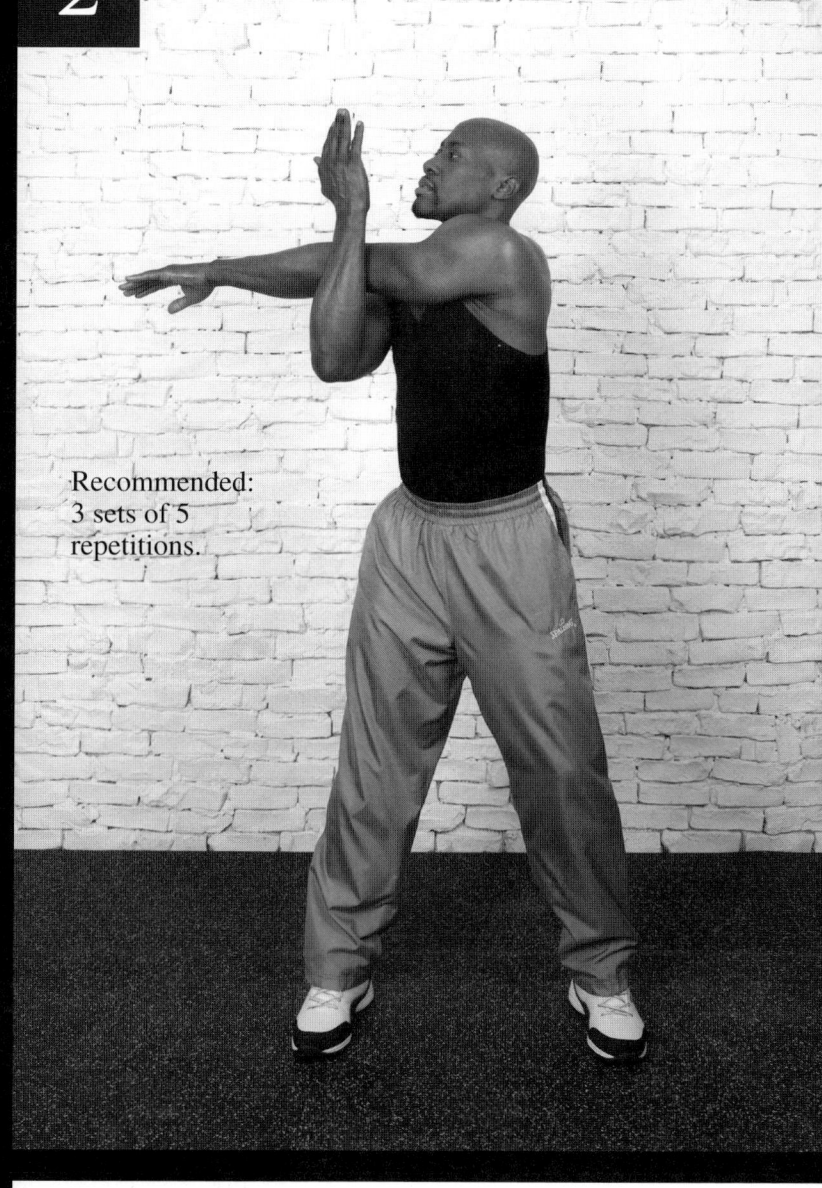

Recommended: 3 sets of 5 repetitions.

The feet are more than shoulder-width apart. The opposite forearm should rest in the junction of the opposite elbow and the torso should be twisted slightly to the side of the extended arm. This position should be held for 30 seconds before transitioning to the opposite side.

Right and Left Side Bends and Torso Stretch

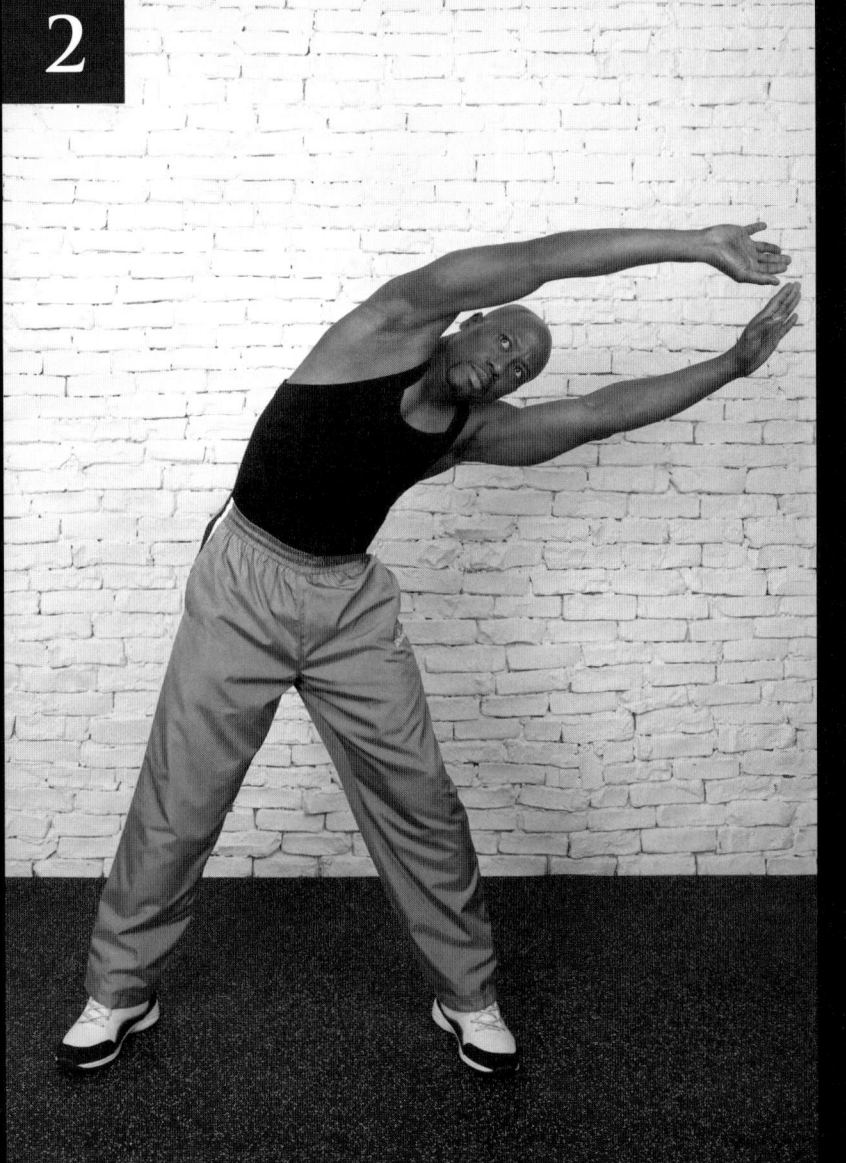

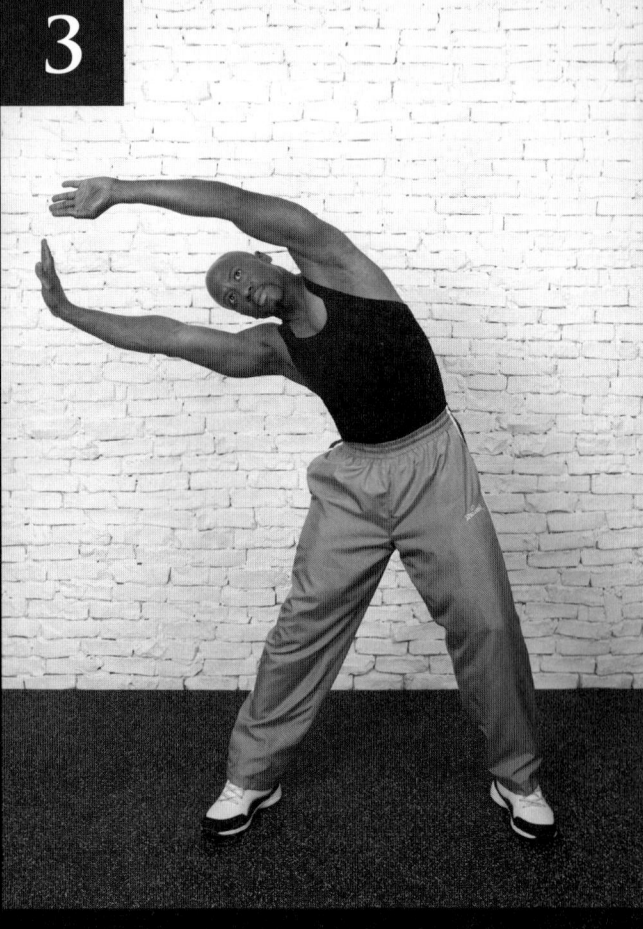

Starting position: Hands are high above the head and palms open. Lift your shoulders then bend to the right and bend to the left. Each side should be held with the hands and palms open to that side for 30 seconds.

FIT TIP:
Breathe throughout this exercise.

Deep Lateral Side Bends and Torso Stretch

1

Start with the hands high above the head and palms open. If you are bending to the right side, the right leg should be straight, and drop your body and torso in the sideways position to the left.

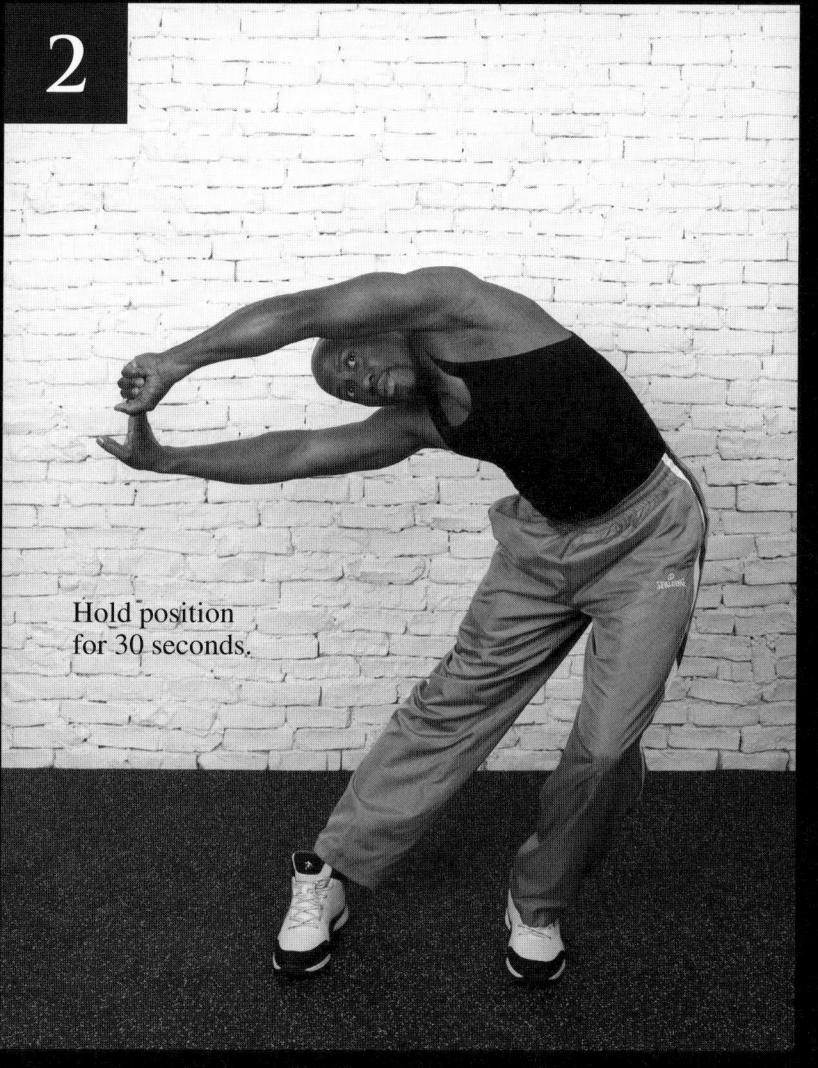

2 Hold position for 30 seconds.

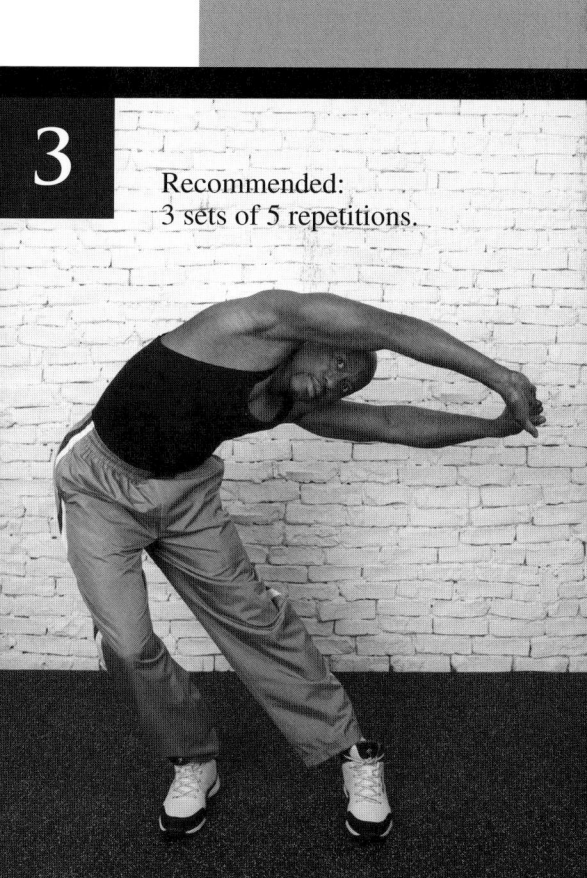

3 Recommended: 3 sets of 5 repetitions.

Trapezius and Neck (Cervical) Stretch

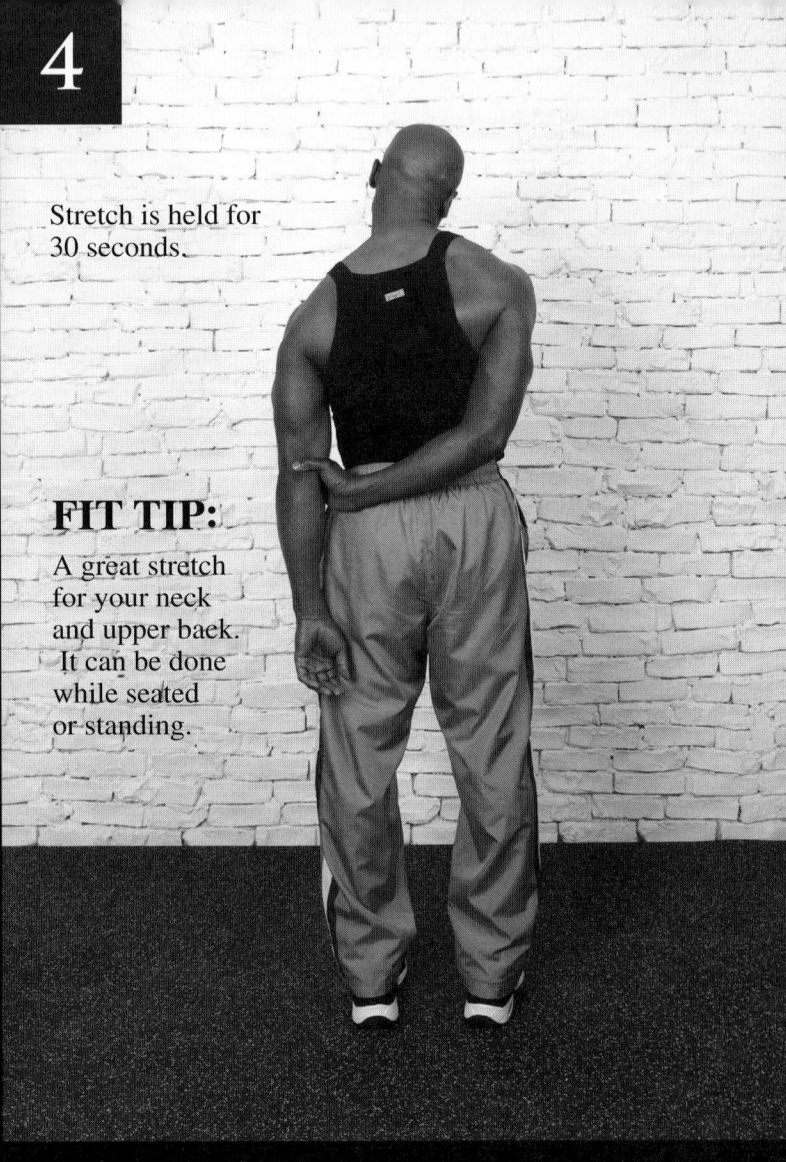

Stretch is held for 30 seconds.

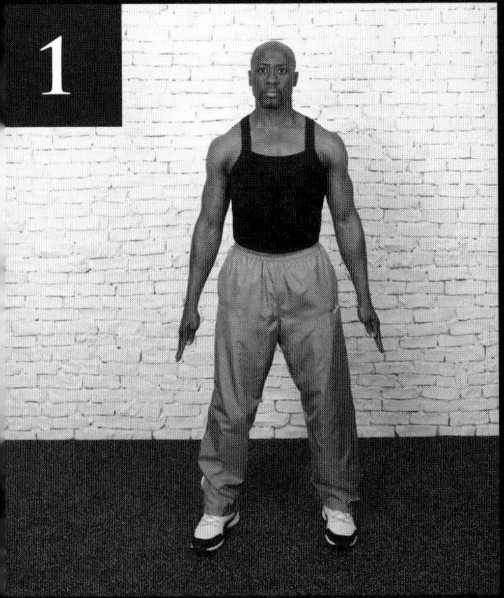

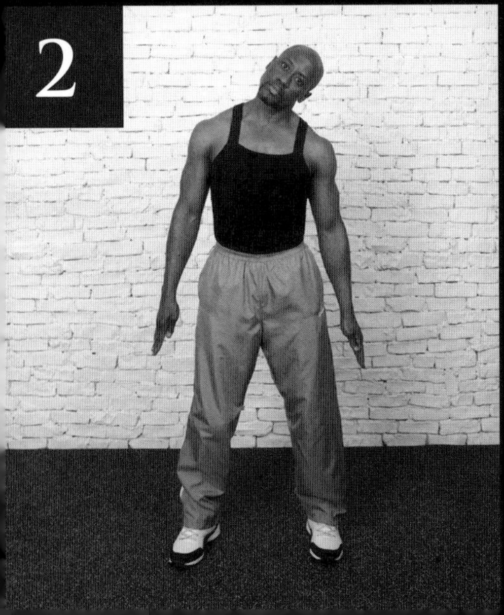

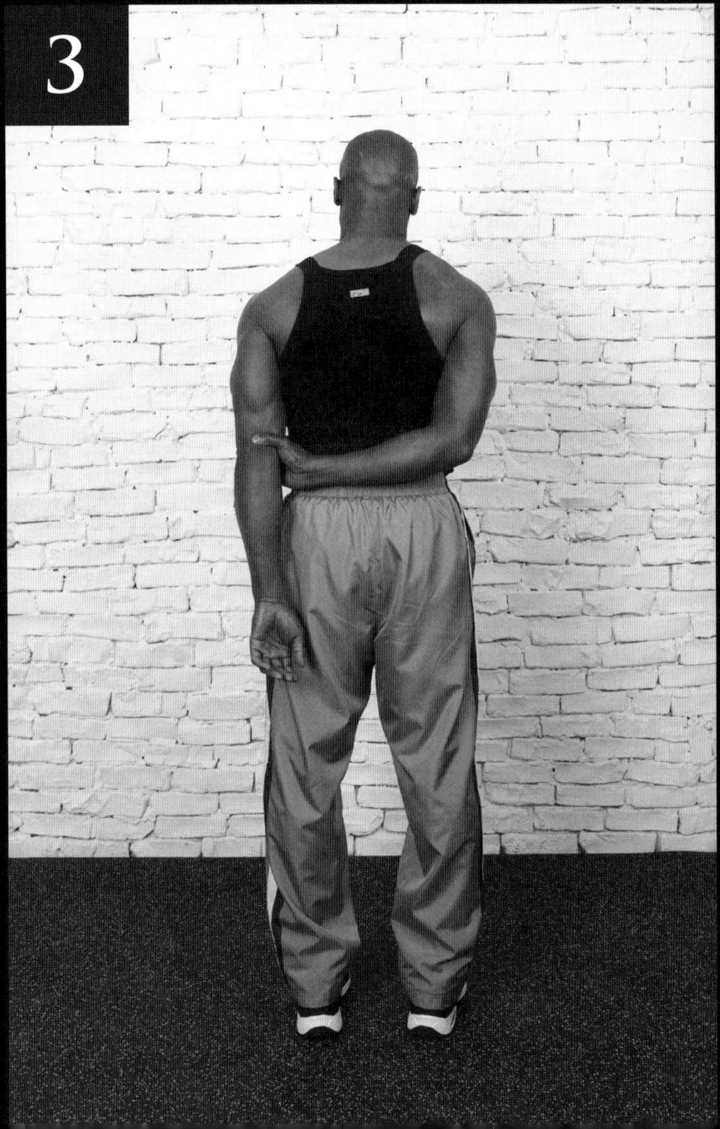

FIT TIP: A great stretch for your neck and upper back. It can be done while seated or standing.

From a standing upright, neutral position for the right side, the head should be tilted to the right side. Use the right arm to grasp the left arm from behind. Pull the left arm downward right above the elbow and bend your neck to the right side. The knees should be slightly bent.

Quadriceps, Hamstrings and Calf Stretches Combined

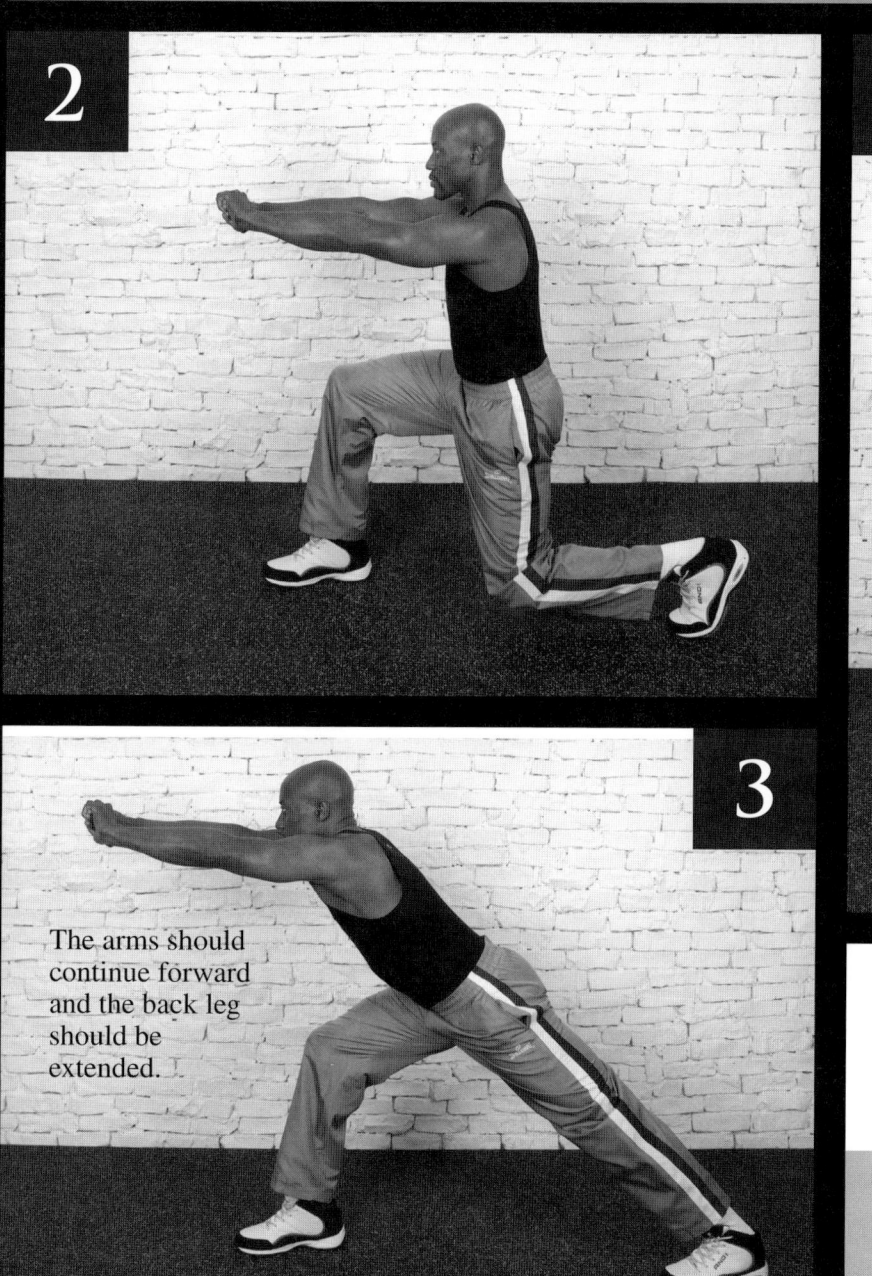

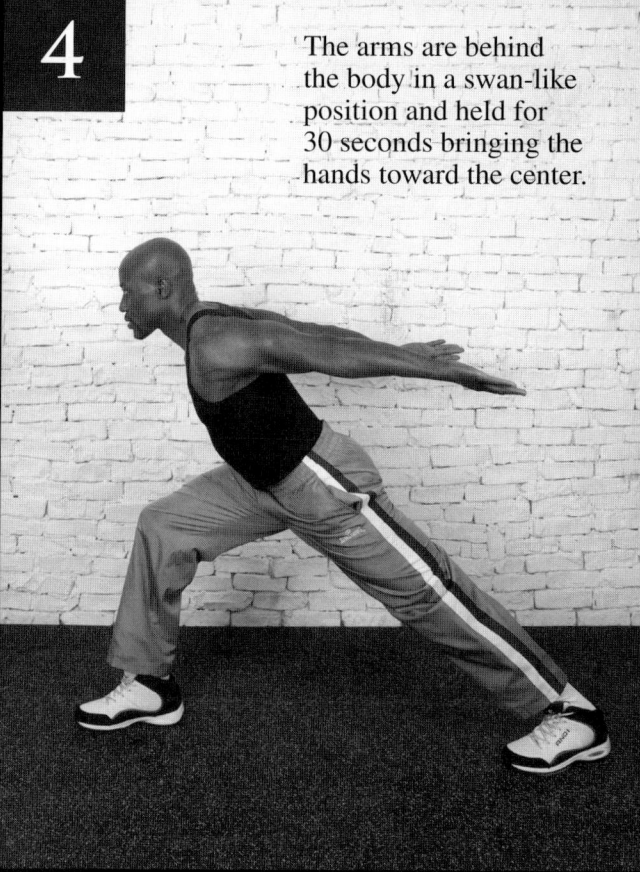

2. The arms should continue forward and the back leg should be extended.

4. The arms are behind the body in a swan-like position and held for 30 seconds bringing the hands toward the center.

The starting position is standing in neutral position. One leg should be brought posteriorly and the knee should be flexed and dropped downward. However, the forward leg and knee should remain directly over the ankle. This position should be held for 30 seconds with the hands in front of your body; palms open, lift the back heel, and hold for 30 seconds.

Recommended:
3 sets of 3 to 5 repetitions.

TORSO AND OBLIQUES STRETCH
Serratus Anterior

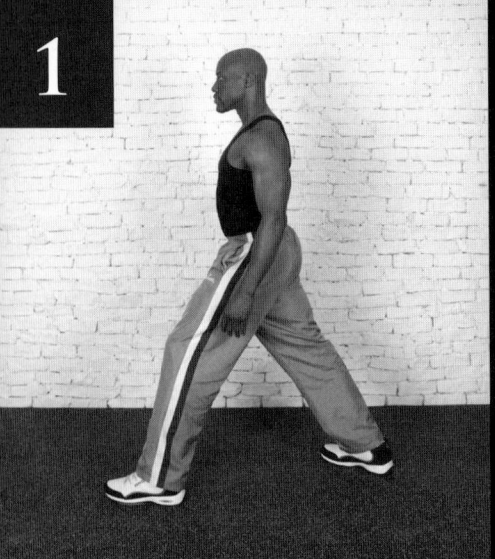

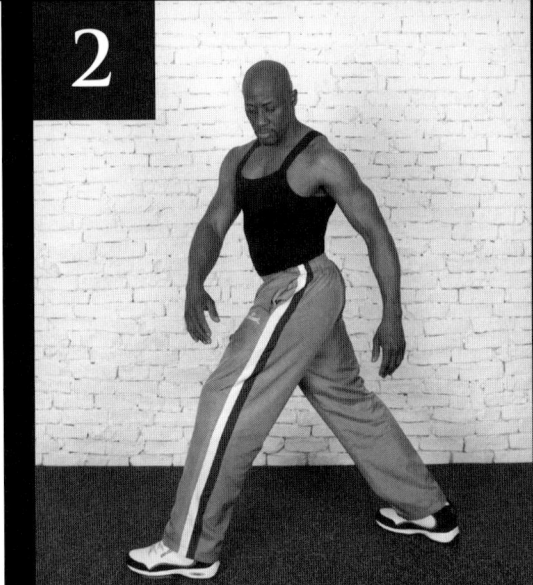

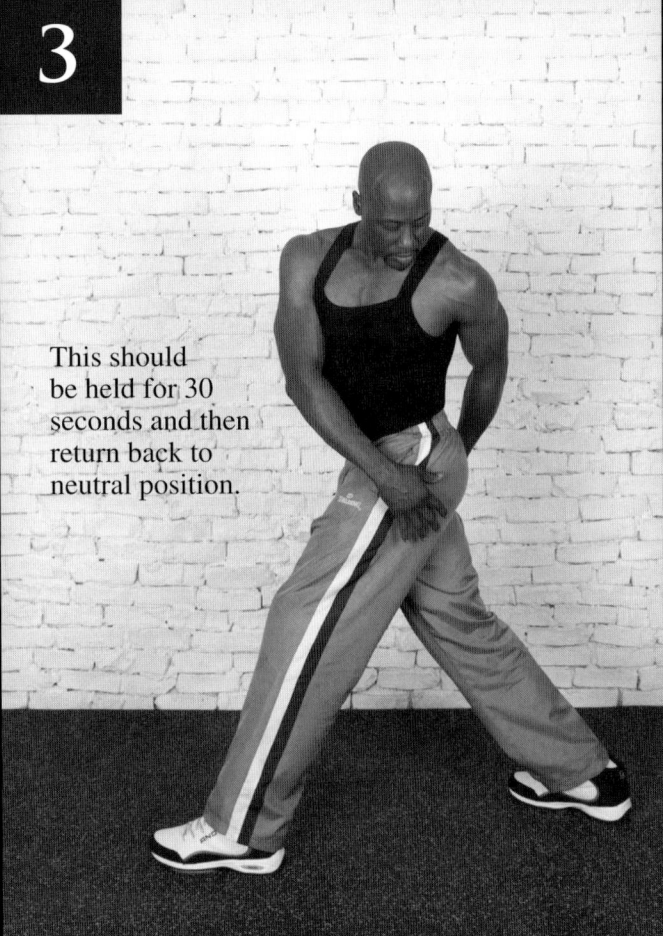

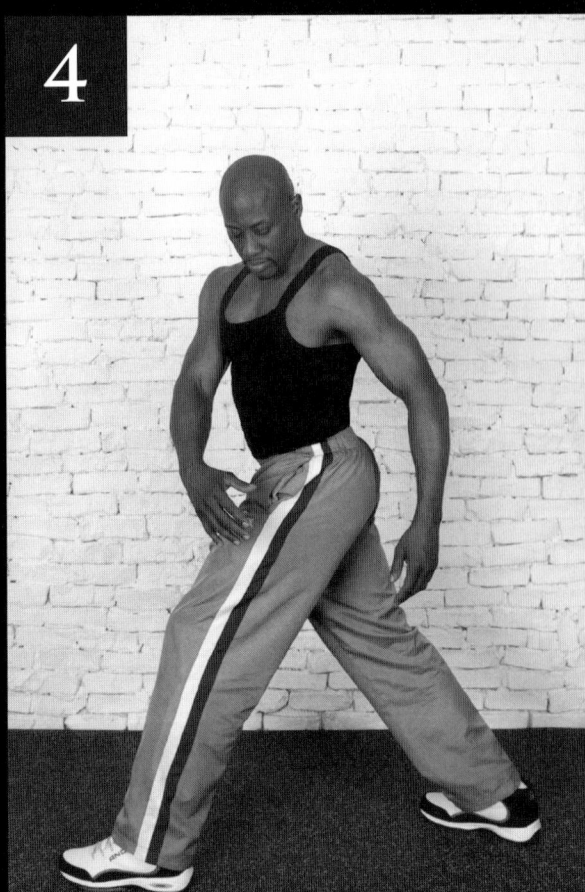

The stretch is done by starting in neutral position with one foot behind the other (more than 2 feet behind the other forward foot). The body is gently turned toward the leg that is forward and the opposite hand holds the side of the hip of the forward leg.

This should be held for 30 seconds and then return back to neutral position.

FIT TIP:
Keep the knee bent on the forward leg.

Squats and Seated Calf Raises

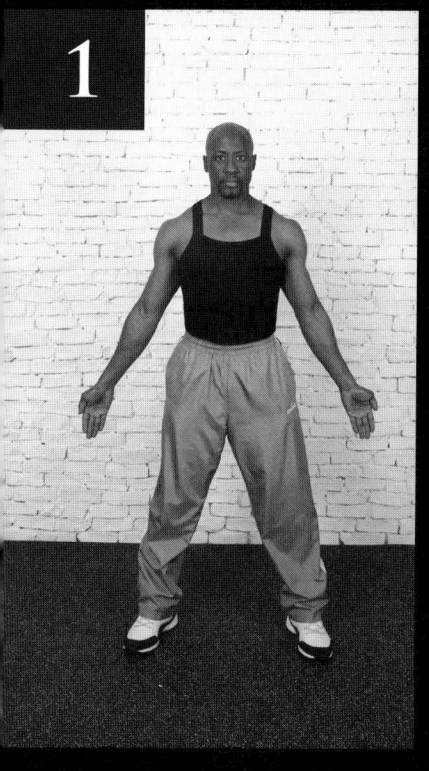

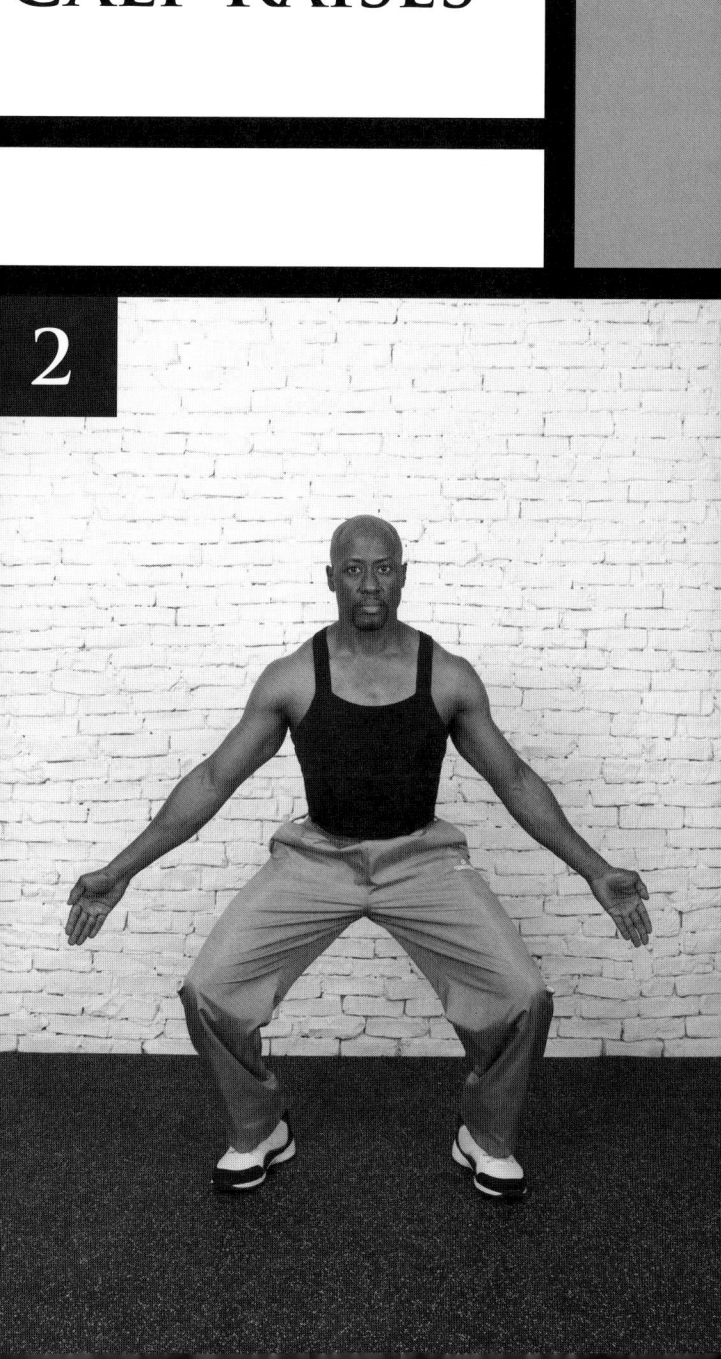

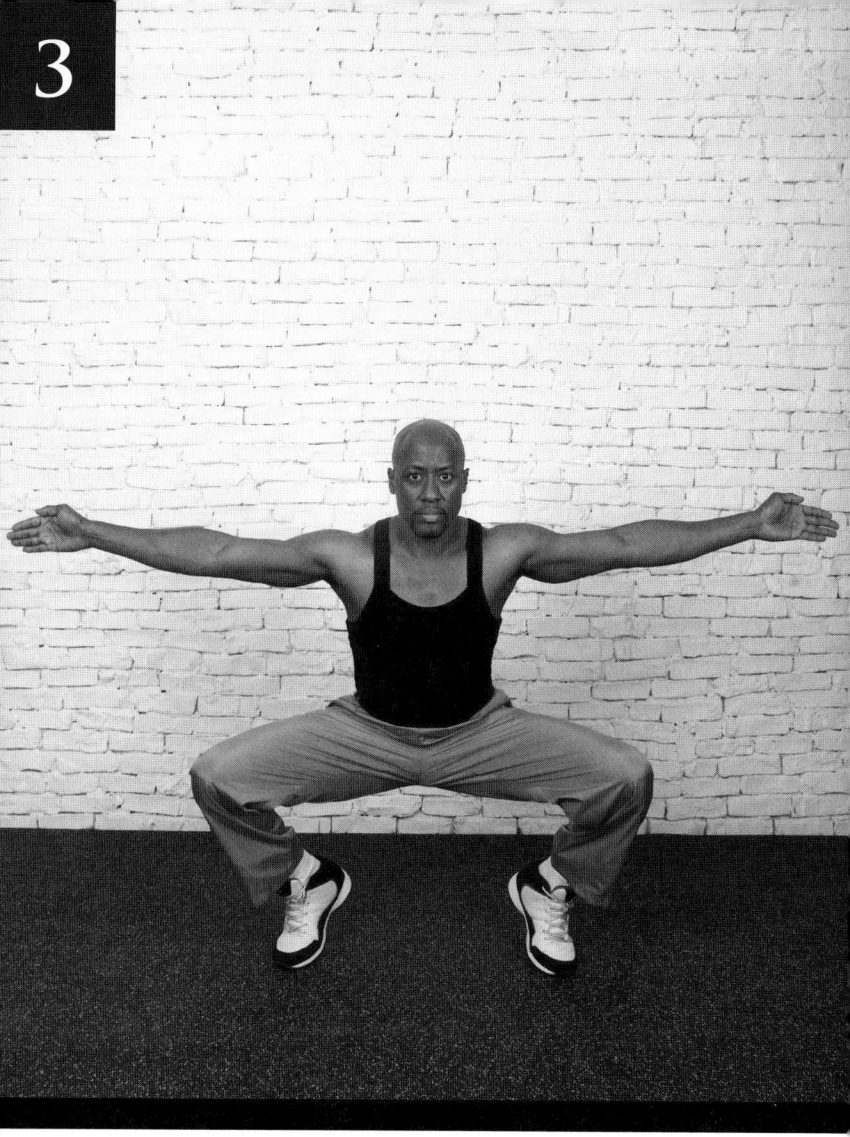

FIT TIP:

Keep back straight and abdomen tight. Avoid leaning forward.

Recommended: 3 sets of 3 to 5 repetitions.

This exercise is done by dropping your body downward with your back straight, bending your knees. As your knees are bent, you lift up on your toes and hold the squatting position for 30 seconds.

Hamstrings and Quadriceps Stretch and Balance

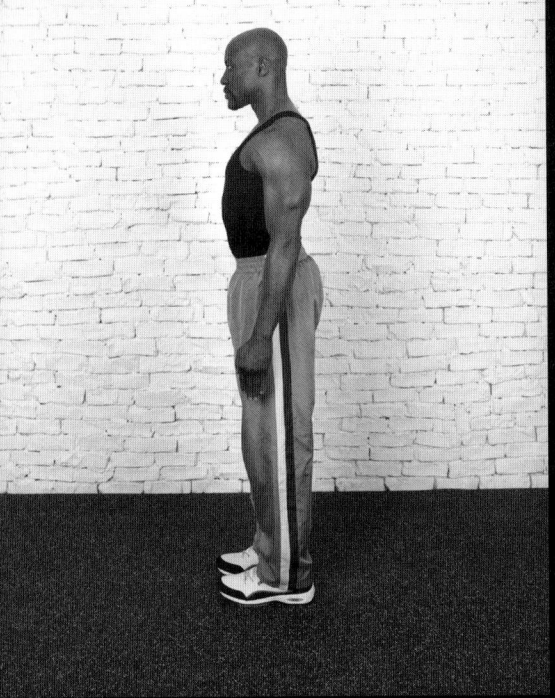

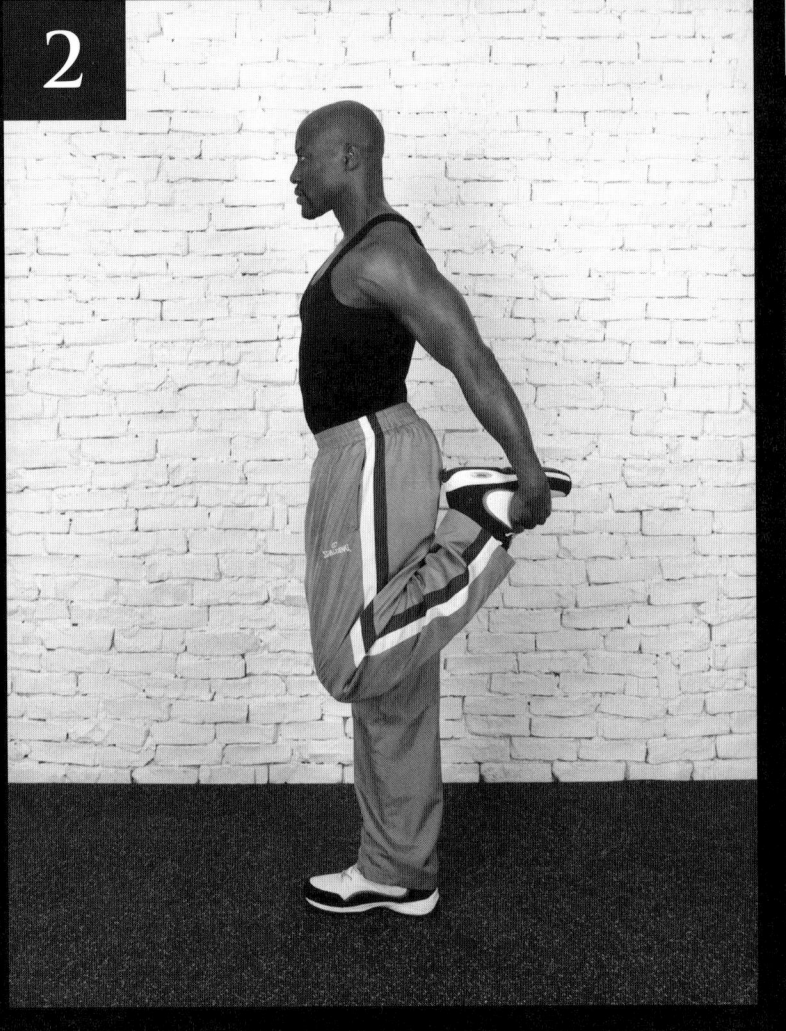

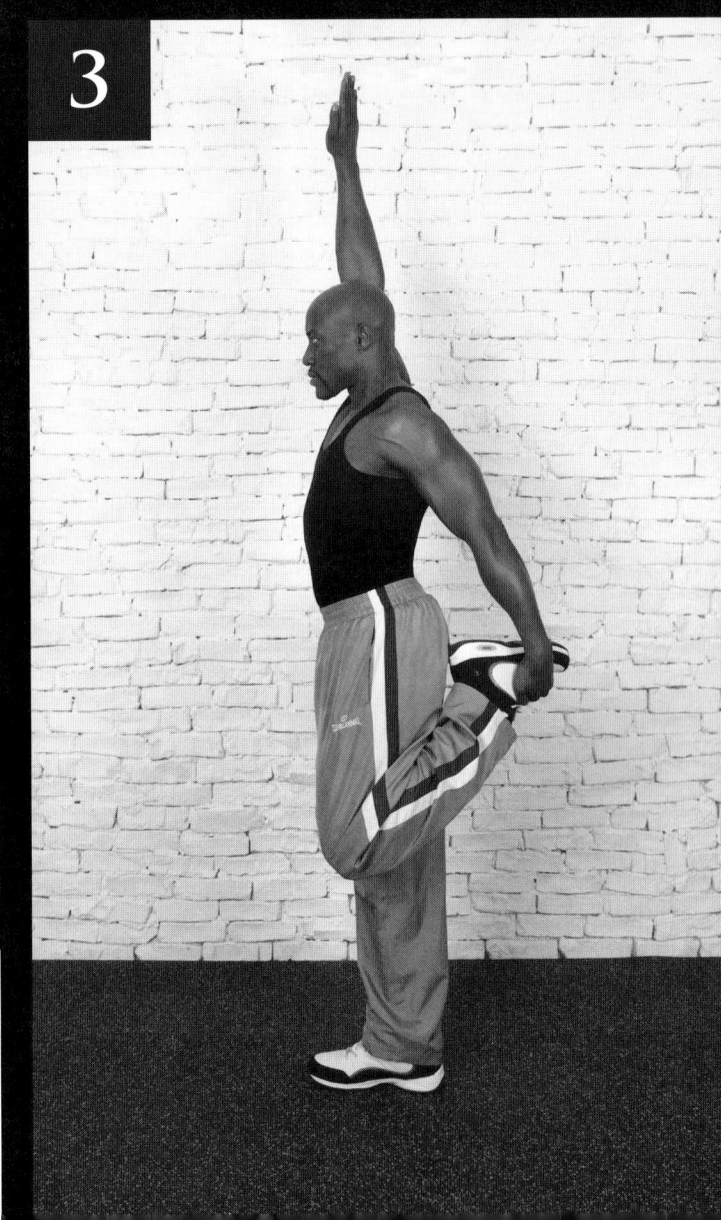

The execution of the exercise is starting from the neutral standing position.

Part 1: The feet are shoulder-width apart. Starting with the left side, the left foot should be grasped by the left hand and held with the knee flexed with the right hand held high above the head.

FIT TIP:

Keep back straight.

Recommended: 3 sets of 5 repetitions.

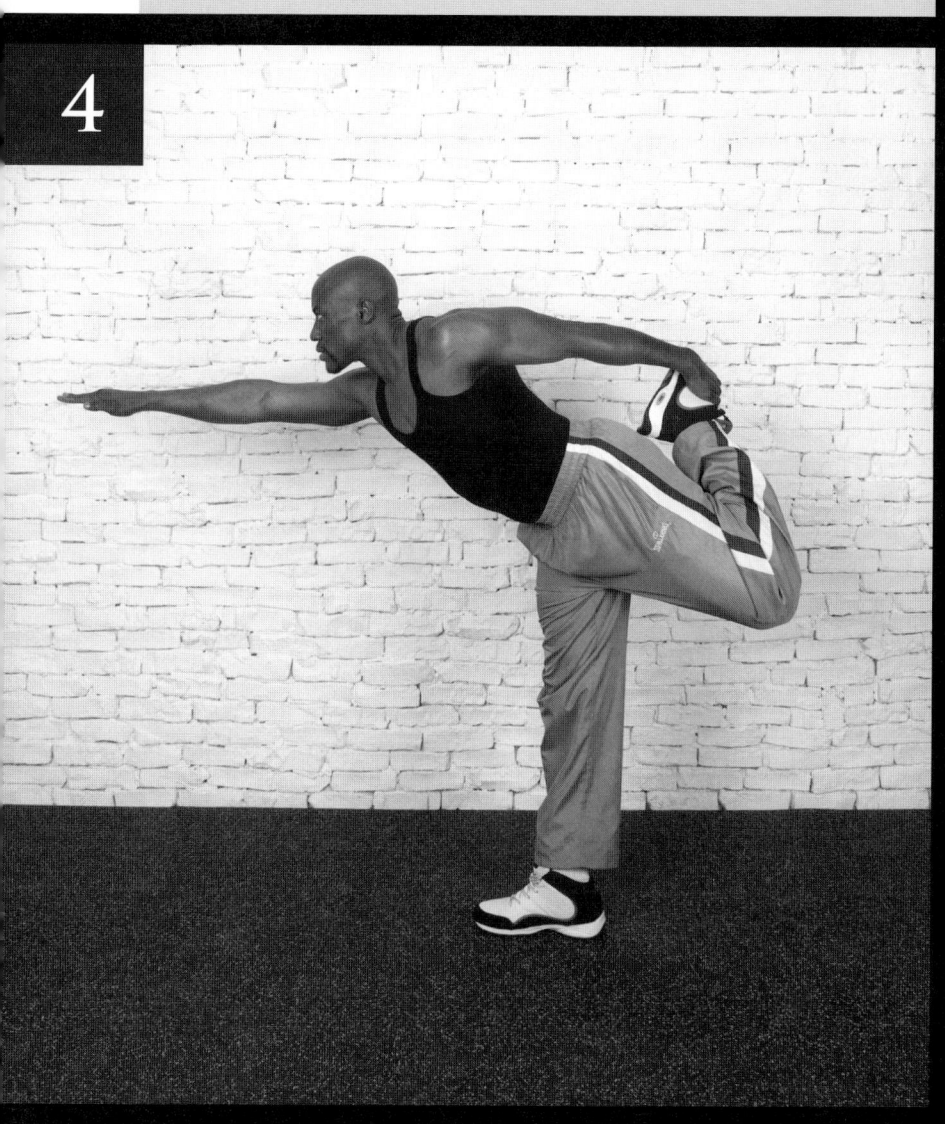

4

5

This should be held for 30 seconds.

Part 2 of the exercise: The torso should be tilted forward while holding the left leg and balanced. Again, hold for 30 seconds. Part 3 of the exercise: The left leg should be extended posteriorly and the body dropped forward with the right arm forward, the left arm behind, and the left leg behind. This should be held for 30 seconds.

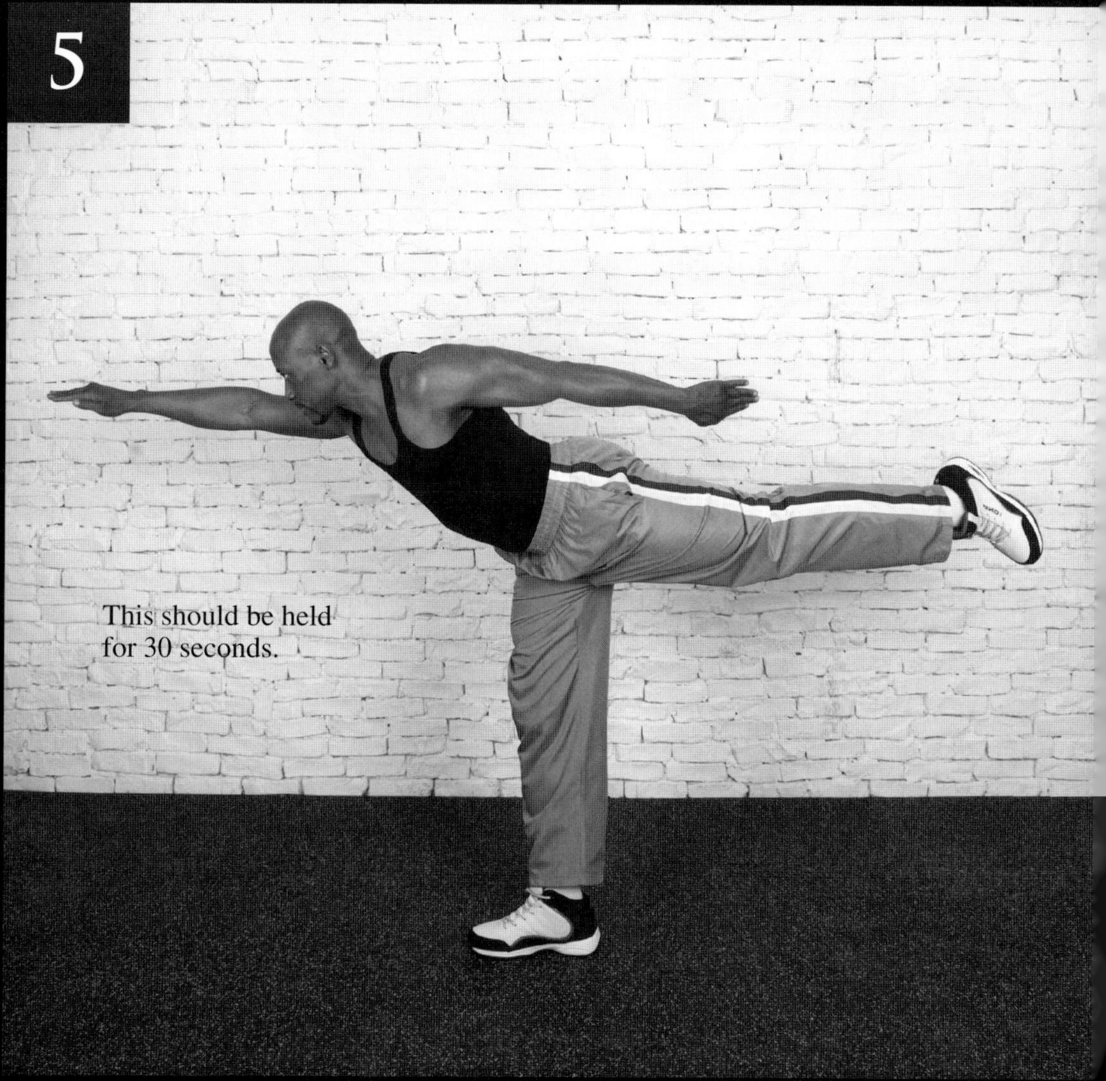

TOE TAP, BUTTOCKS TONE, AND BALANCE EXERCISE

1

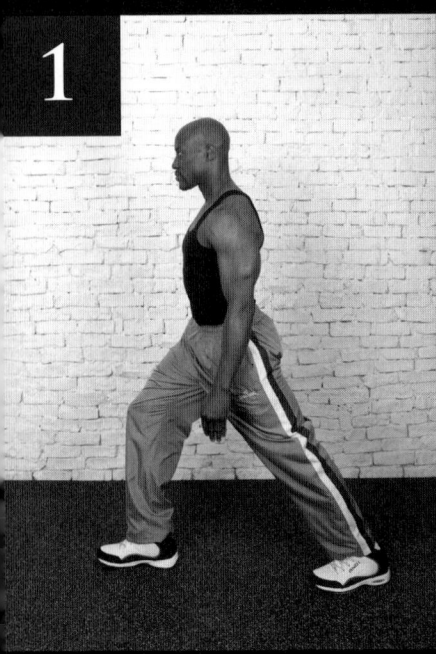

Stand with the right leg forward and the left leg behind you as seen in photo. Lean forward with the hands clasped together with the palms open.

2

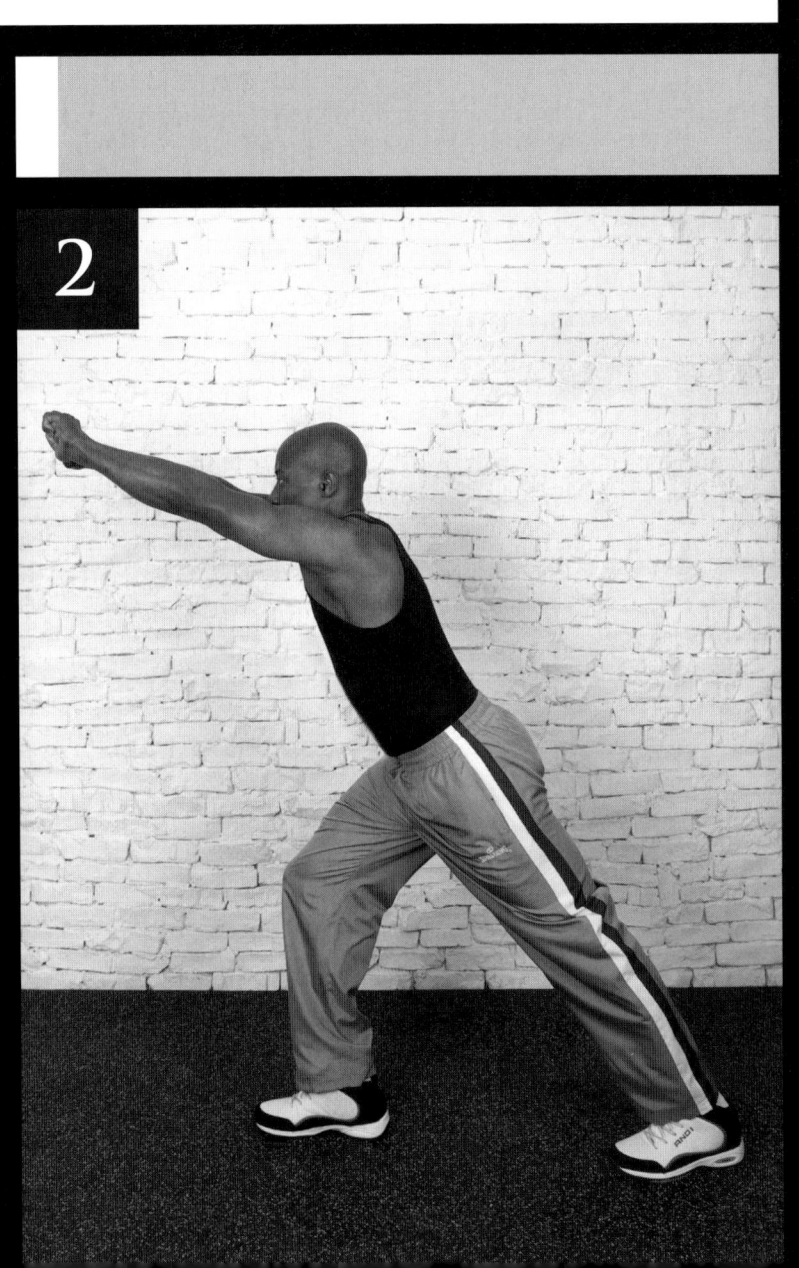

3 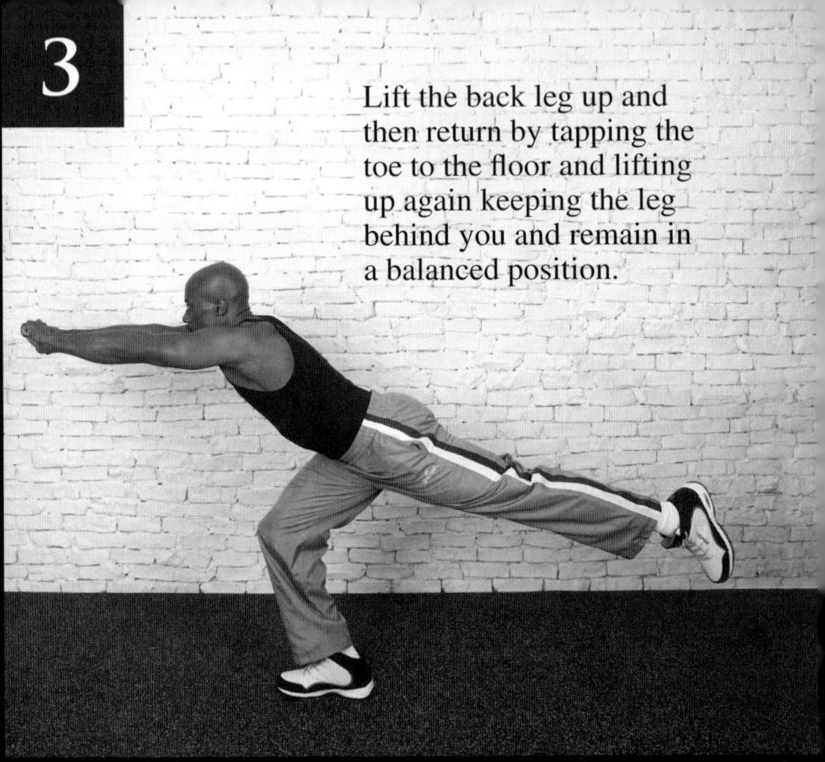 Lift the back leg up and then return by tapping the toe to the floor and lifting up again keeping the leg behind you and remain in a balanced position.

4 The toe should be tapped to the ground for a total of 10 to 15 times. With every tap of the toe of the foot that is behind you, you should lift up and then go back down to touch and then lift up.

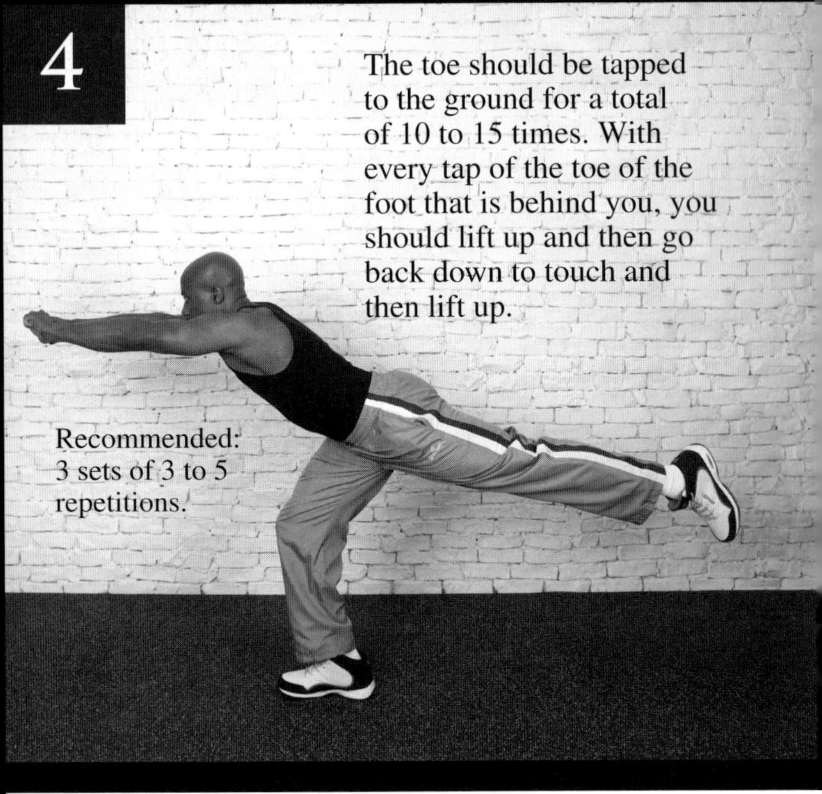

Recommended: 3 sets of 3 to 5 repetitions.

Calf & Hamstrings Stretch and Balance Exercise

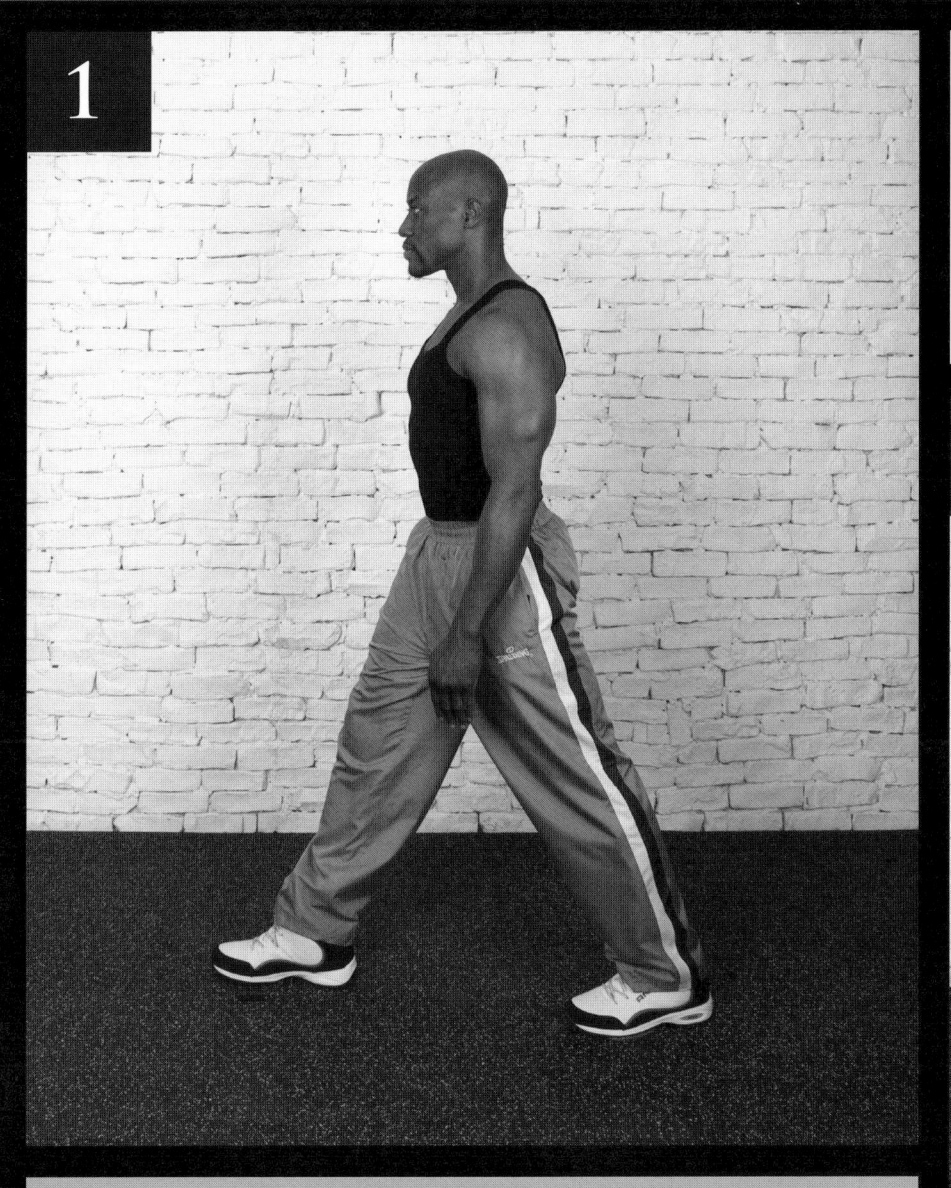

This exercise is executed starting from the neutral position with the feet apart and with one leg behind in a stride position. The body/torso should be dropped forward grasping the right foot with the right hand while bending the left knee and holding this position for 30 seconds.

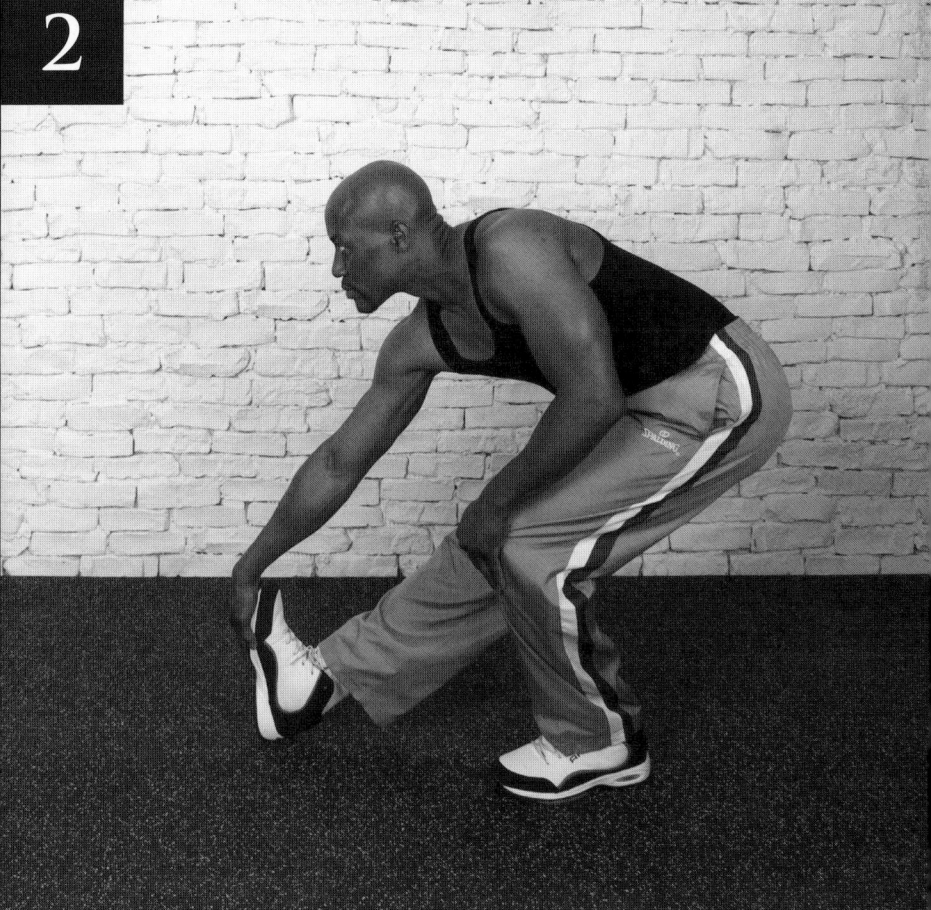

Hamstring Stretch

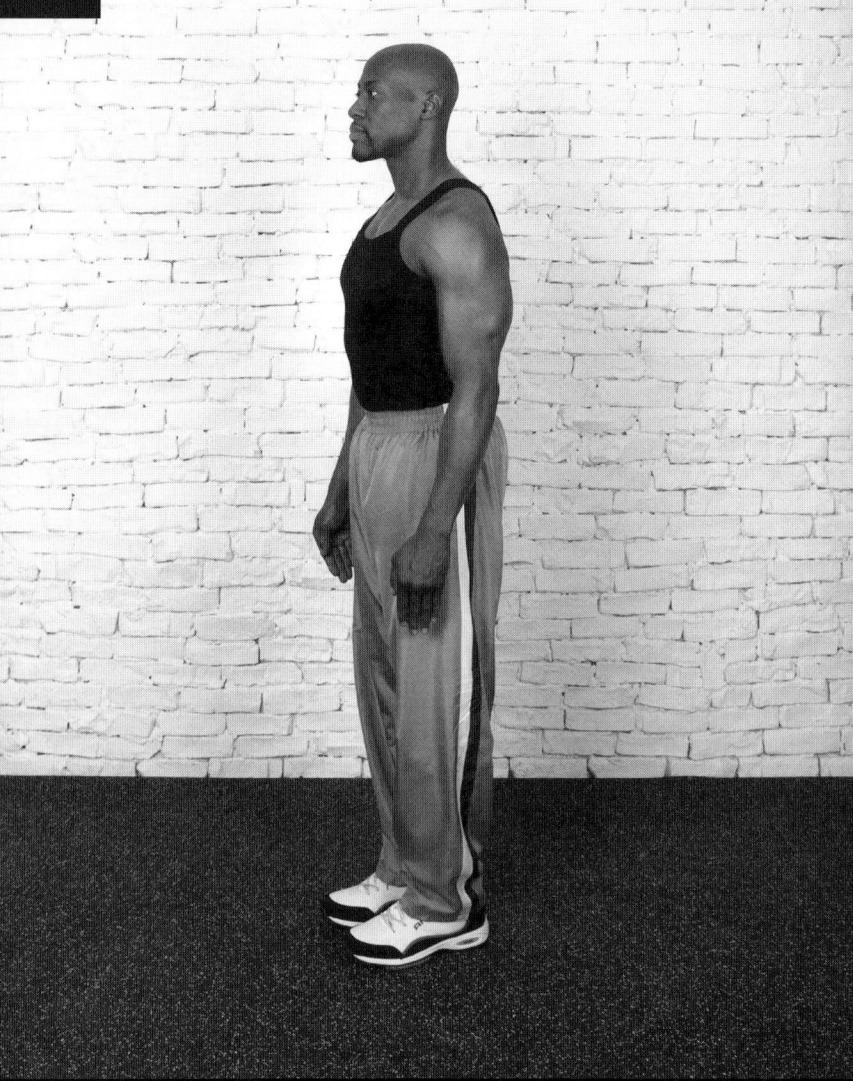

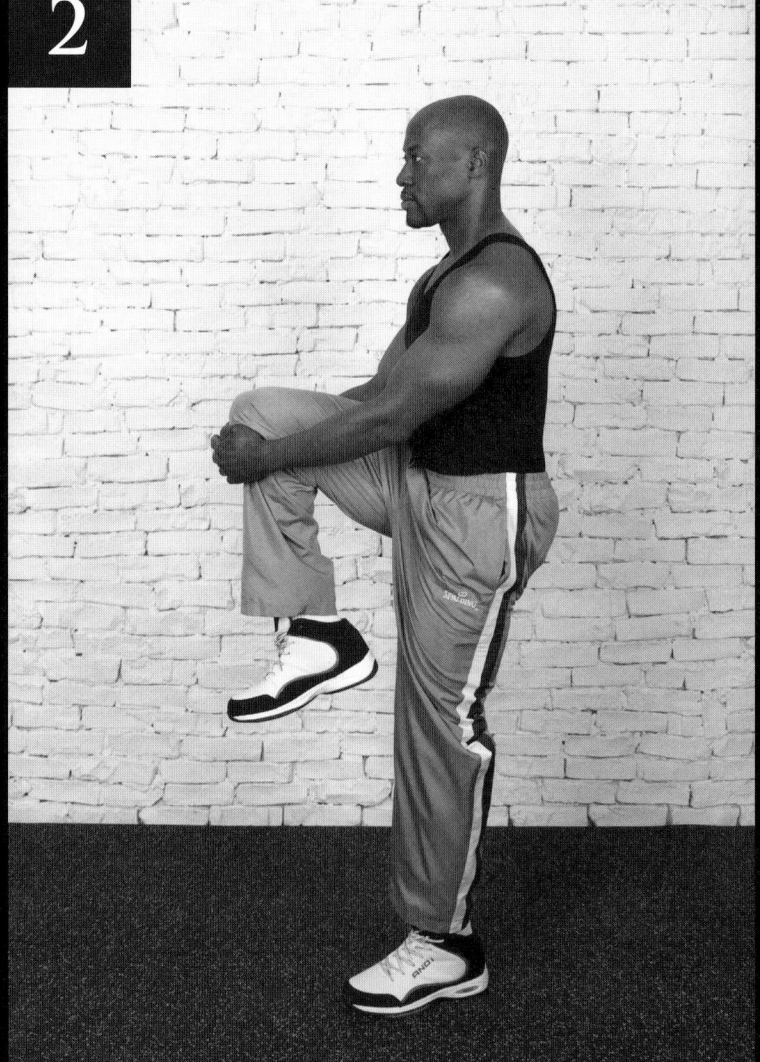

Start from the standing position with the feet slightly apart. Lift one leg forward and hold with the hands and hold this position for 30 seconds bringing the knee upward toward the chest.

FIT TIP:

Bring your knee up as high as comfortable initially. Do this stretch slowly. This can be done with the back against a wall for more stability and balance.

Hamstrings Super Stretch & Balance

Also Called Forward Hamstring Stretch and Balance

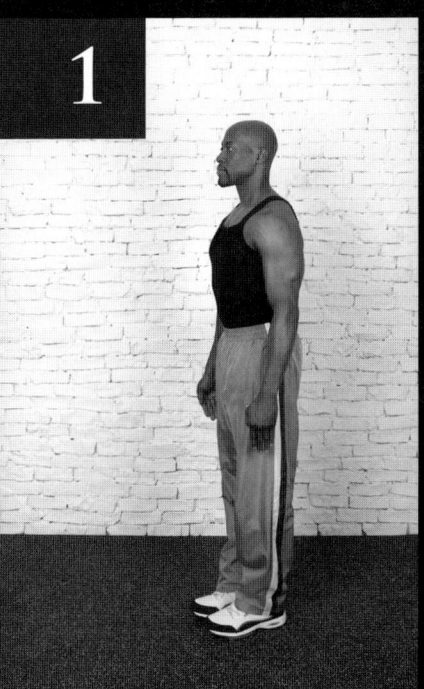

Stand with the feet shoulder-width apart. Starting with the right side, lift the right knee up. Grab and hold the foot of the elevated right leg. Extend the right knee and hold upright.

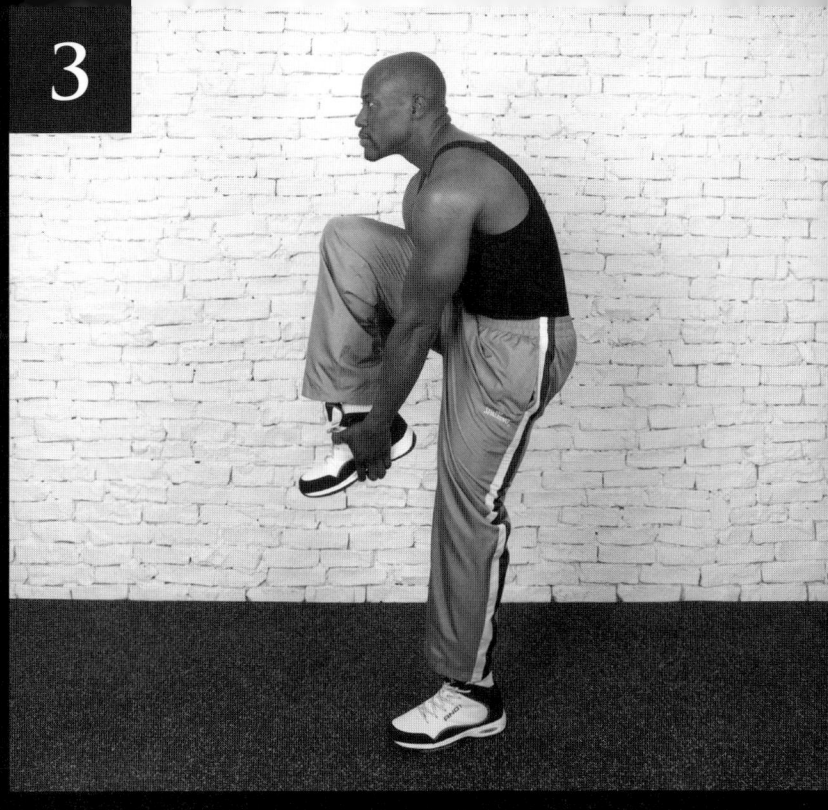

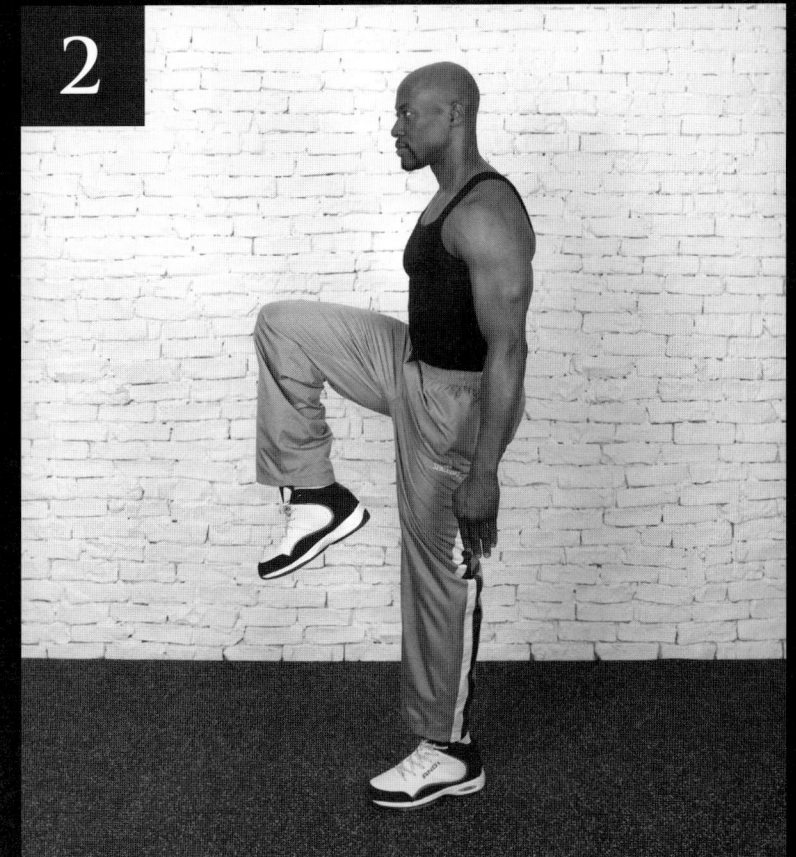

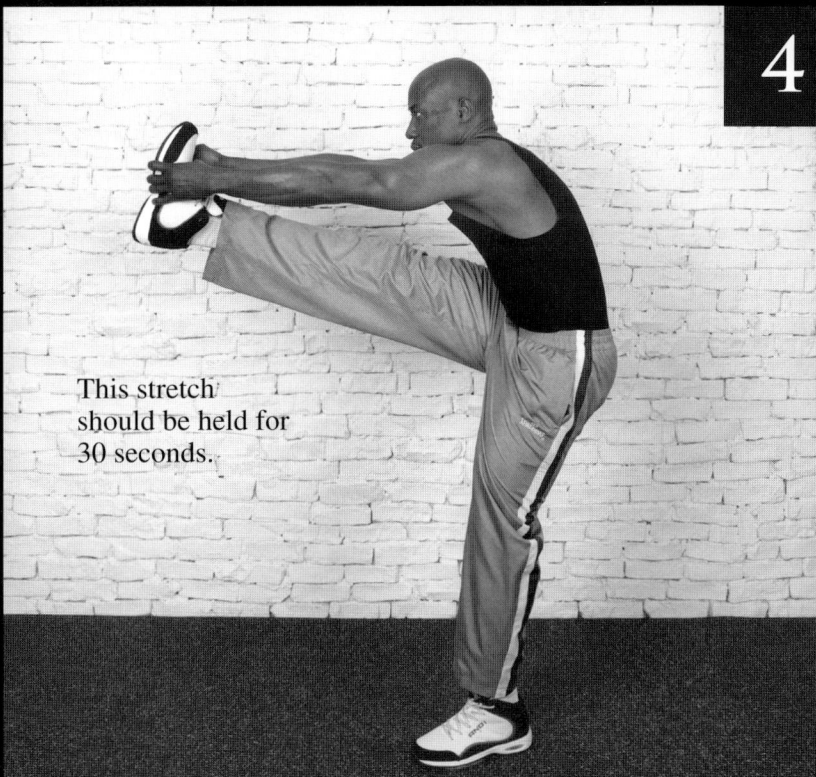

This stretch should be held for 30 seconds.

FIT TIP:

It is recommended doing this with your back against a wall for support initially.

Recommended: 3 sets of 5 repetitions.

Lateral Hamstrings Super Stretch & Balance

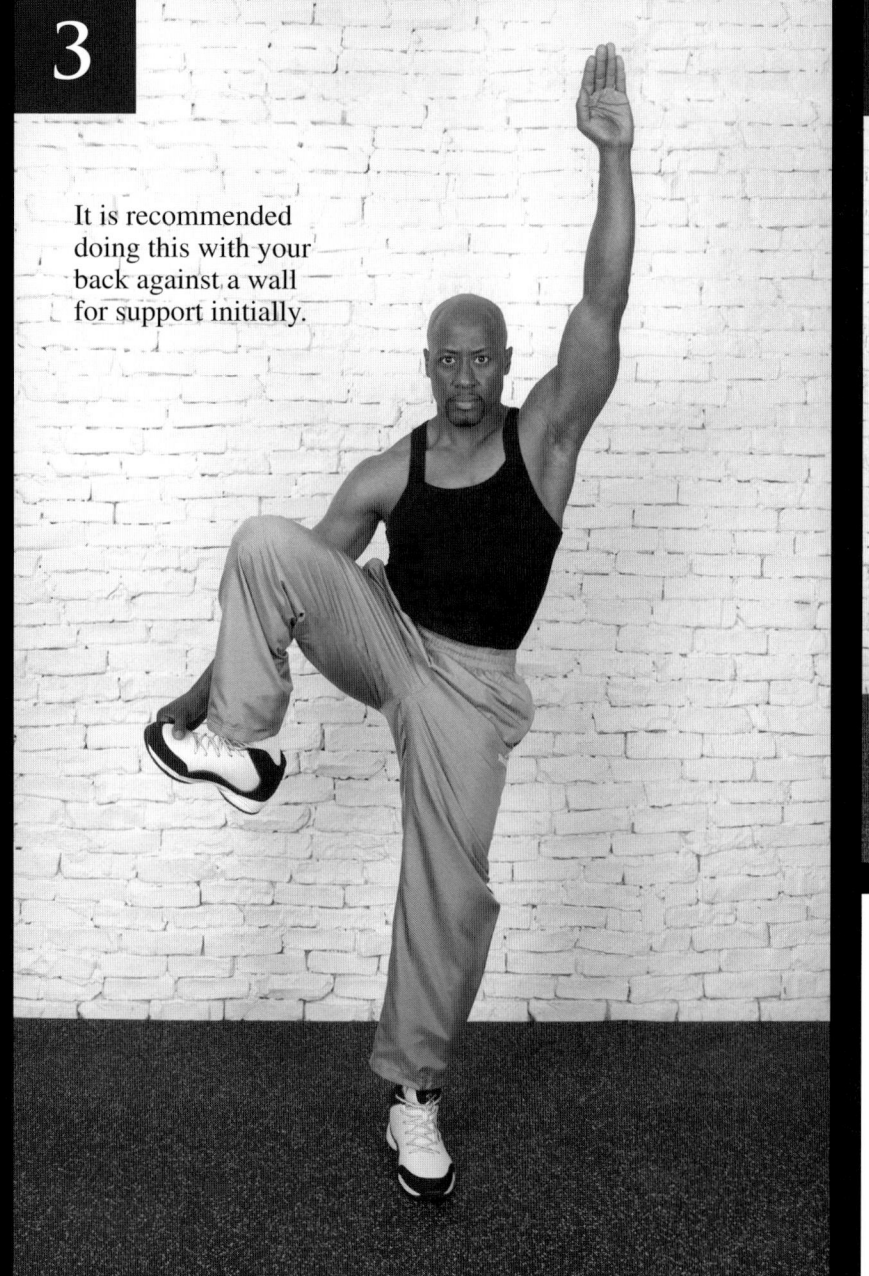

It is recommended doing this with your back against a wall for support initially.

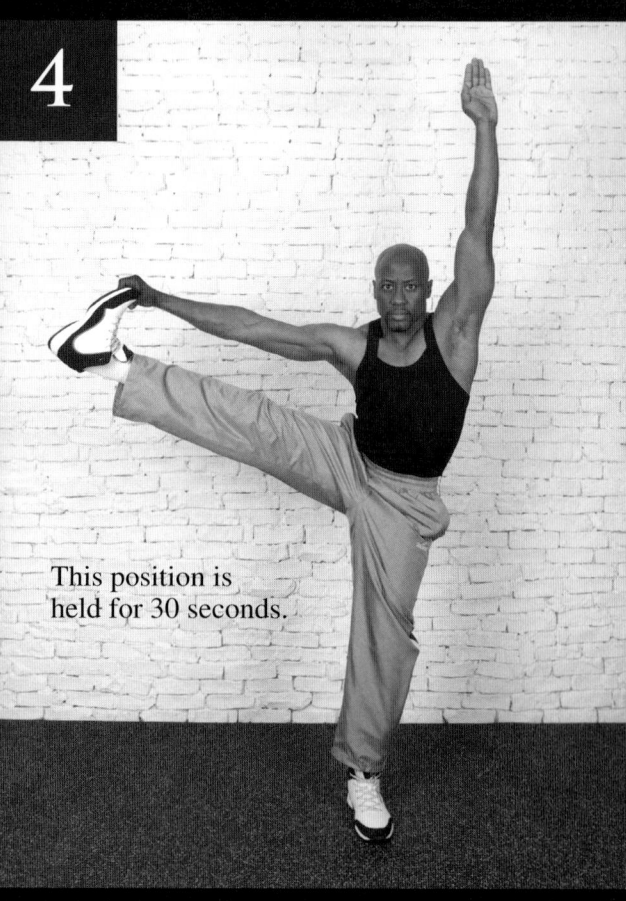

This position is held for 30 seconds.

Start from the standing neutral position. Starting with the right side, the right foot is grasped with the right hand. The outside of the foot is grasped and the knee is extended. While facing forward, the knee and leg are extended outward laterally with the left arm above the head.

BACK STRETCH

1

Starting from the seated position, the toes should be flexed forward and the hands are open with palms reaching for the toes. This is a static stretch. There should be no bouncing. Hold position for 30 seconds.

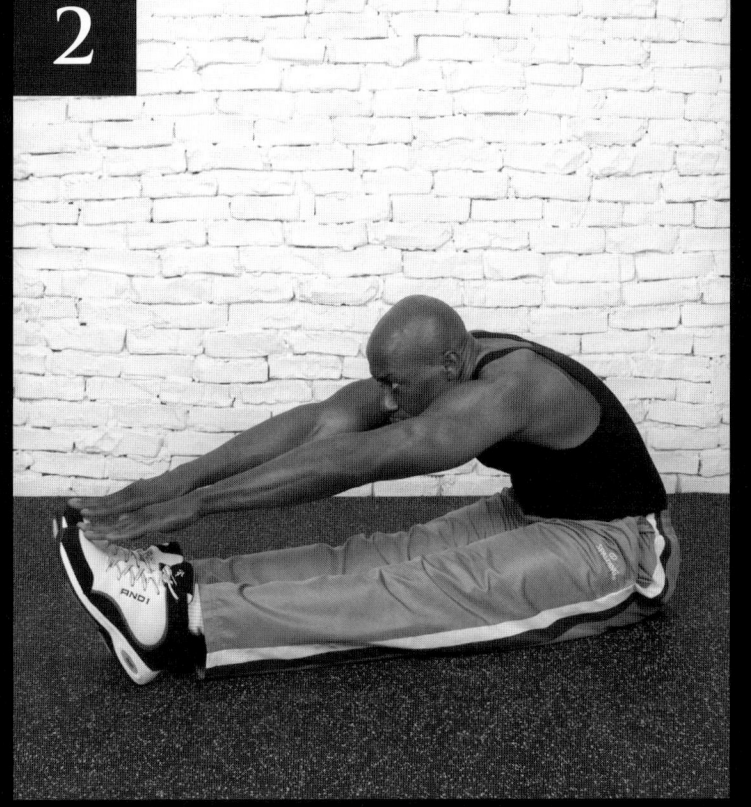

2

3

This should also be done with the toes now pointing toward you.

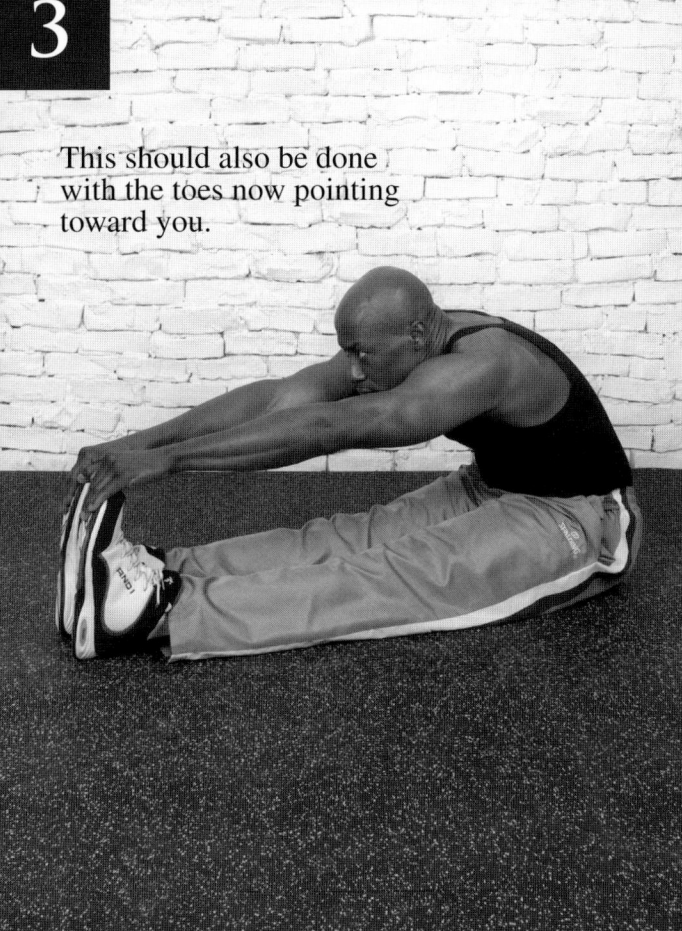

FIT TIP:

Exhale when reaching forward.

Recommended: 3 sets of 3 to 5 repetitions.

Seated Hamstrings & Calf Stretch

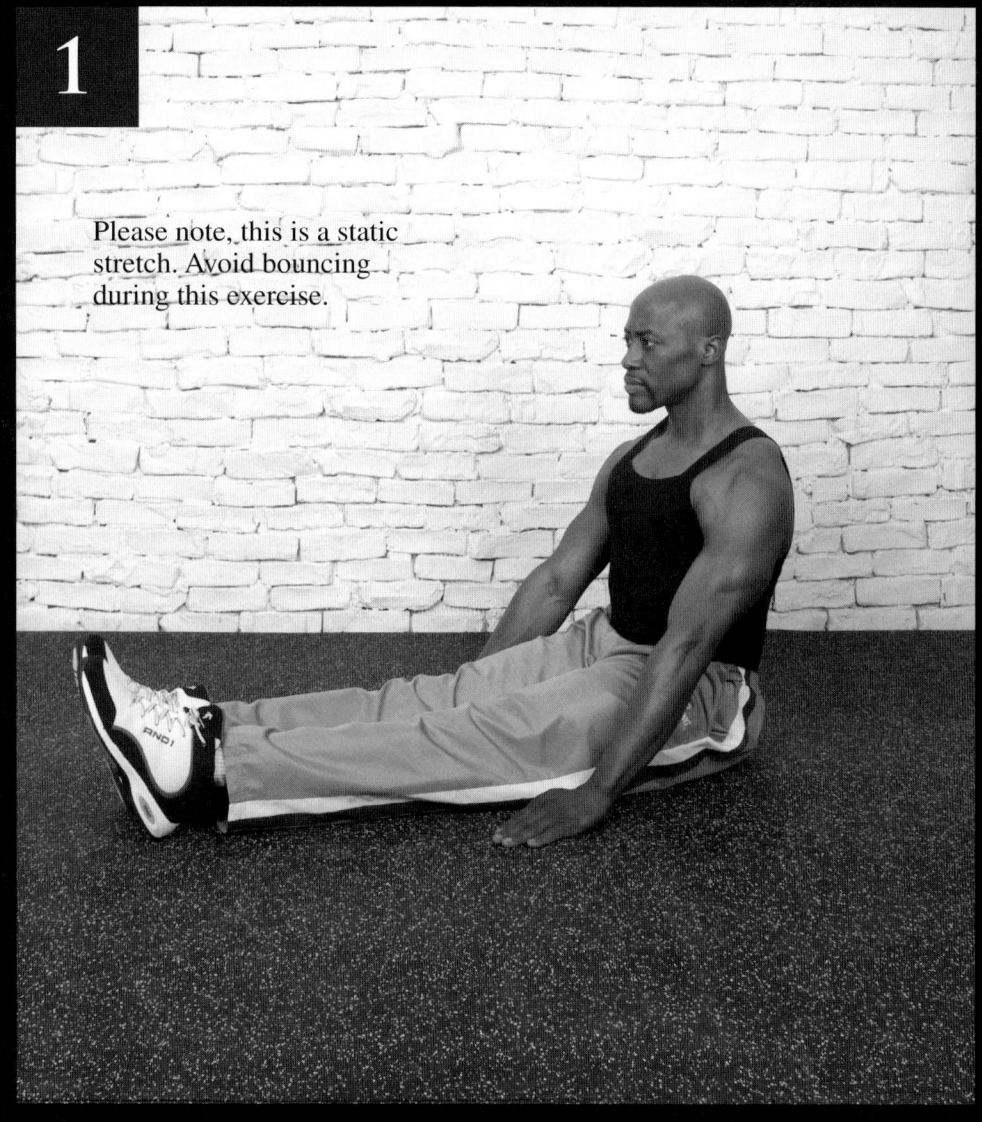

Please note, this is a static stretch. Avoid bouncing during this exercise.

FIT TIP:
Exhale when leaning forward
Recommended: 3 sets of 3 to 5 repetitions.

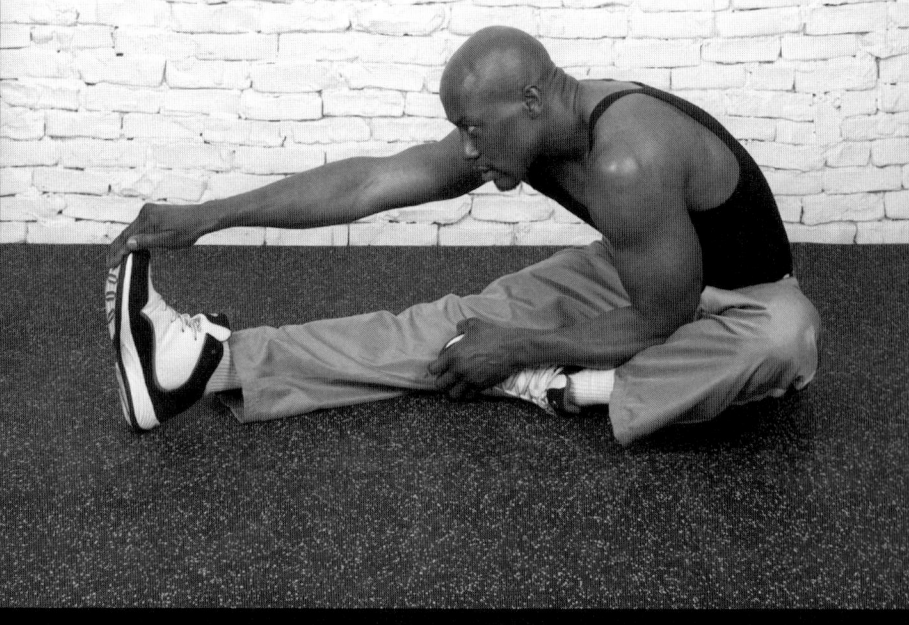

From the seated position, the right leg is extended. The left knee is bent with the left foot facing toward the right inner thigh and the right hand grasping the right foot with the back tilted forward.

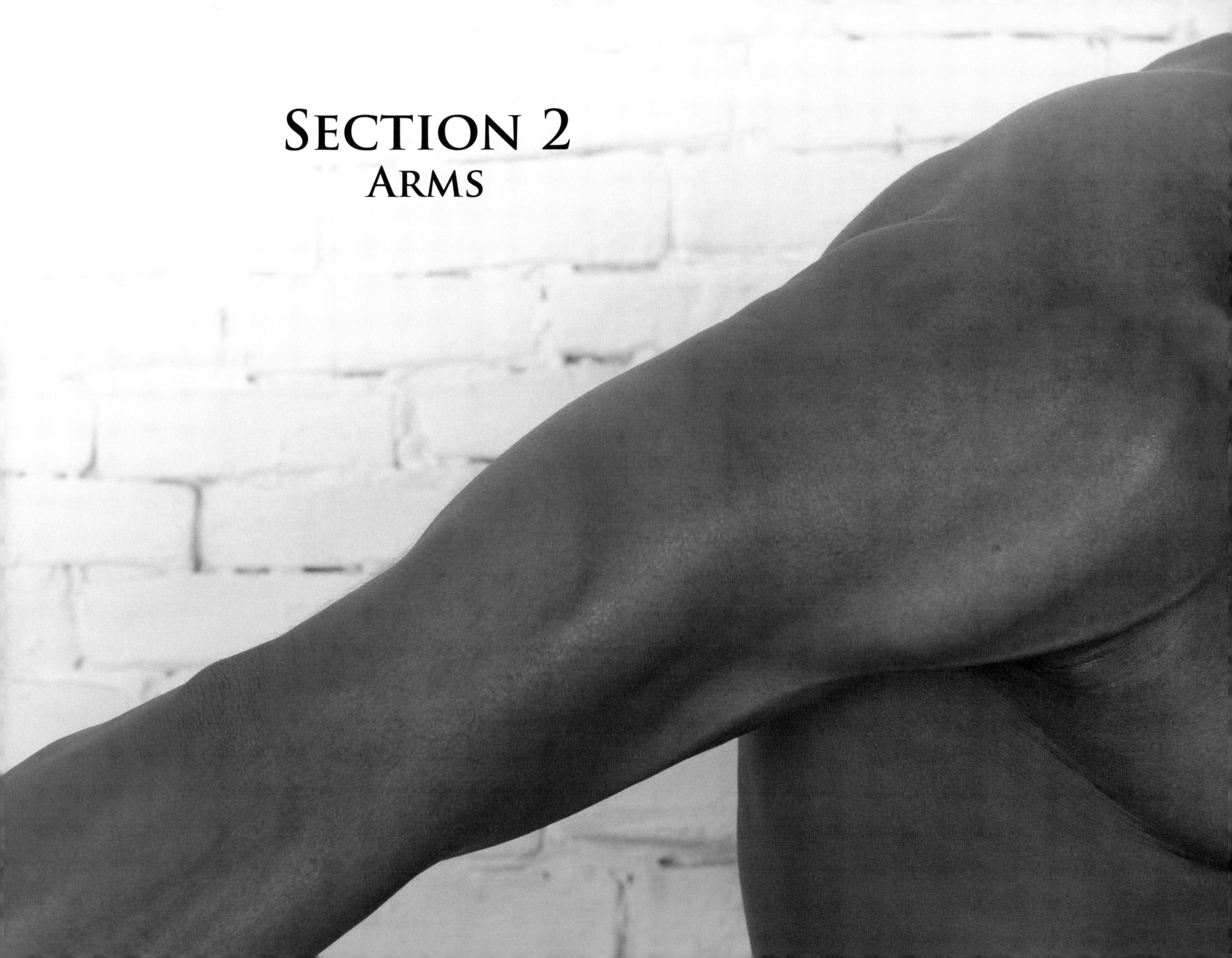

SECTION 2
ARMS

Standing Pulley Squats and Shoulder Press
Military Style

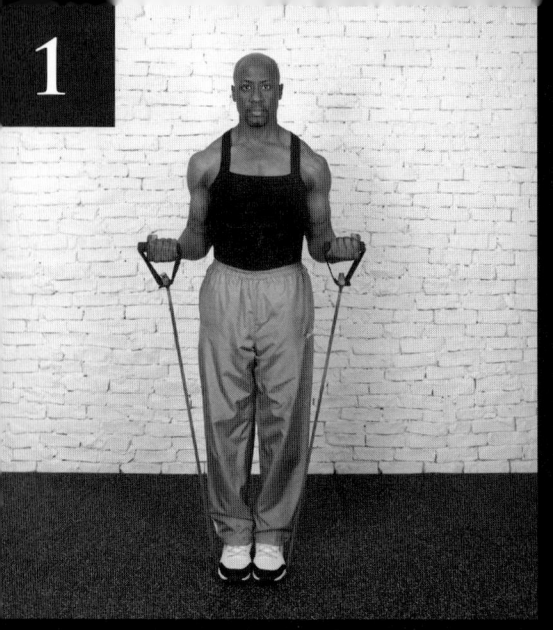

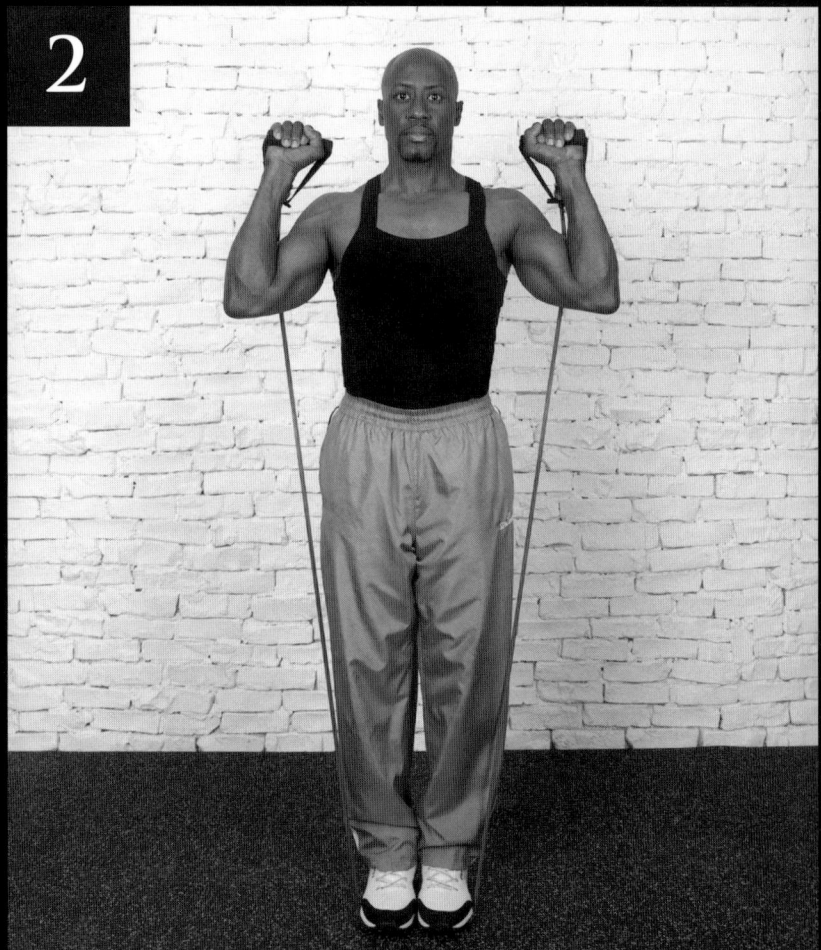

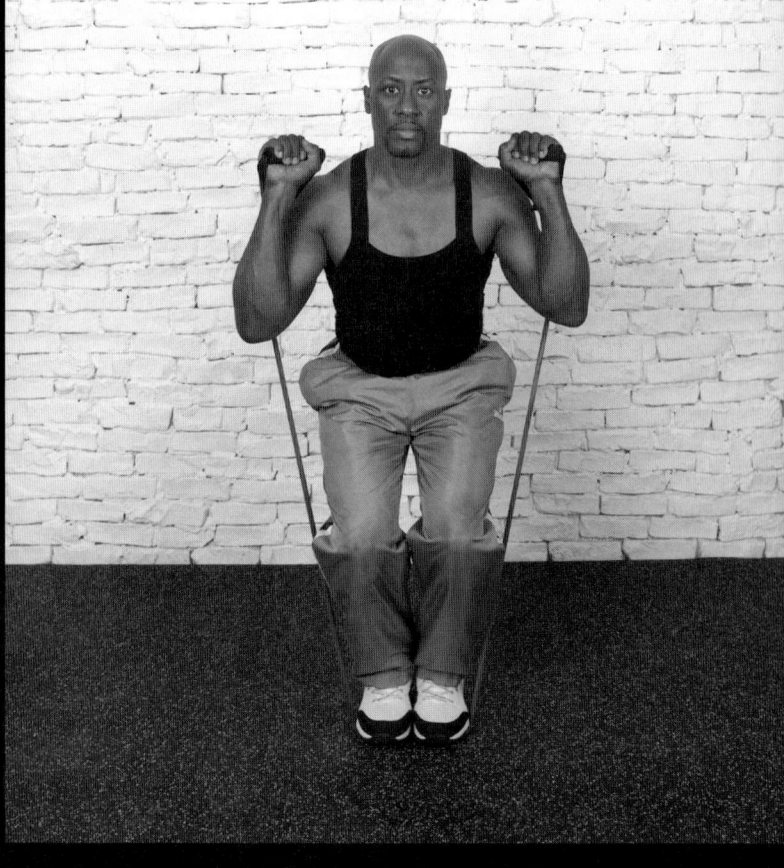

Starting from the biceps position, a biceps curl is done. Note: This is a twisting biceps curl and the palms are to face upward. The hands are brought up to the shoulders. A squat is done and the hands are lifted above the head.

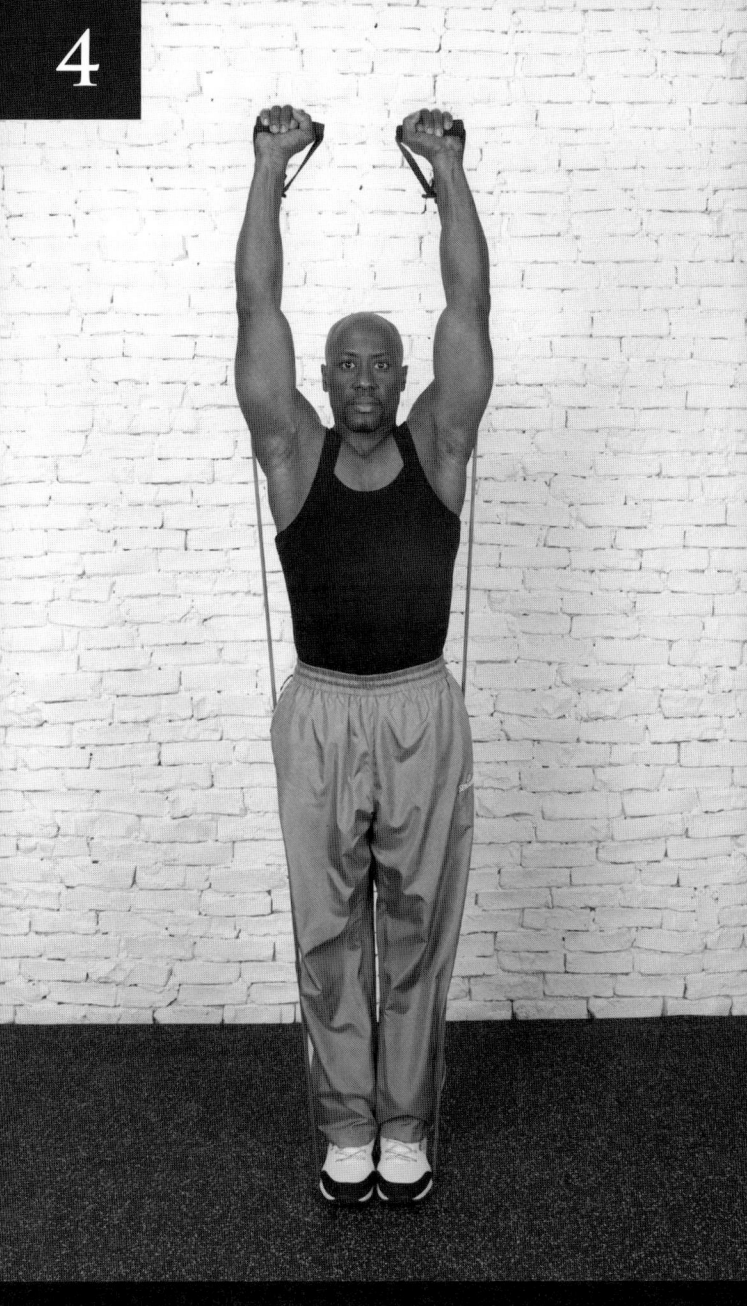

4

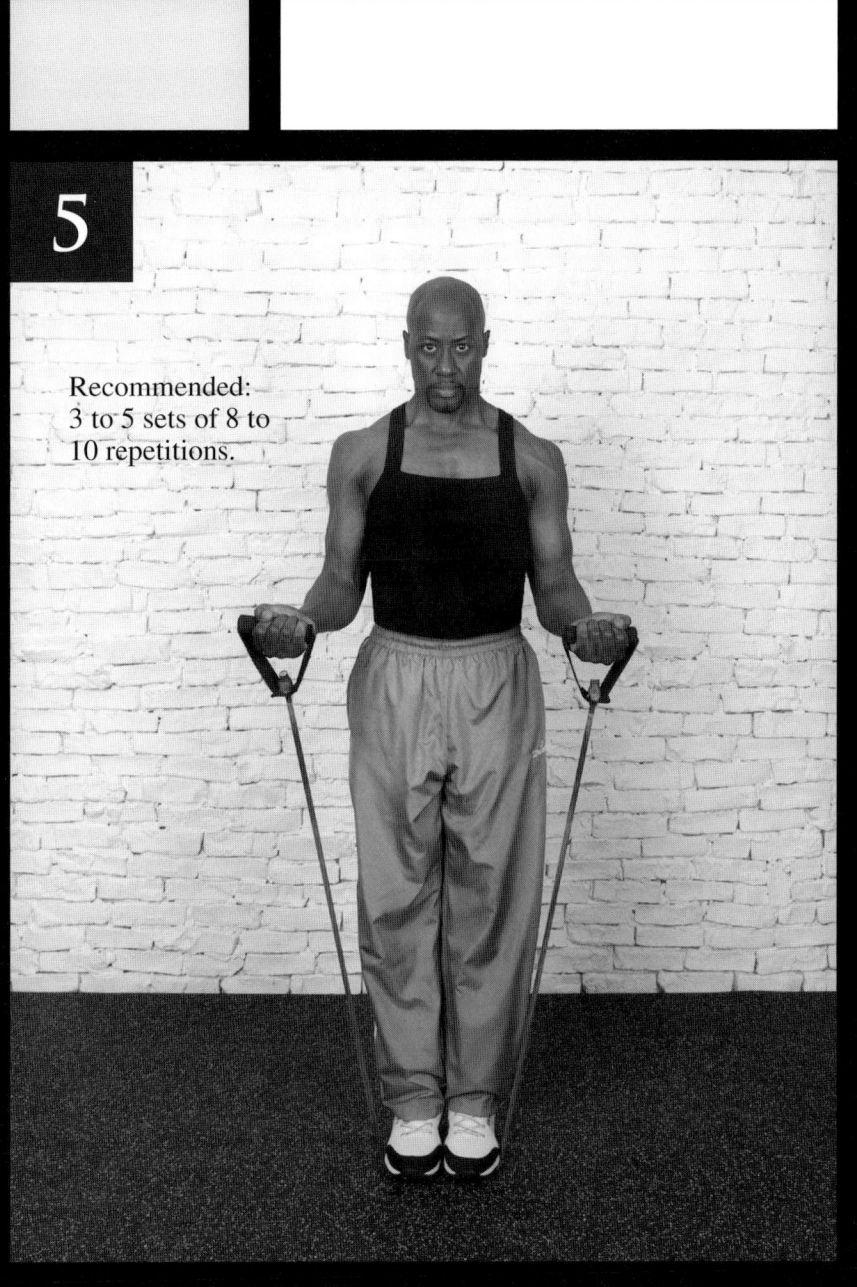

5

Recommended: 3 to 5 sets of 8 to 10 repetitions.

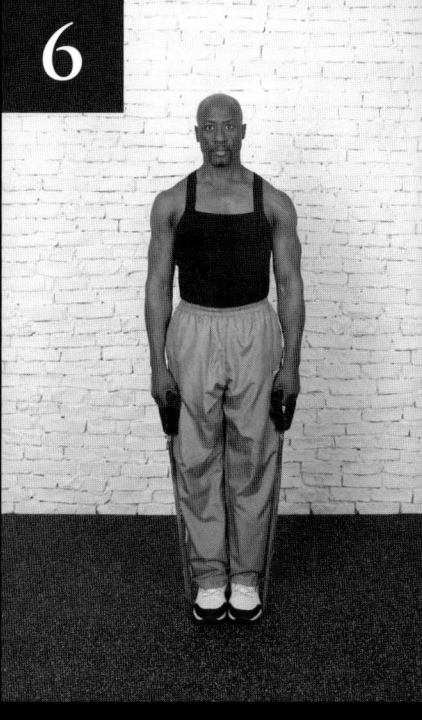

6

The exercises are completed by bringing the hands back to shoulder position, back to the half biceps curl position, and then extend the elbows.

STANDING PULLEY BICEPS CURLS

FIT TIP:
Exhale when lowering the pulley.

This position should be held for 5 seconds and then the pulley is slowly lowered downward.

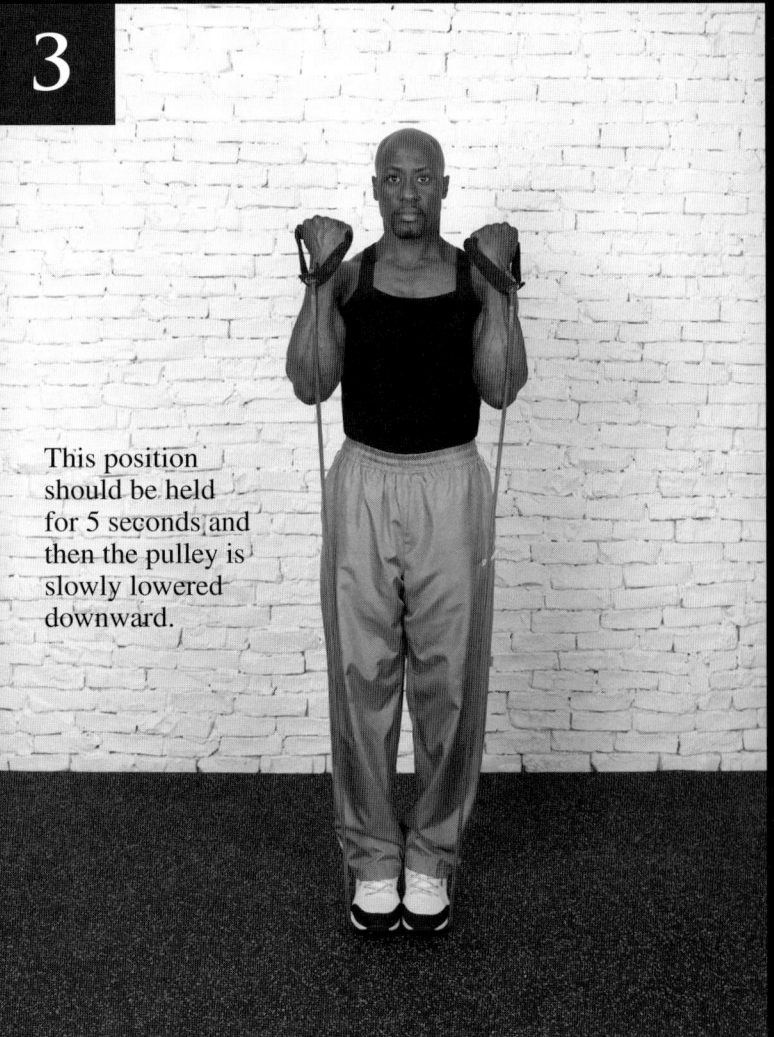

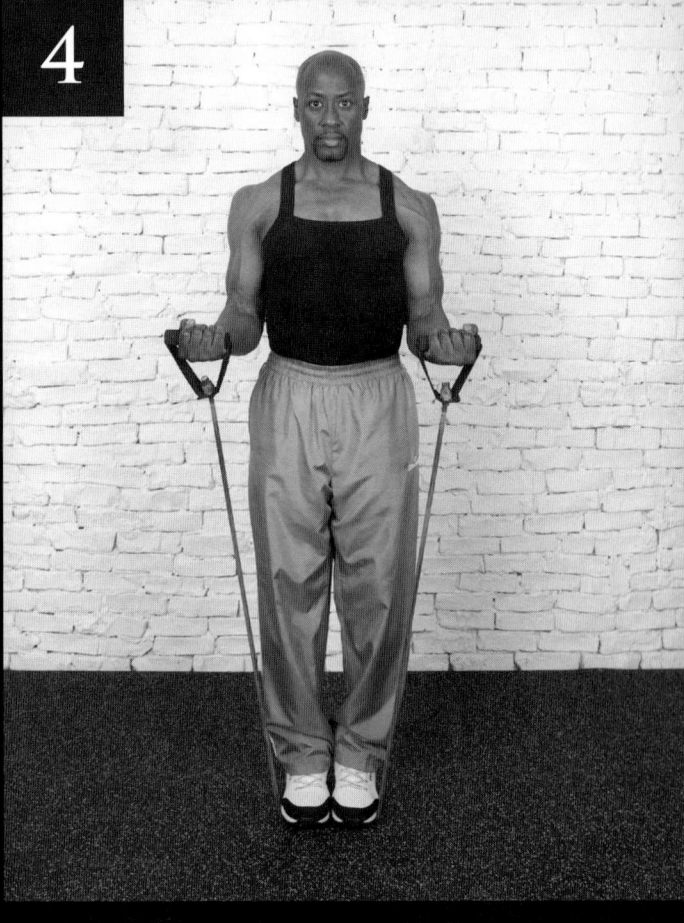

This exercise is done by stepping on to the pulley with the feet together. Knees slightly bent, grasp the pulleys, flex at the elbow, and bring the hands upward toward the shoulder. Complete the exercise by bringing the hands downward and then extending the elbows.

Standing Forward Flexion Lateral Deltoid Raises

For Rhomboids, Lateral Deltoids, and Latissimus Dorsi

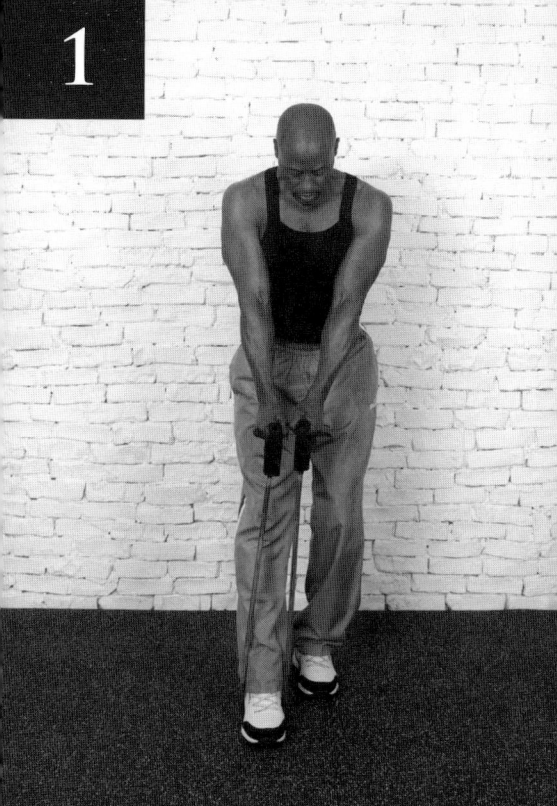

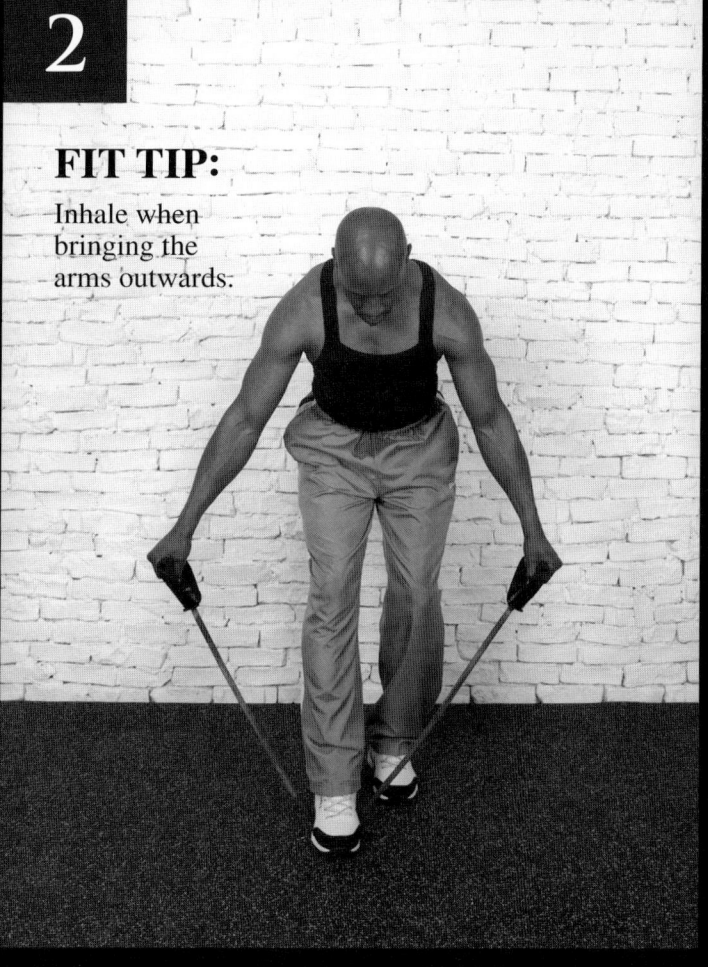

FIT TIP: Inhale when bringing the arms outwards.

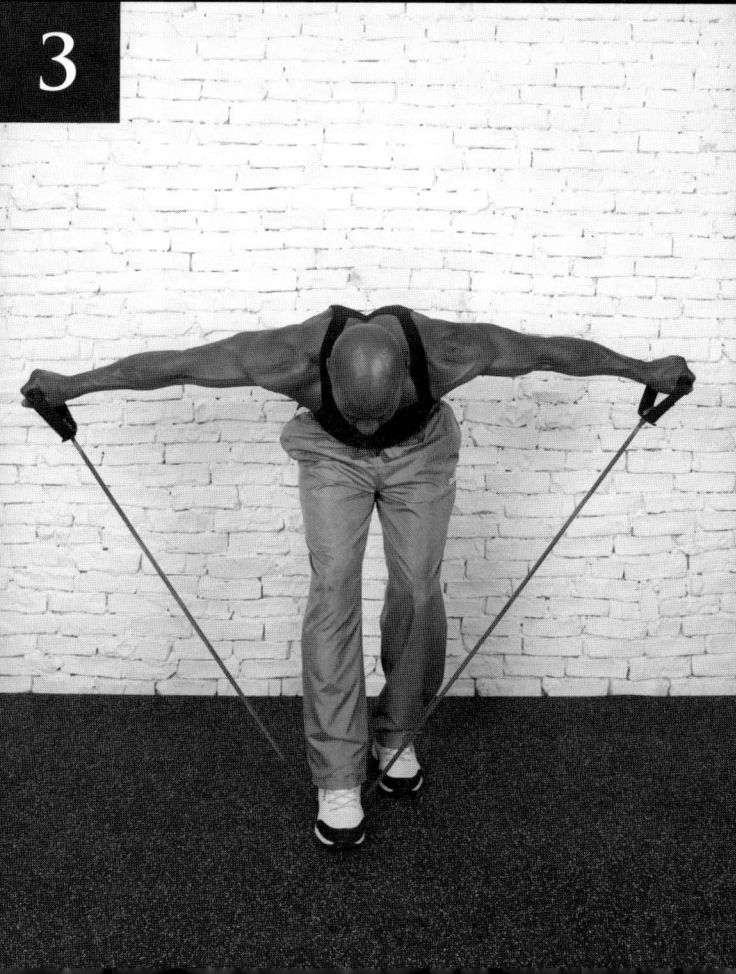

Stand upright with one leg behind you. Hold the pulley down with the forward leg and lean forward. The arms are elevated to the sides laterally pulling the pulley upright to 90 degrees with the arms straight out to the sides.

Recommended: 3 to 5 sets of 8 to 10 repetitions.

ANTERIOR DELTOID RAISES
With Pulley

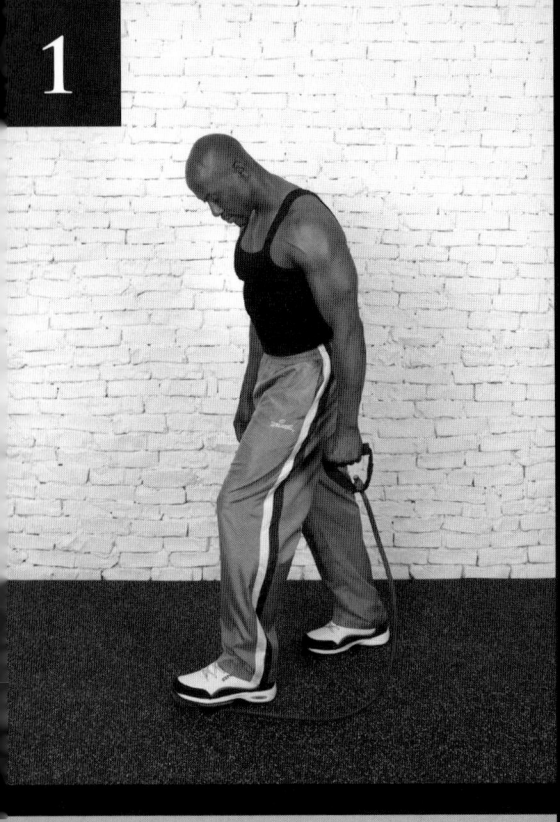

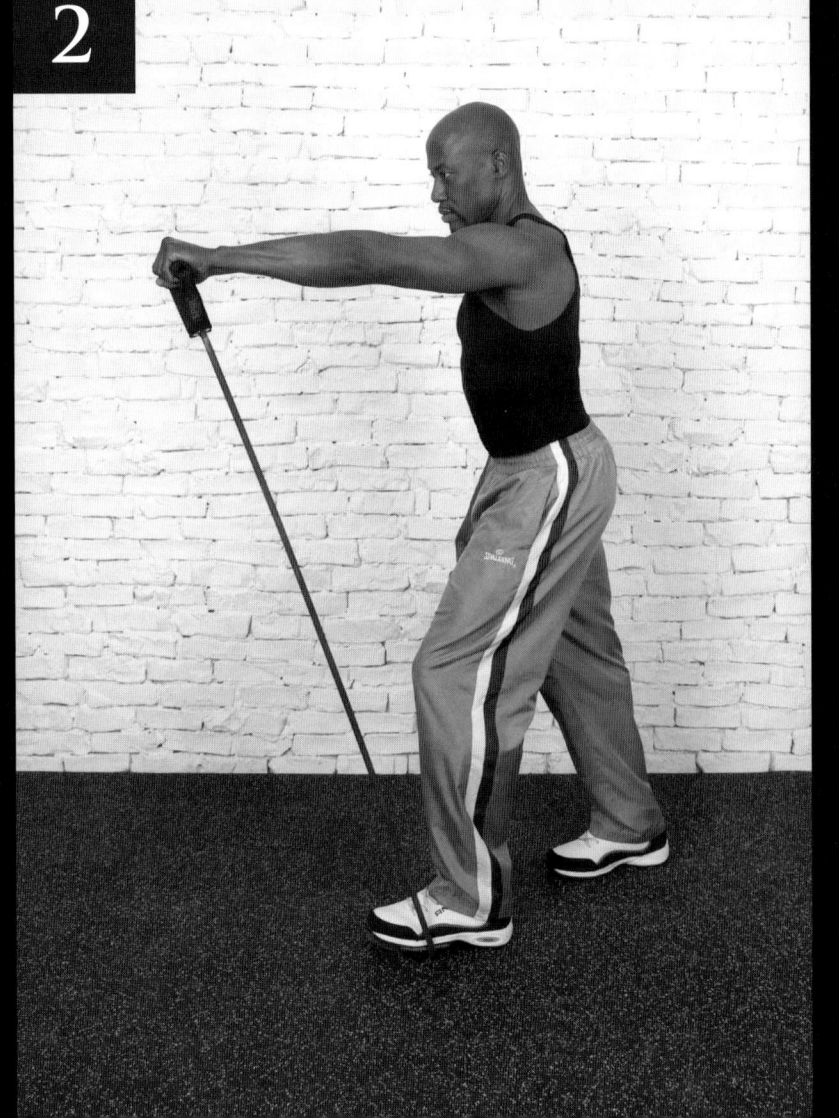

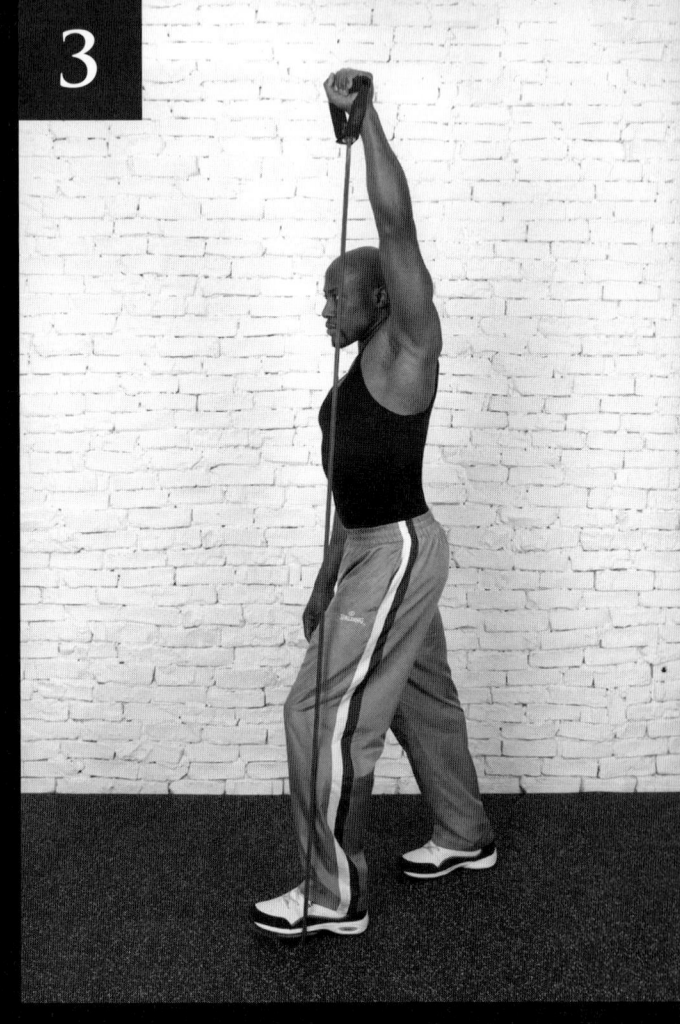

Stand starting from the neutral position. The pulley should be stepped on at slightly less than a halfway point. The palm is facing backwards. The feet are apart and the arm should be lifted above the head while leaving the pulley extended forward. The pulley should then be brought to the halfway point in front of your face and then brought up again above the head, then back to the halfway point and then back down to the side of your body.

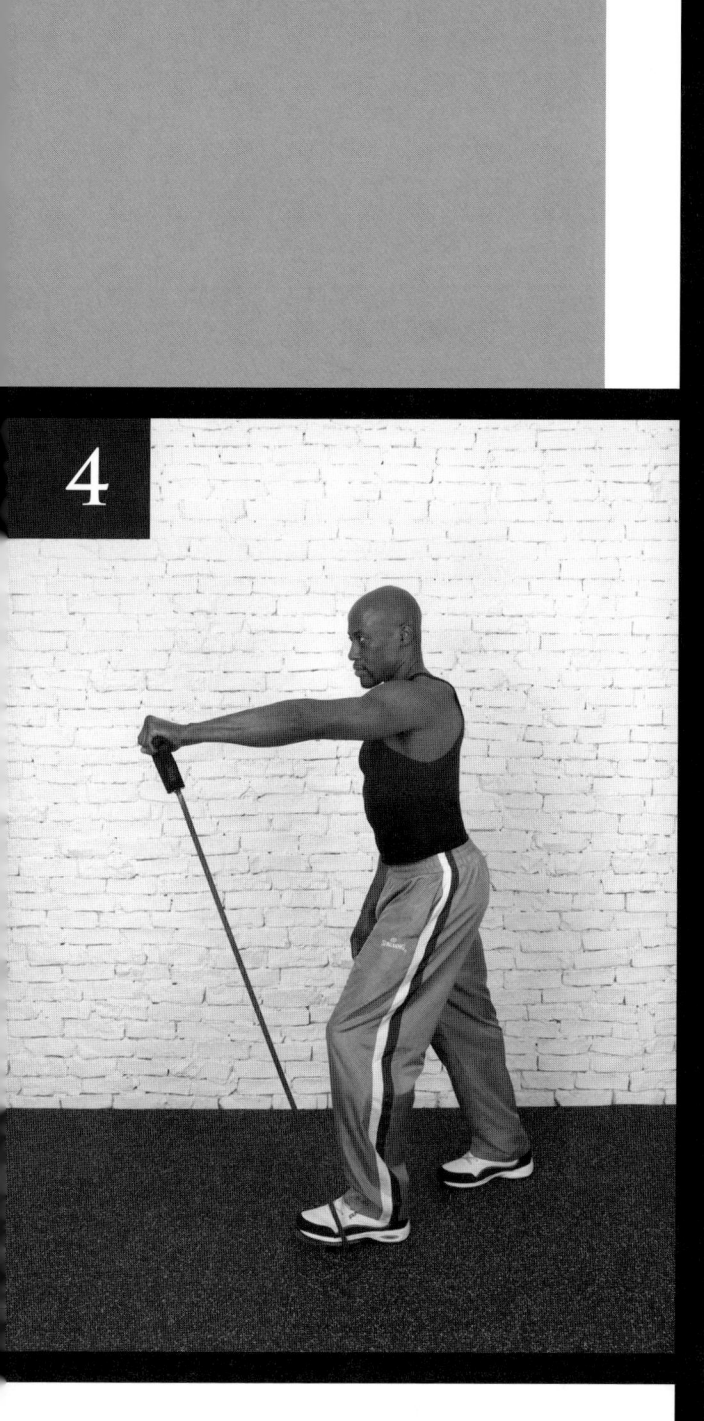

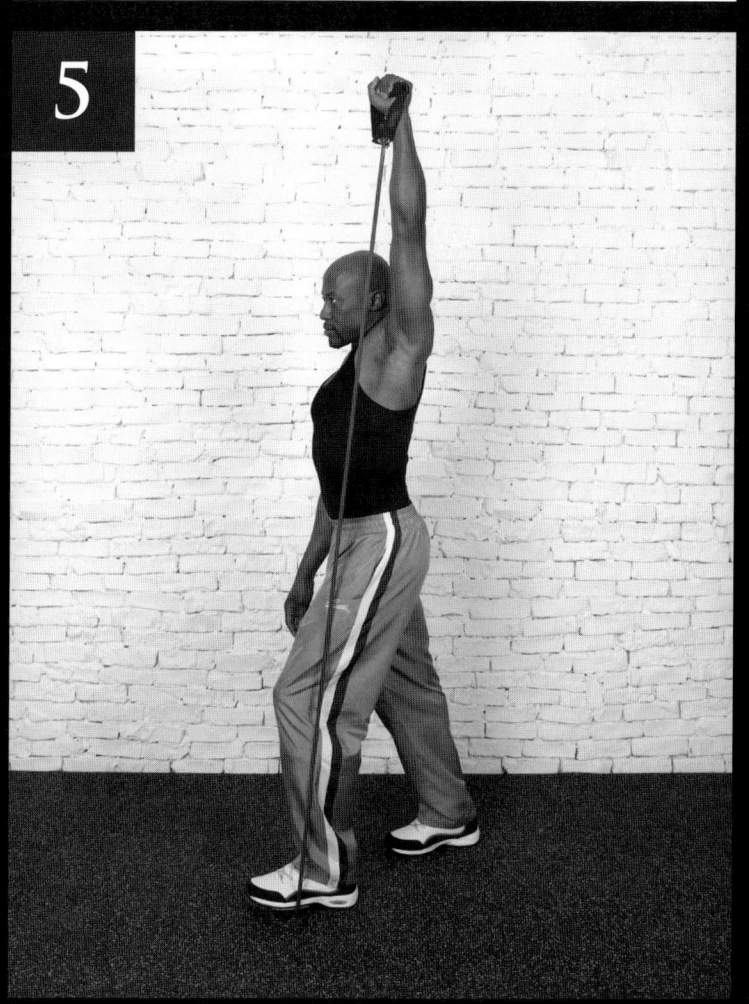

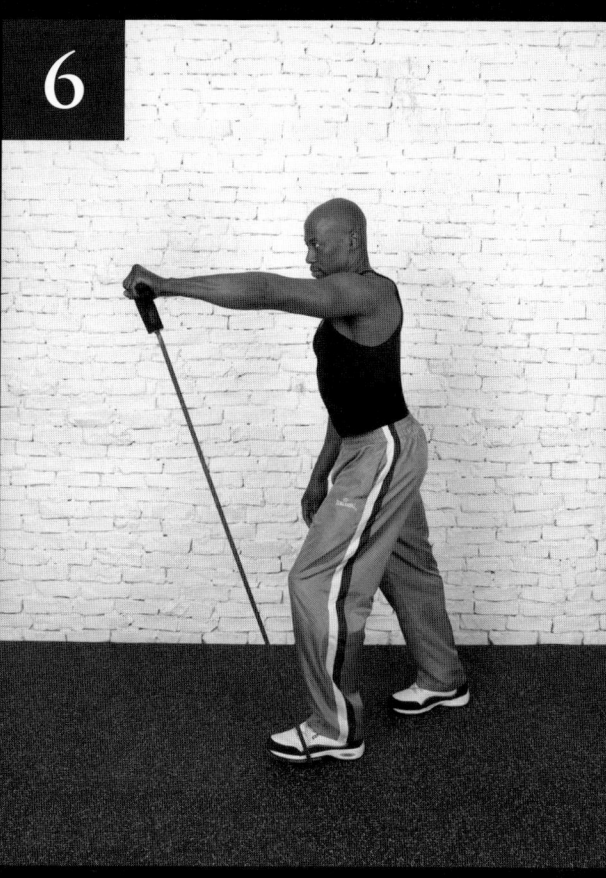

FIT TIP:

Keep your back straight and inhale when lifting hand overhead.

Recommended: 3 to 5 sets of 8 to 10 repetitions.

Posterior Deltoid Raises

With Pulley

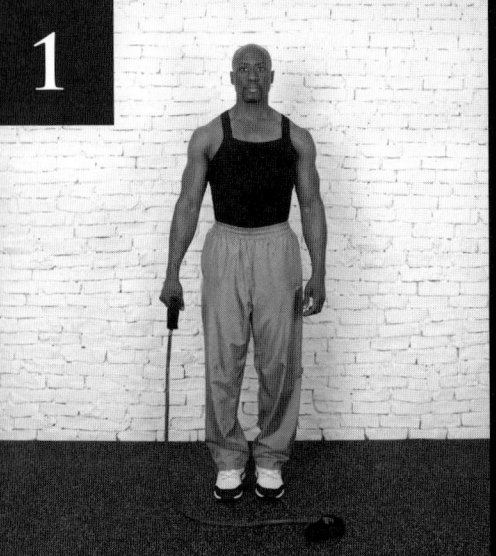

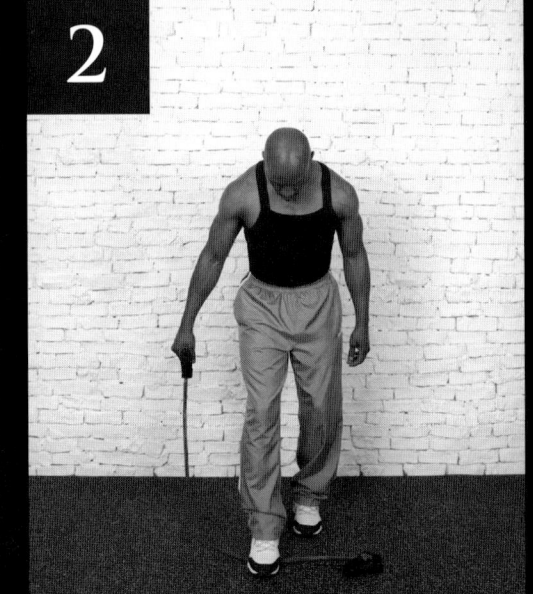

Starting from the neutral position, feet slightly apart, one foot should hold down the pulley at slightly less than the halfway point. Please note the palm should be facing the thigh. The arm should be lifted upward and posterior, not simply lateral but actually posterior with the elbow straightened.

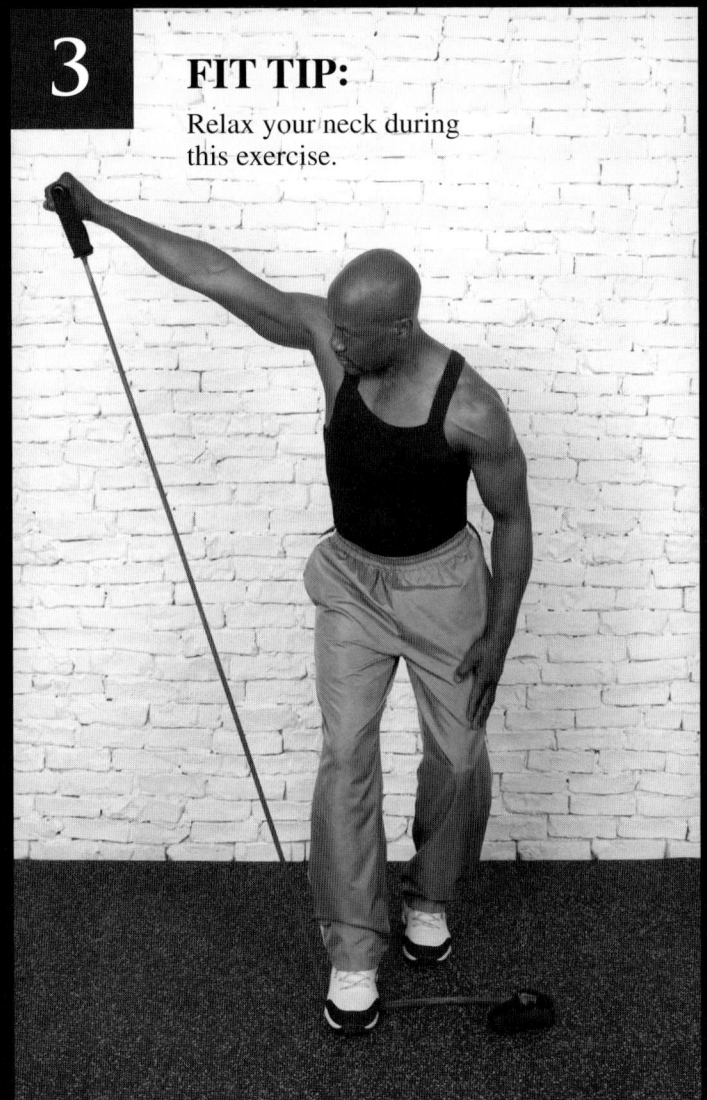

FIT TIP: Relax your neck during this exercise.

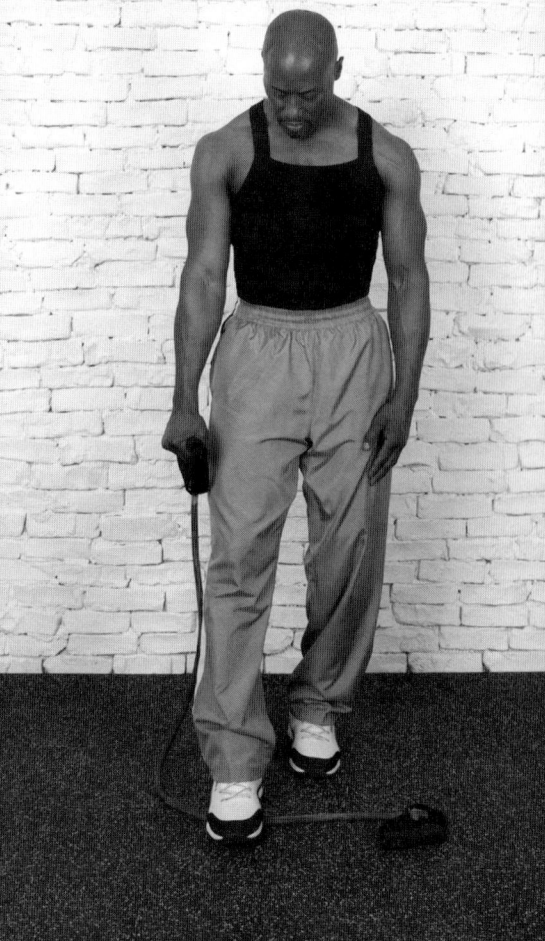

Recommended: 2 to 3 sets of 10 to 15 repetitions.

Seated Biceps Hammer Curls

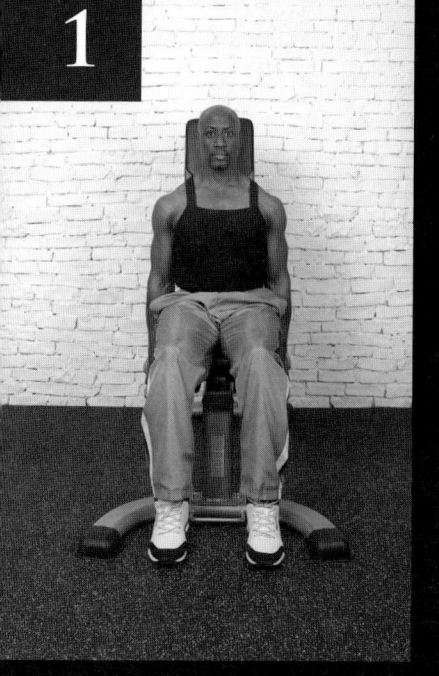

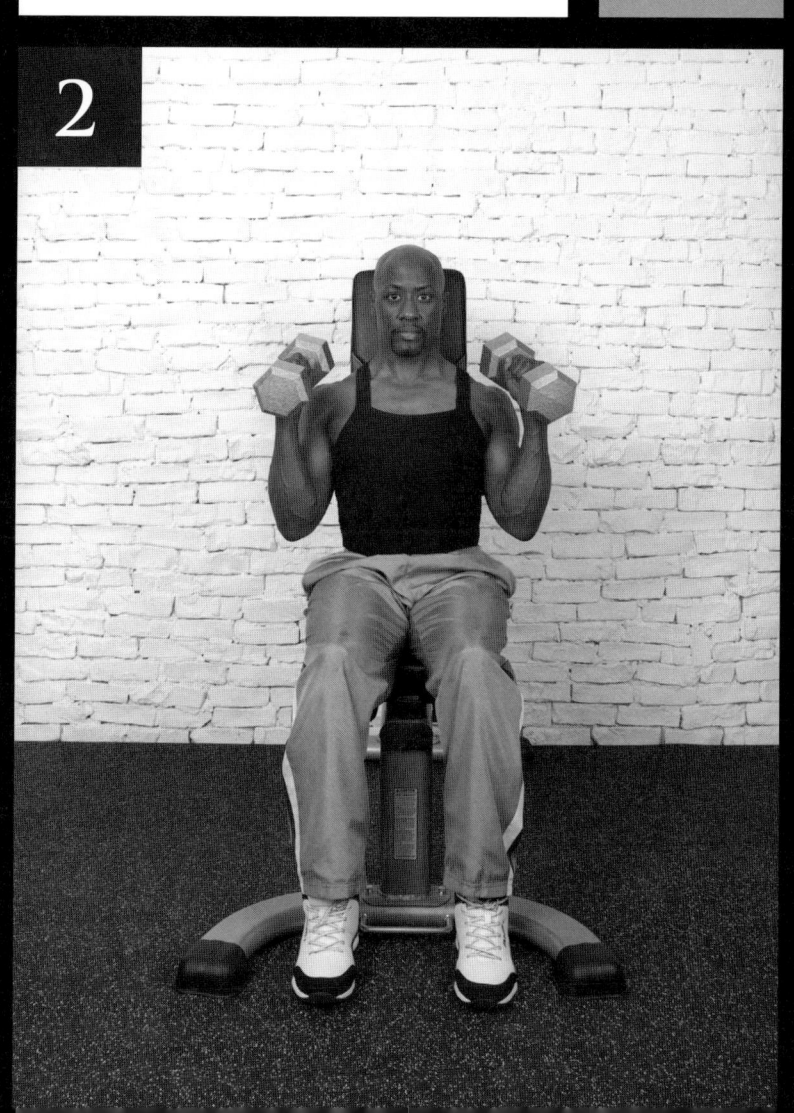

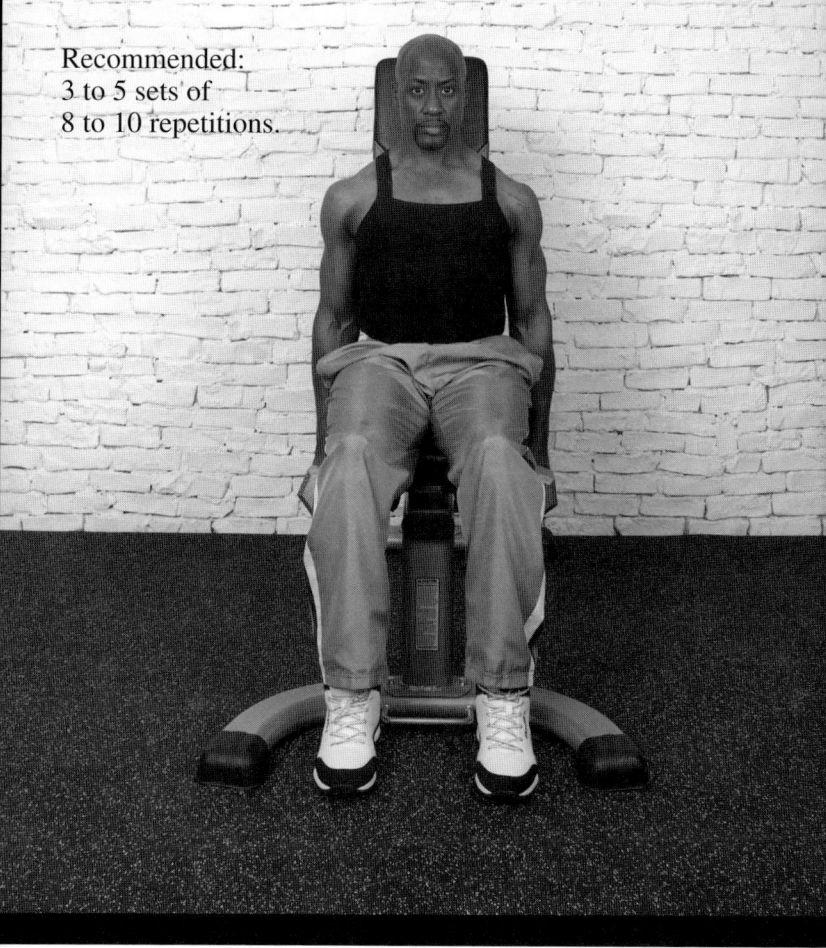

Recommended:
3 to 5 sets of
8 to 10 repetitions.

In a seated position hold the weights with the palms toward the thighs, keep the palms facing toward each other and lift the weights up flexing the biceps. Do the biceps curl with the weights in a hammer type position.

Combination Biceps Curls and Shoulder Press

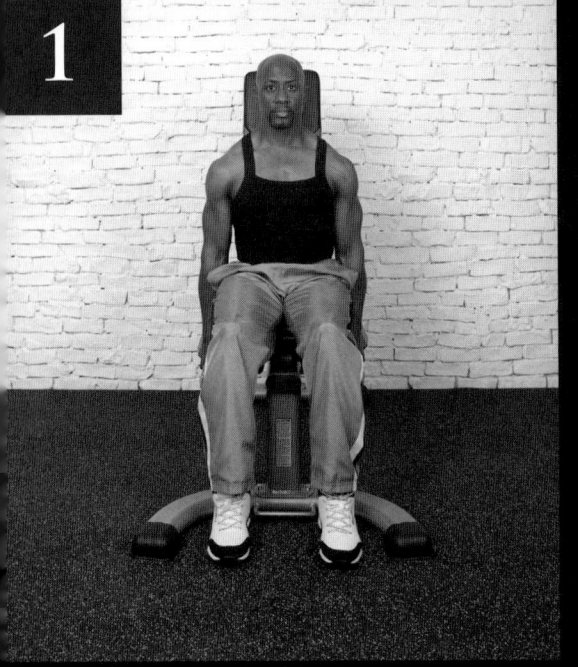
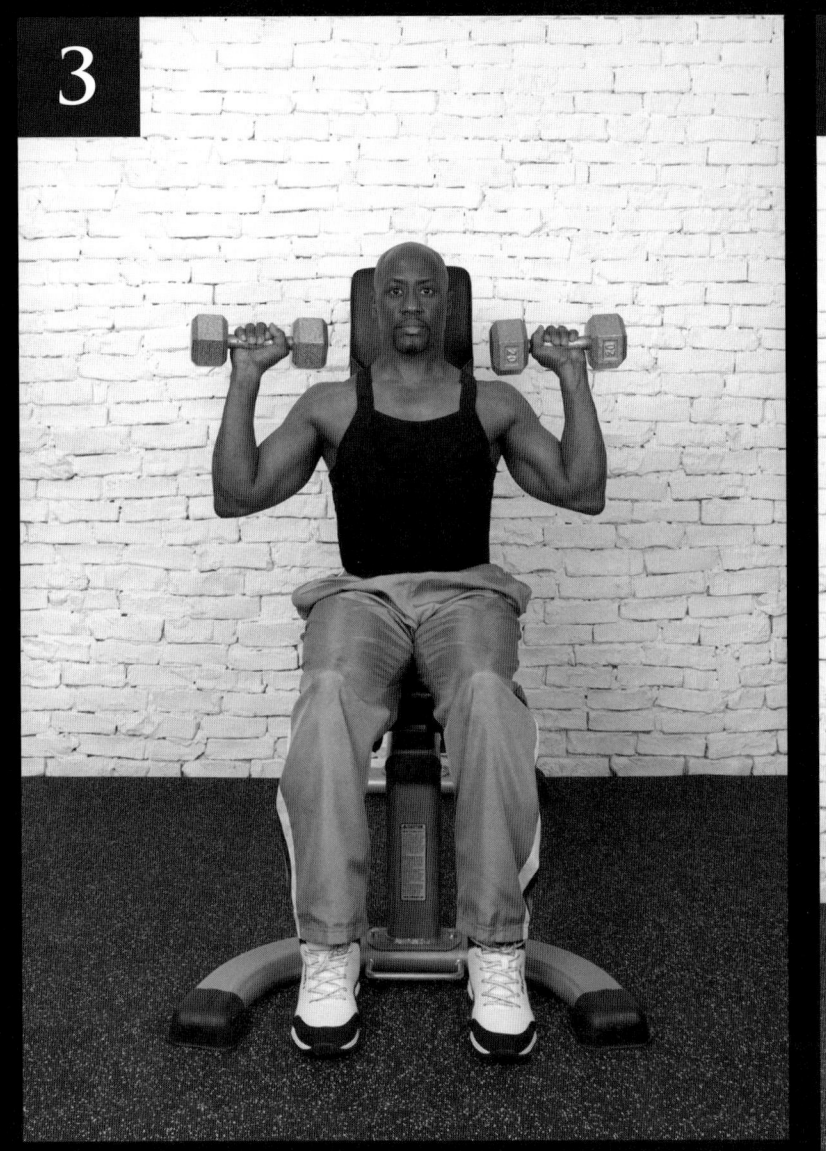
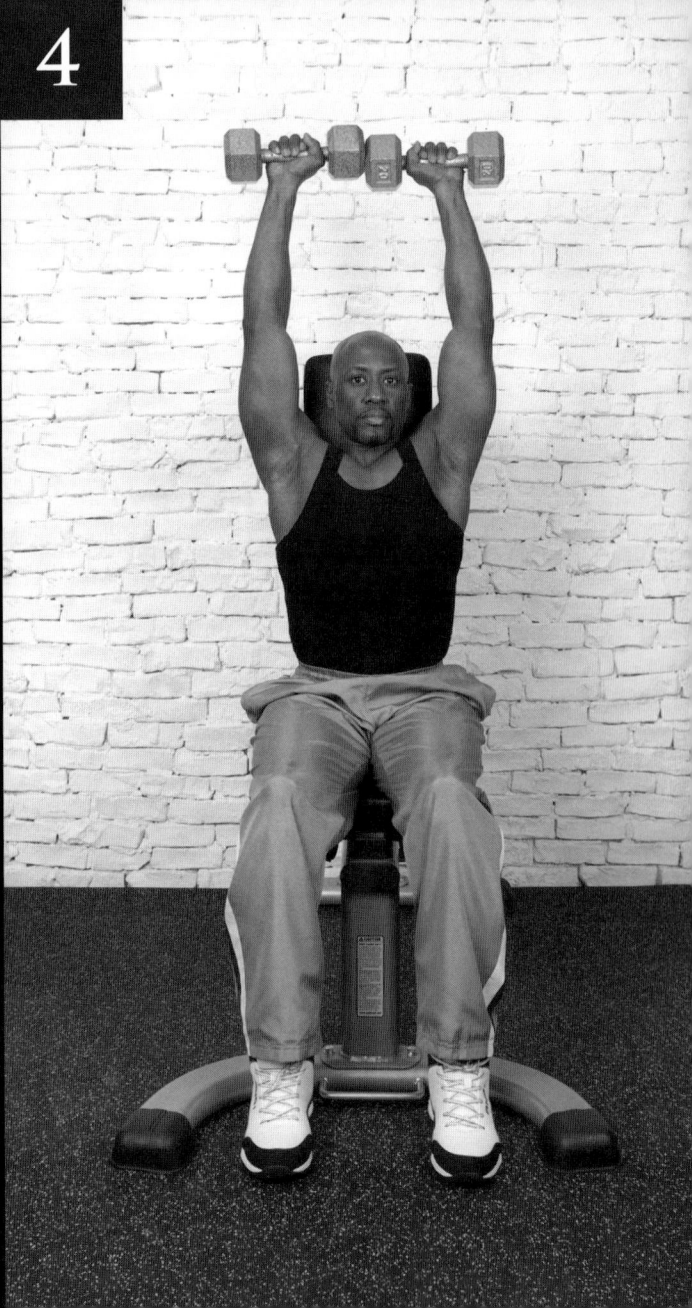

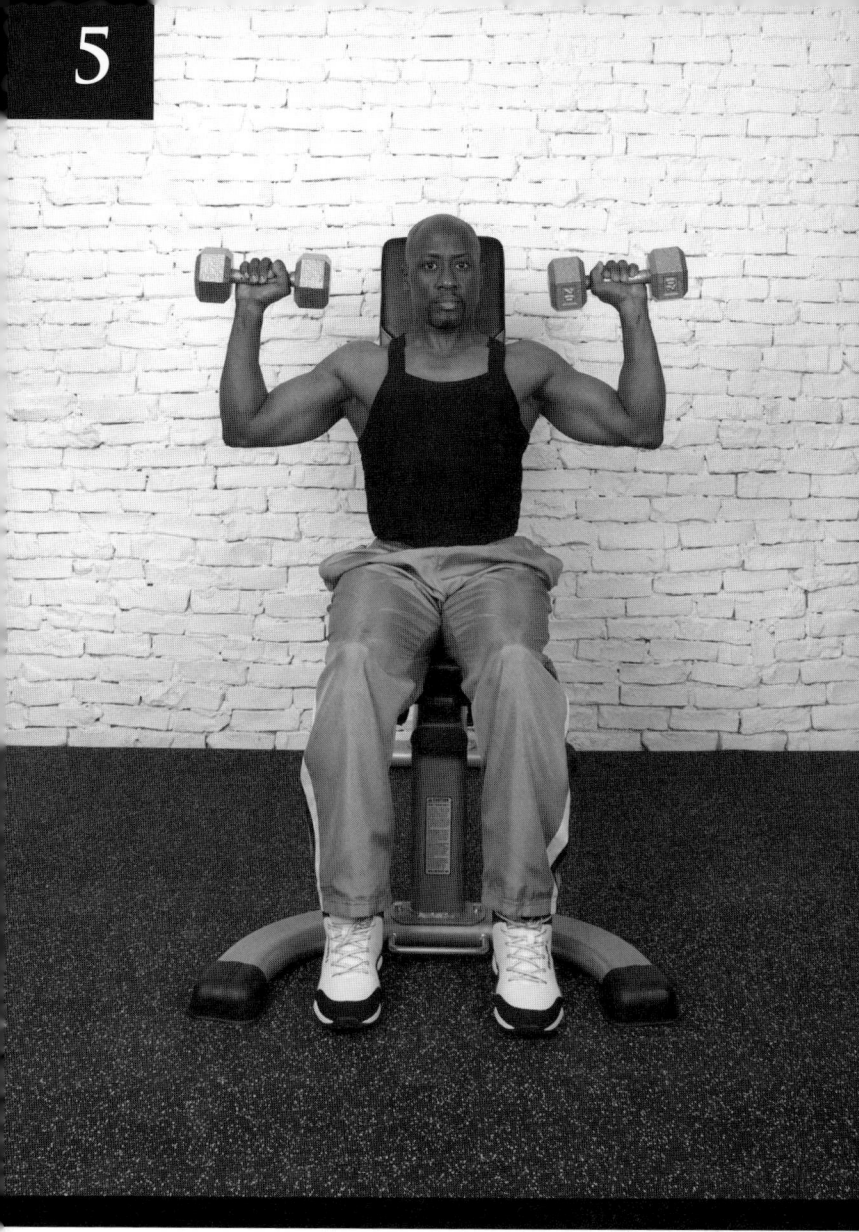
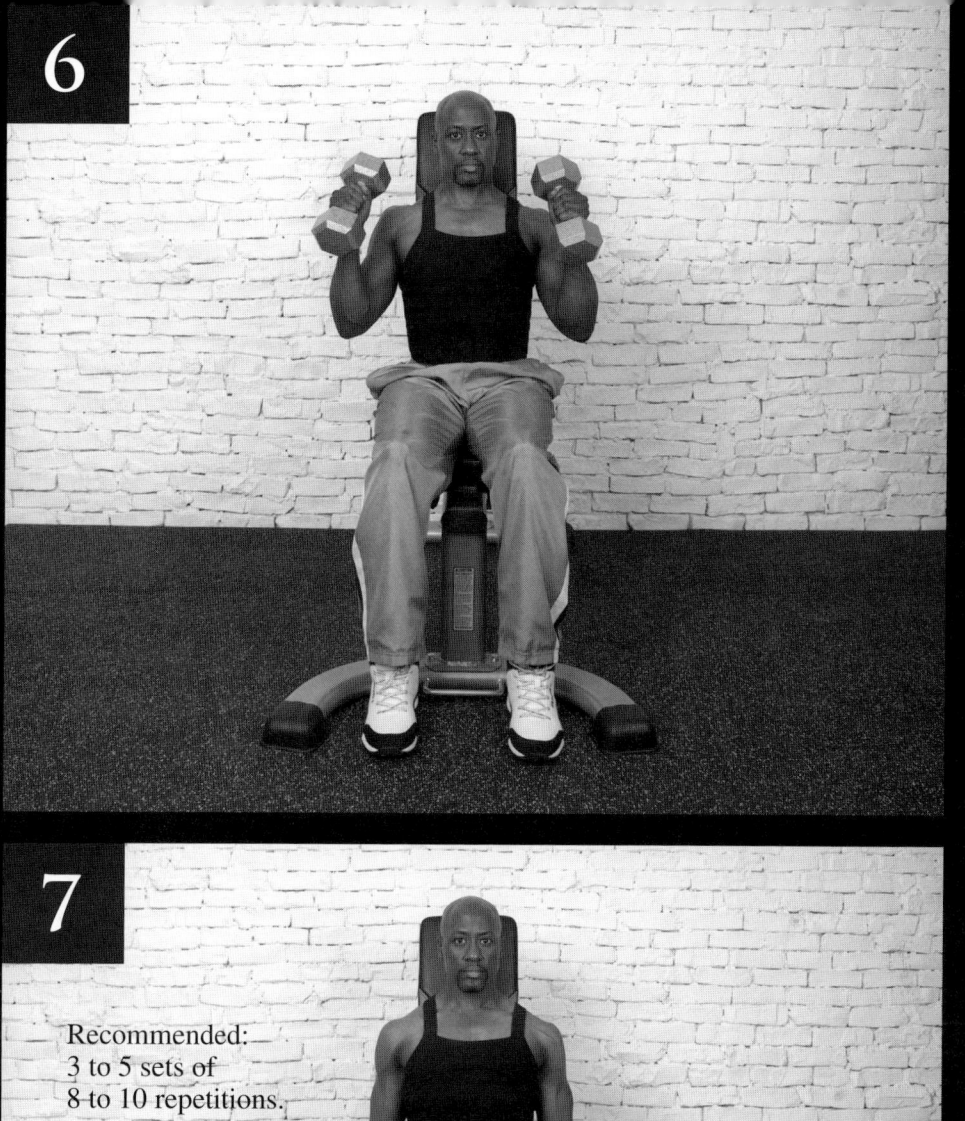
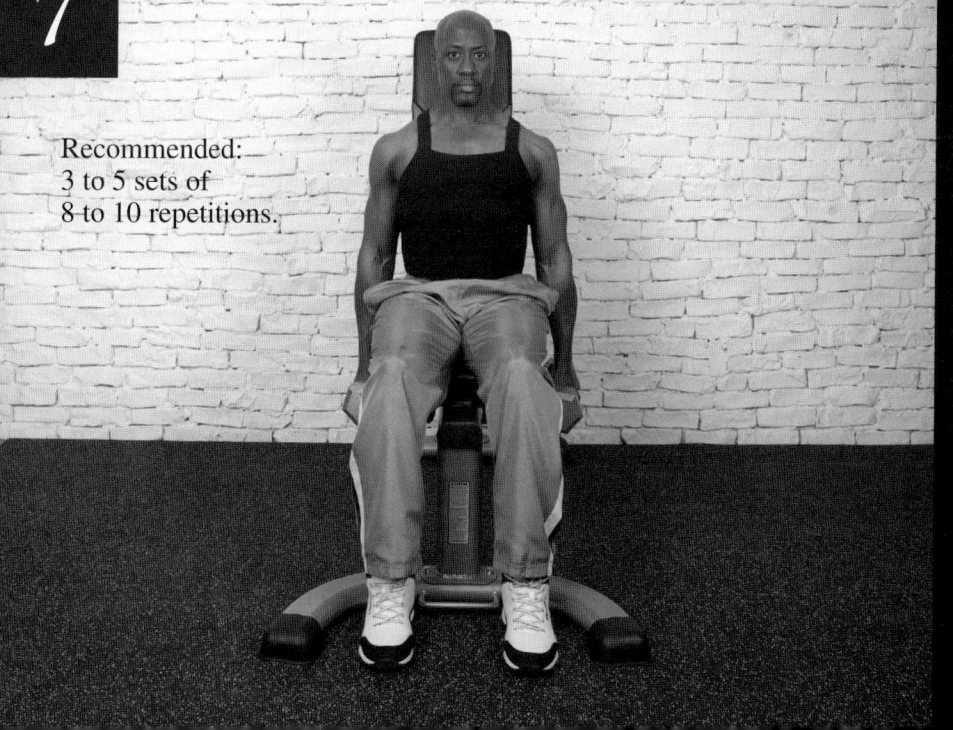

Recommended:
3 to 5 sets of
8 to 10 repetitions.

Starting from the seated position in the chair, the palms are facing toward you holding the weights. Flex the elbows during the biceps curl and bring the weights to the shoulders. Once the hands are at the level of the shoulders with the weights, the weights are lifted above the head. Bring weights down in a controlled manner.

Seated Inner Leg Biceps Curl

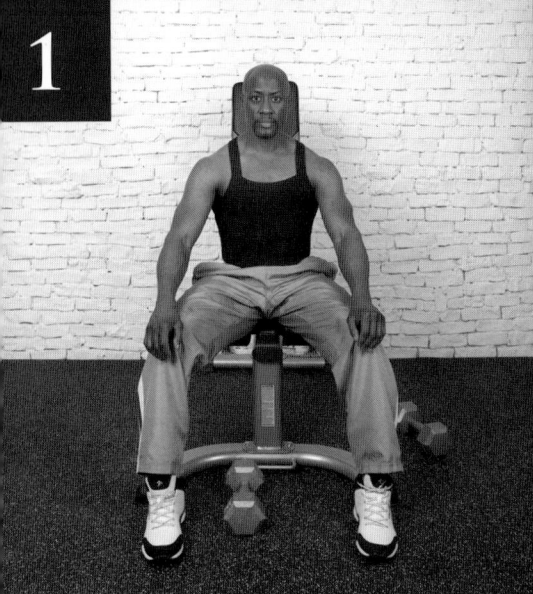

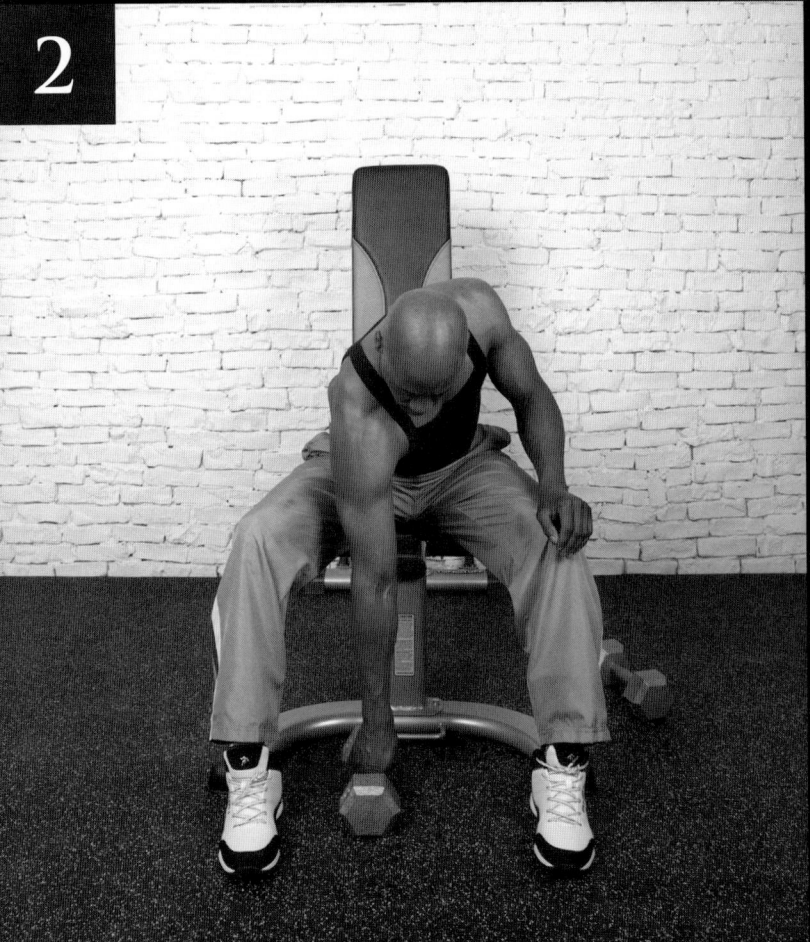

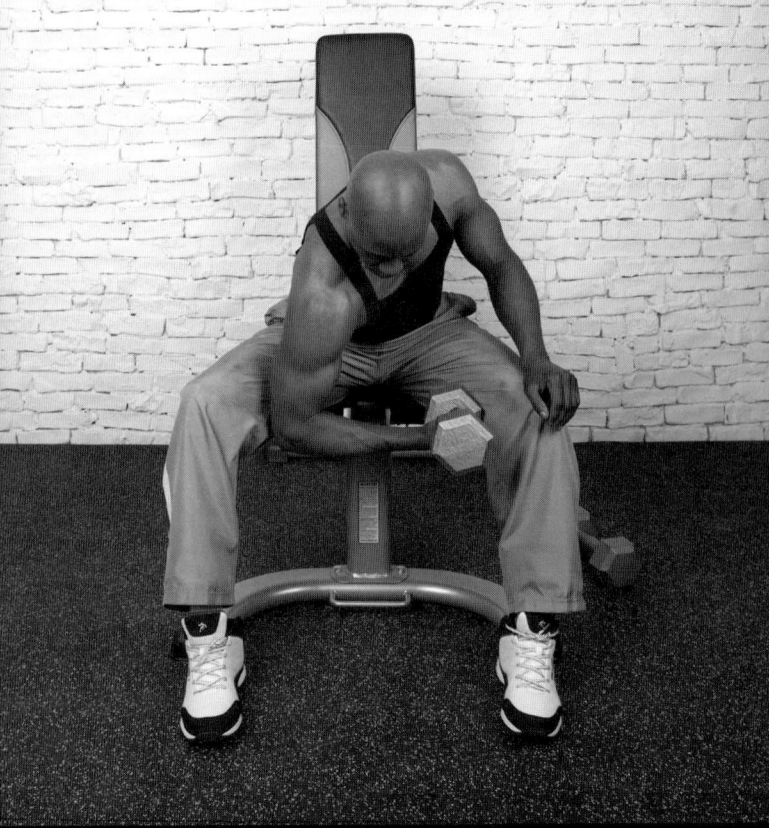

From the seated position, one weight should be inside the thigh on the floor. Keep the elbow adjacent to the thigh and flex the elbow as a regular biceps curl. Bring the weight up to the shoulder without swinging the elbow with the movement.

This should be done in a stable, well balanced movement bringing the weight up toward the shoulder and face, and slightly downward to the halfway position during the biceps curl and back down to the floor.

4

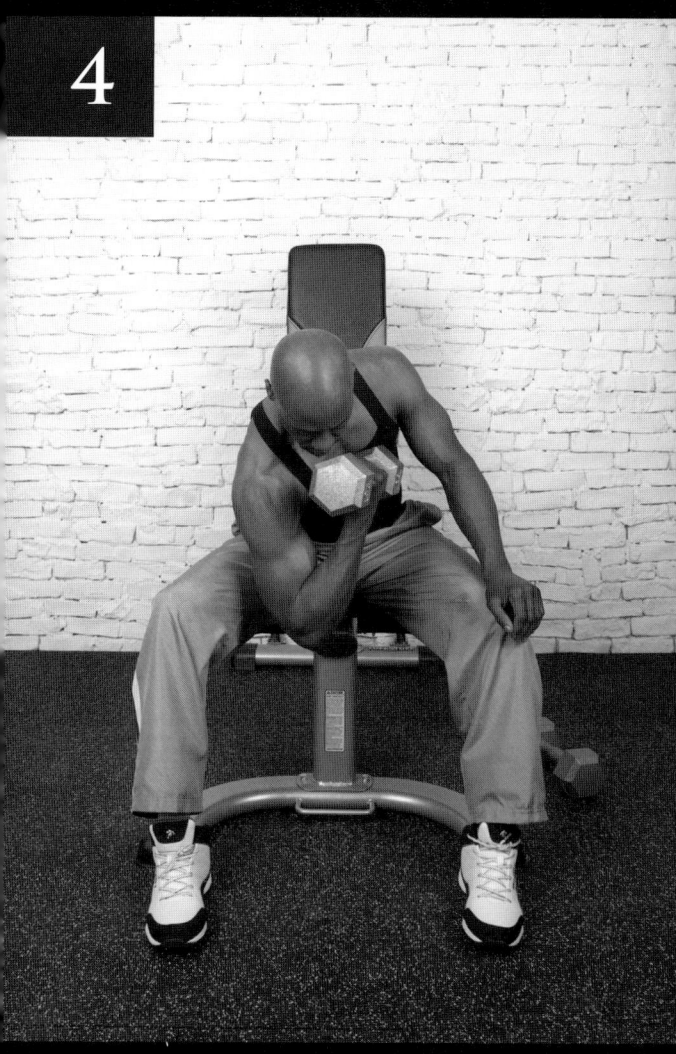

5

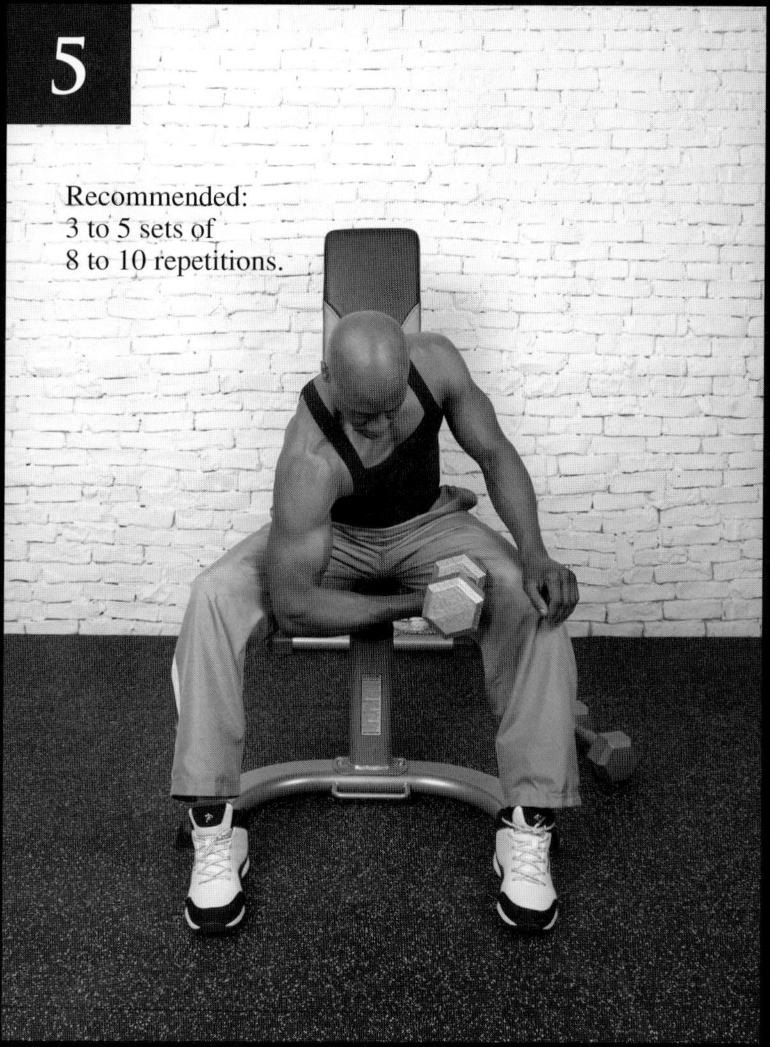

Recommended:
3 to 5 sets of
8 to 10 repetitions.

6

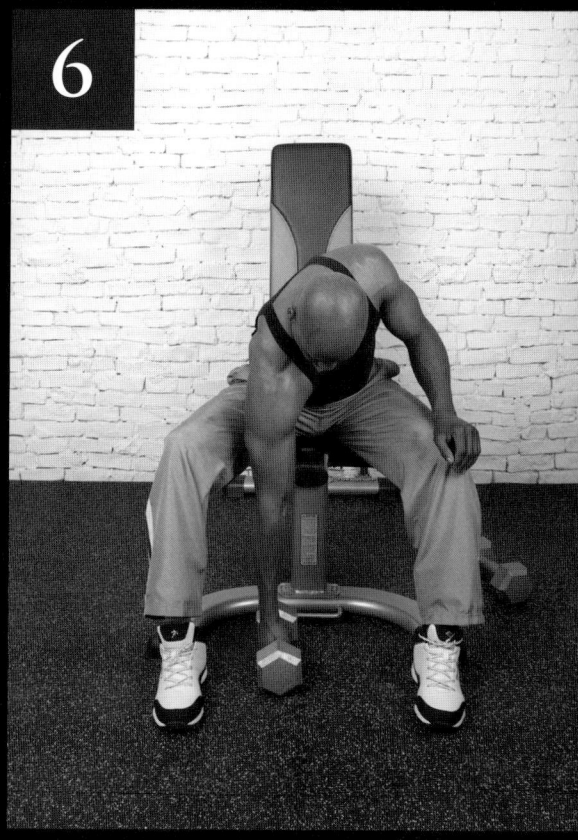

FIT TIP:

Avoid swinging the elbow and keep it against your inner thigh.

CHAIR TRICEPS DIP

FIT TIP:
Avoid swinging the elbows outward. Inhale when dropping downward and exhale when lifting your body up.

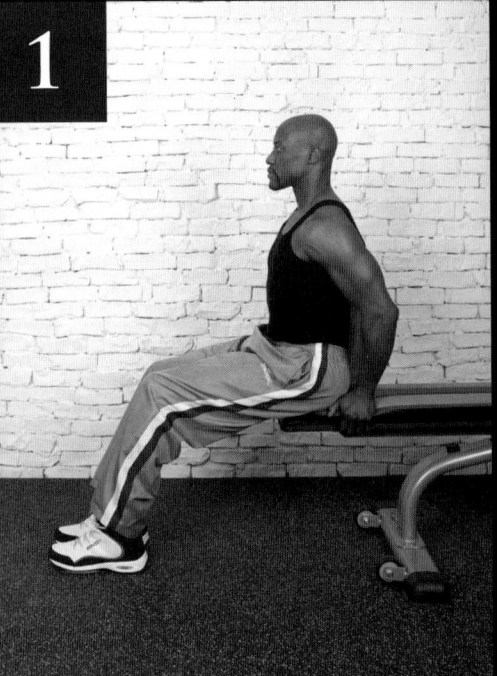

Sit at the edge of the bench with the knees together, feet forward. Slide your body forward off the bench while holding on to the bench. Bend your elbows, keep your back straight against the bench, keep your knees above your ankles, drop your body downward, and push up with your triceps.

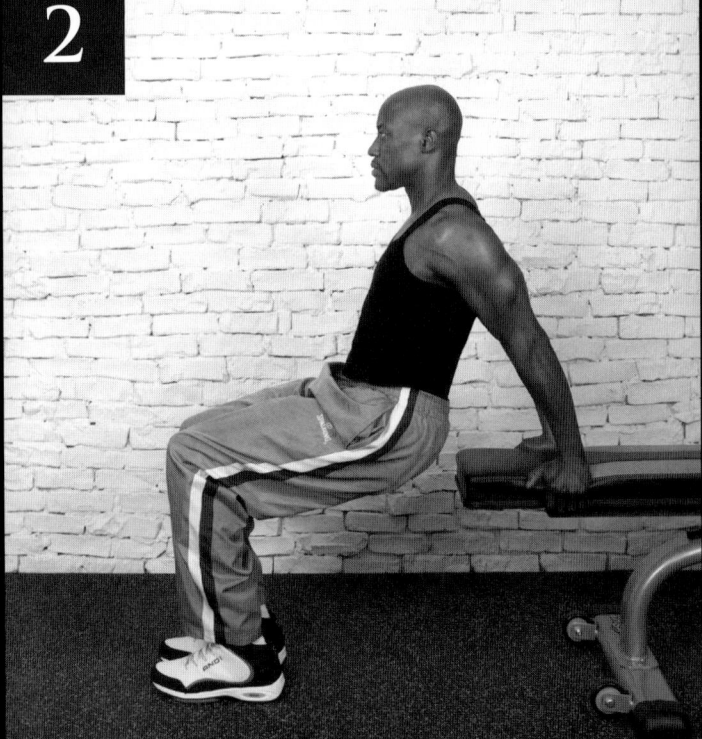

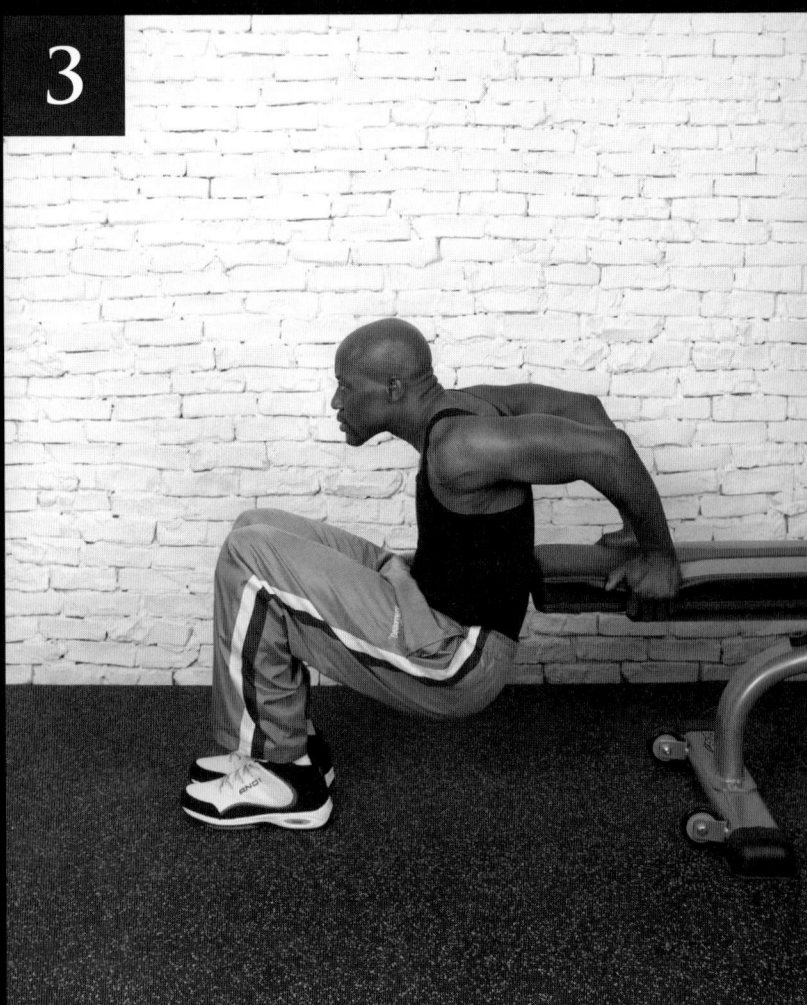

4 Go from a flexed position of the elbows to an extended position of the elbows, keeping the stomach tight and feet together.

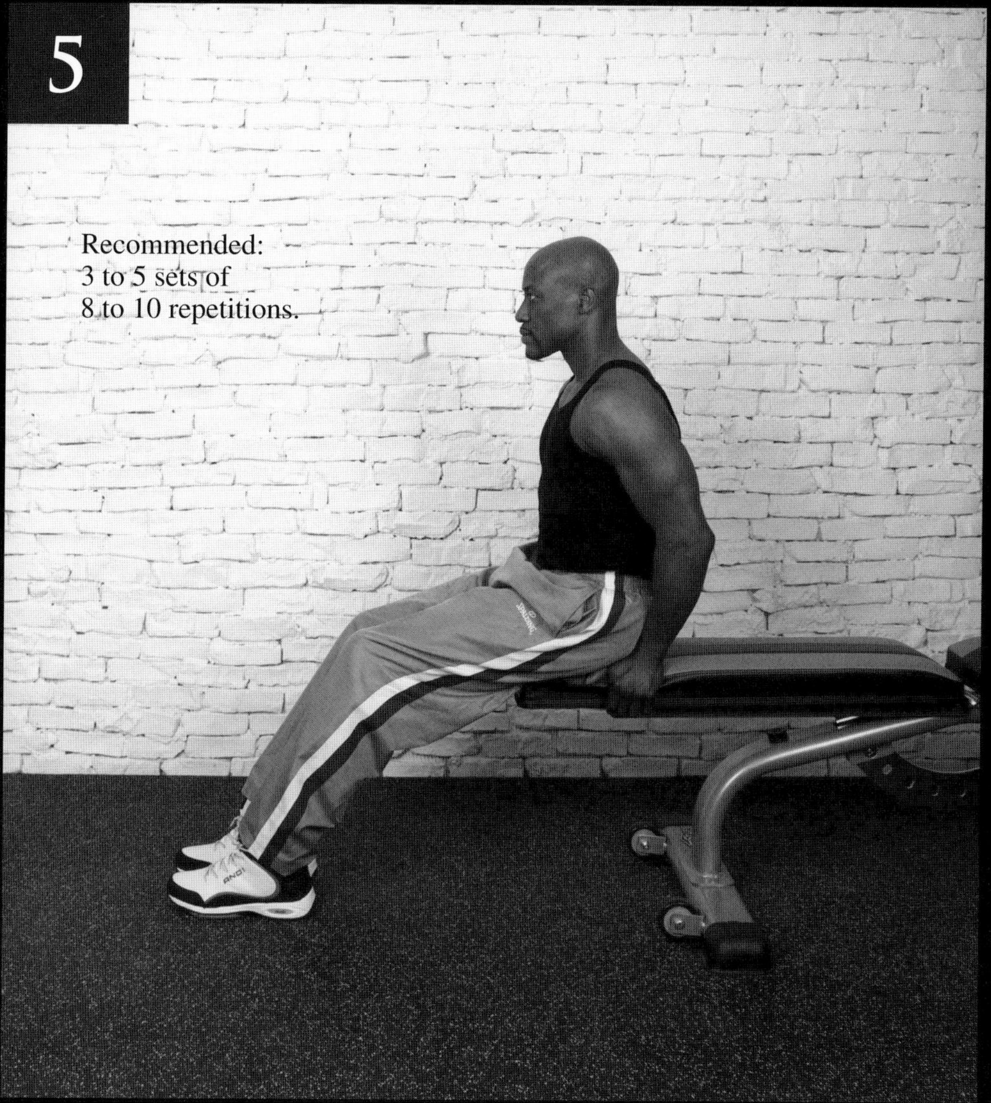

5 Recommended: 3 to 5 sets of 8 to 10 repetitions.

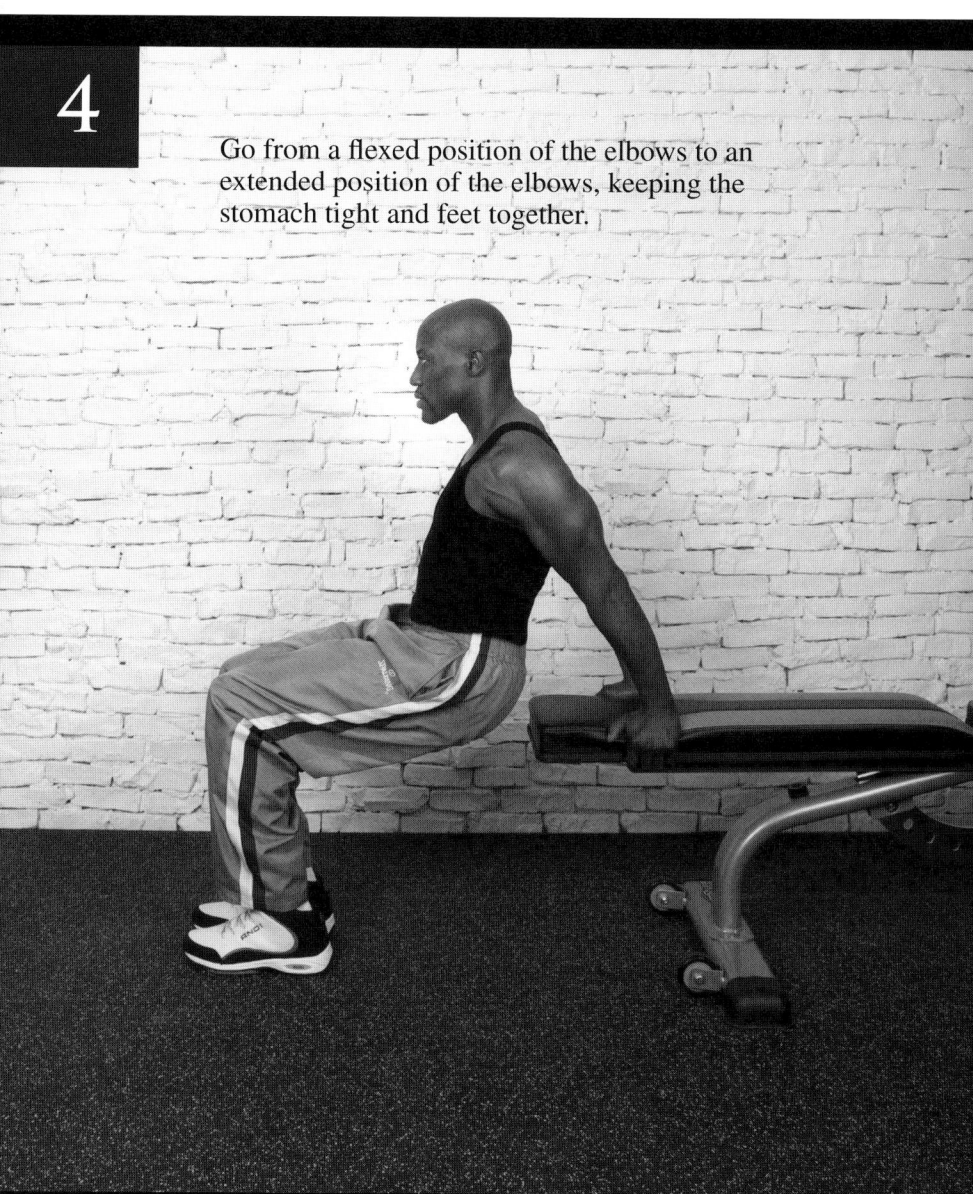

Rotator Cuff Stabilizing Side Raises

External Rotation

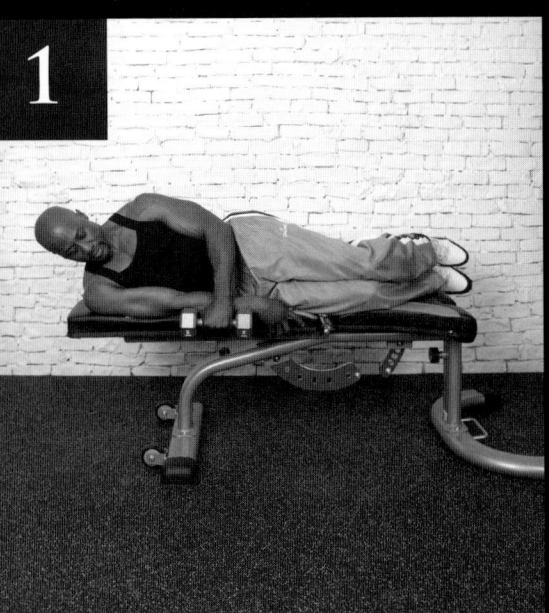

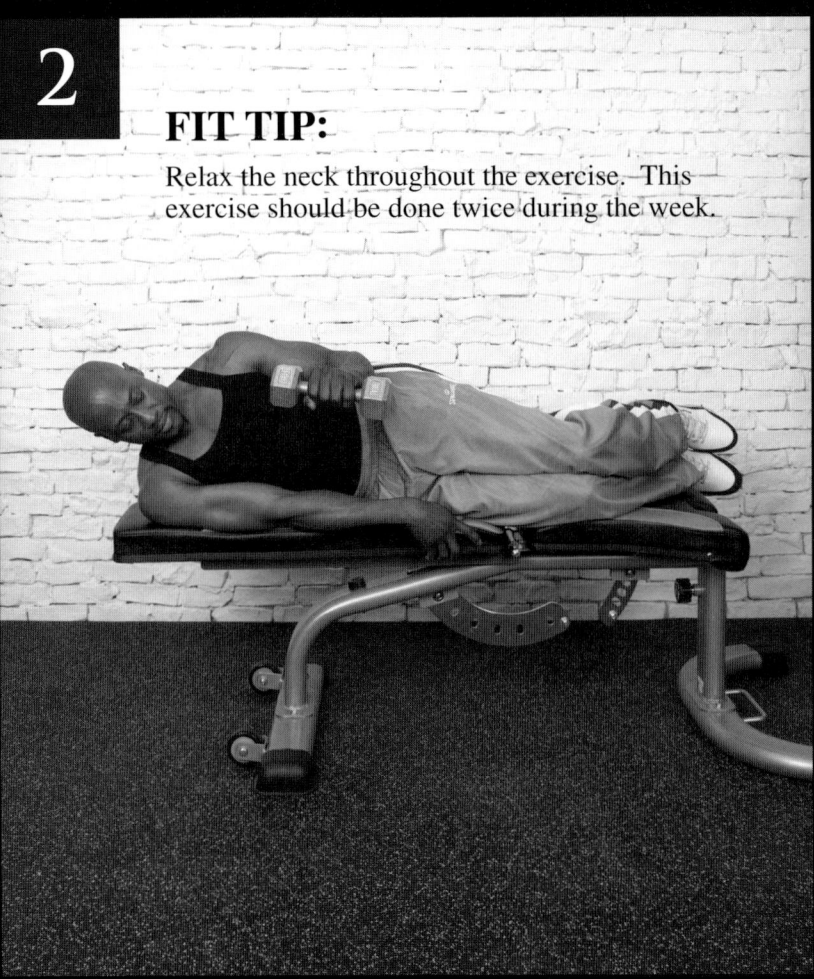

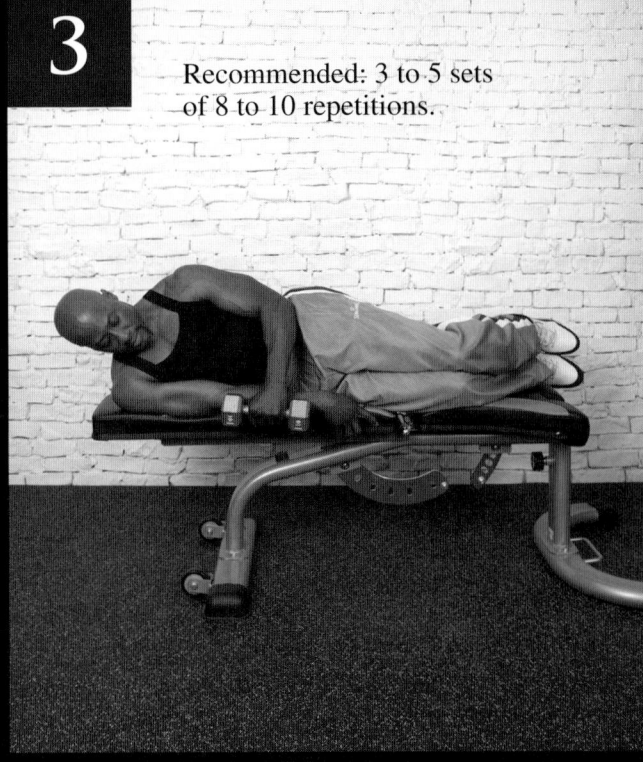

FIT TIP: Relax the neck throughout the exercise. This exercise should be done twice during the week.

Recommended: 3 to 5 sets of 8 to 10 repetitions.

Lie on your side on the bench as shown with the arm that is on top holding the weight in that hand. Keep the elbow at 90 degrees, lift the elbow up while holding on to the bench, relaxing the neck. Externally, rotate the shoulder and lift the weight up.

Rotator cuff exercises will strengthen the rotator cuff muscles and stabilize the shoulder.

Rotator Cuff Stabilizing Side Raises

Internal Rotation

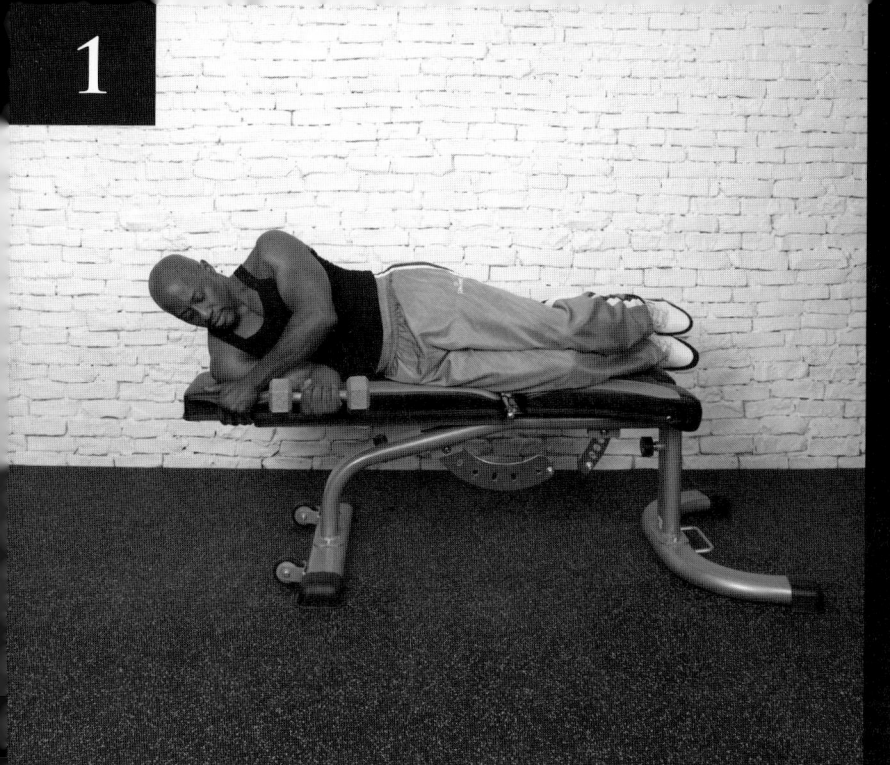

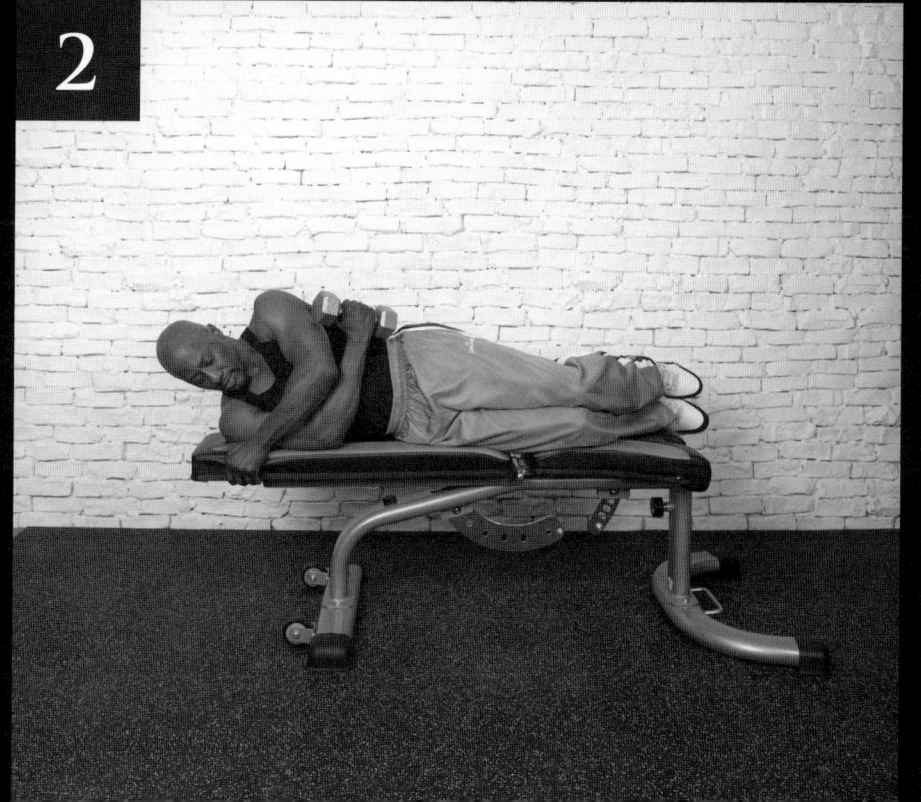

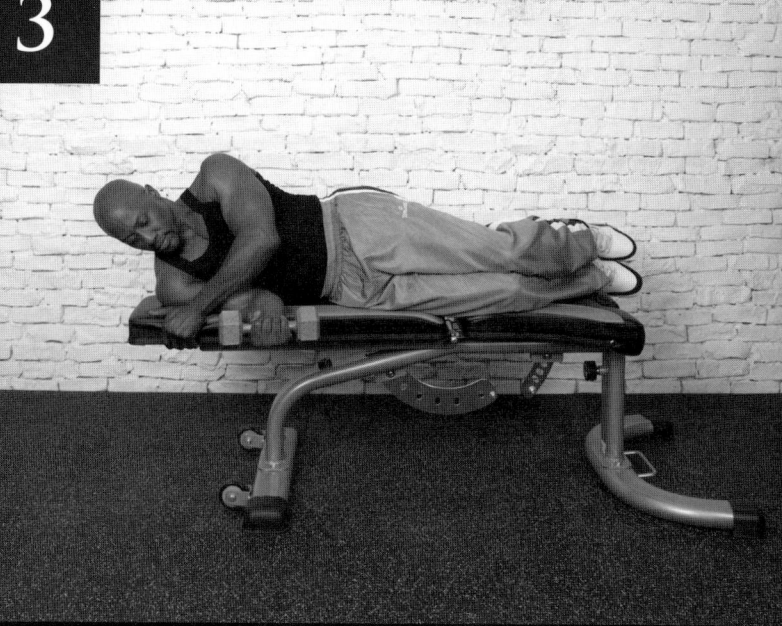

Lying on the side of the bench as shown, hold the weight in the hand of the arm that is against the bench. Lift the weight up across the torso slowly and lower the weight downward at 90 degrees.

Triceps Kickbacks

If this is done on the left side, the left knee and the right hand are placed on the bench. The right foot is planted firmly on the ground. The left elbow is brought up and then extended with the weight in the hand in the hammer position. Keep the back fairly straight without arching during this exercise. Next, the elbow is flexed as you bring the weight back to the starting position.

FIT TIP:
Keep the elbow up and the back flat.

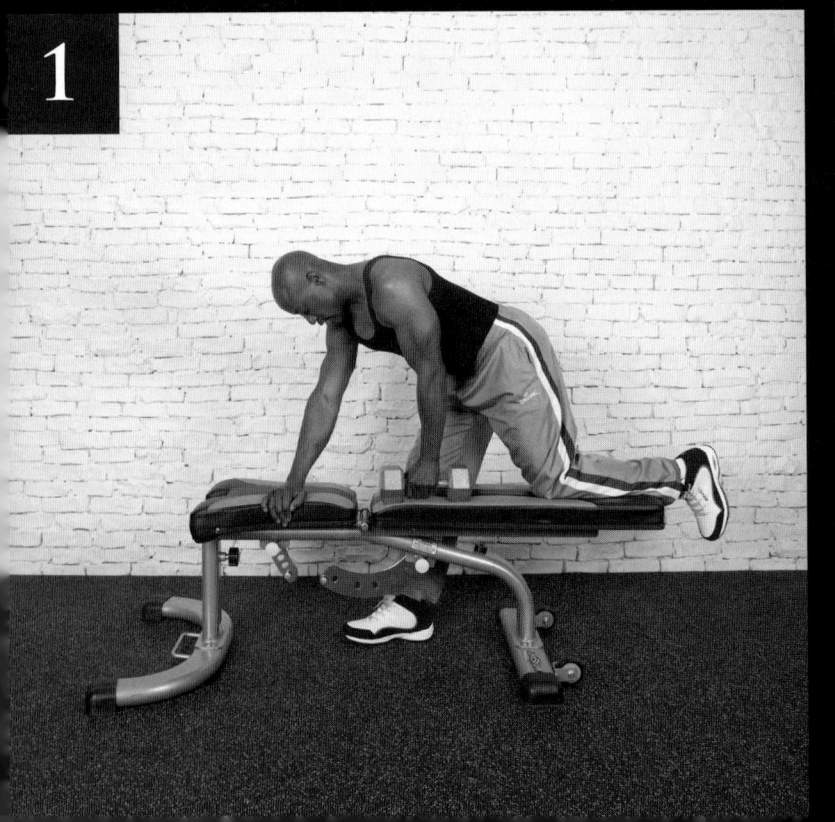

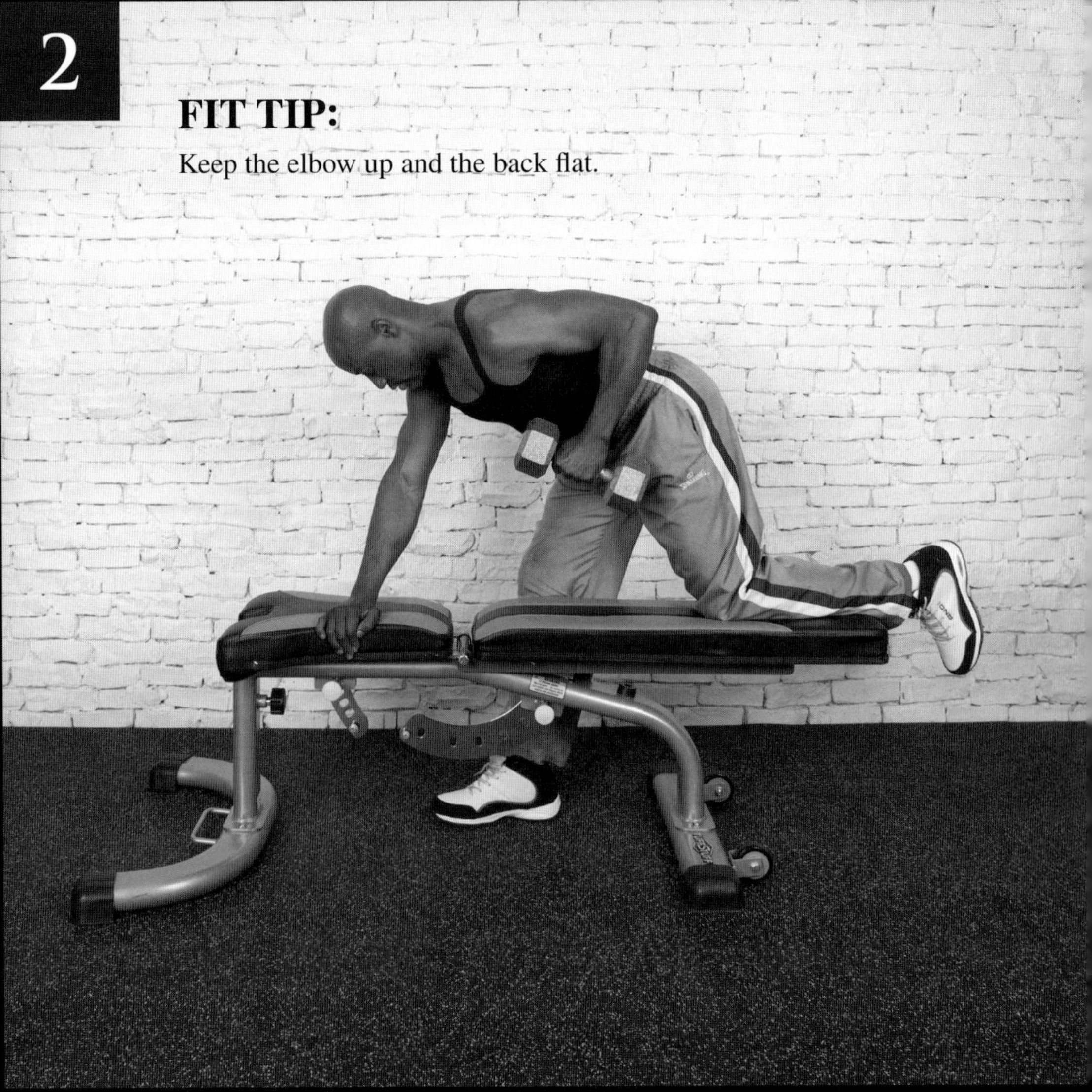

3
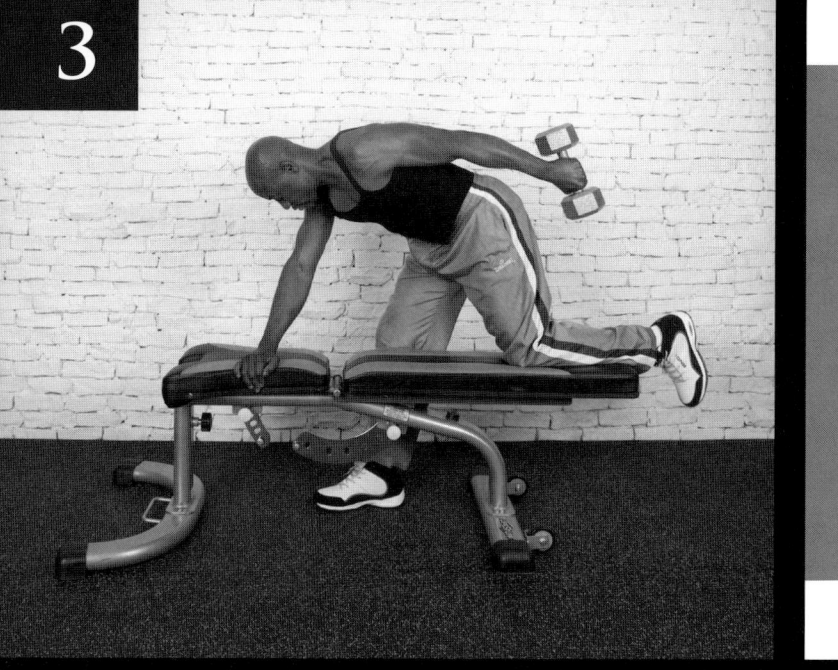

4
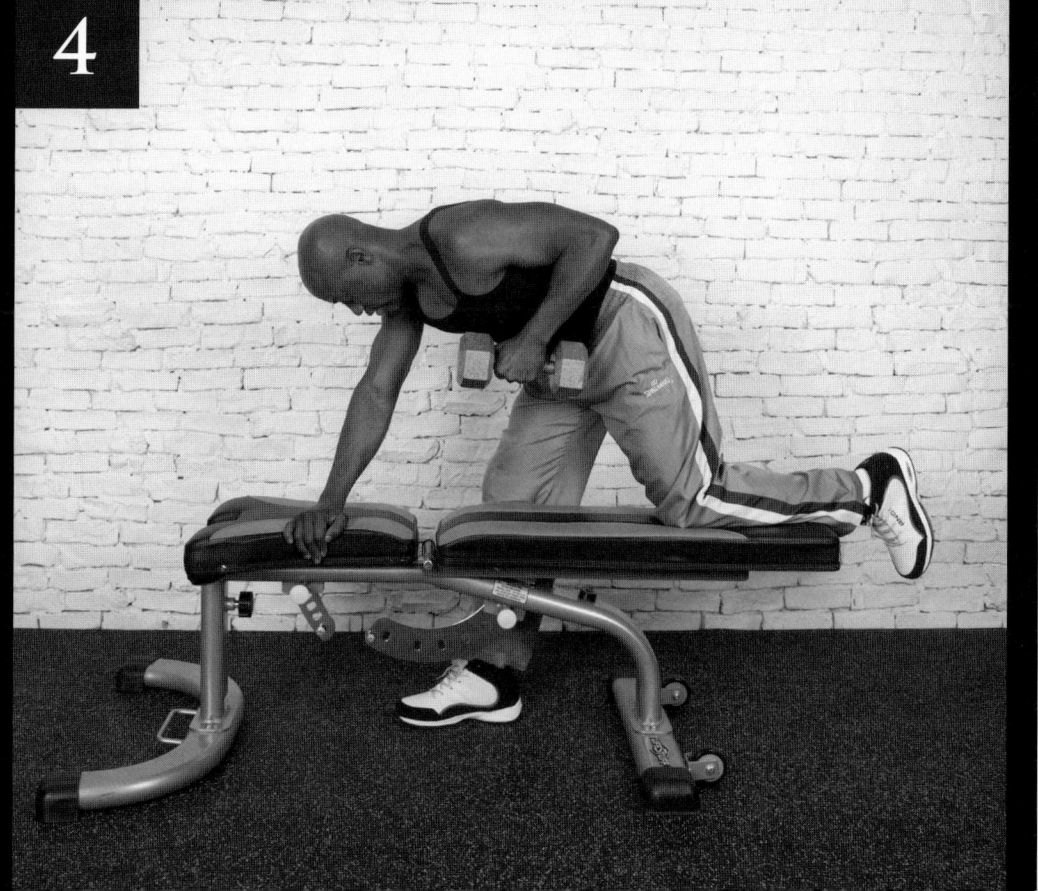

5
Recommended: 3 to 5 sets of 8 to 10 repetitions.

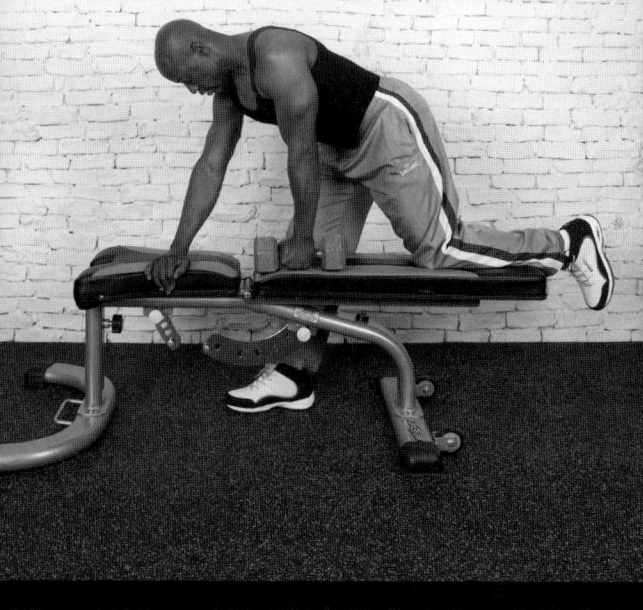

Overhead Triceps Extension

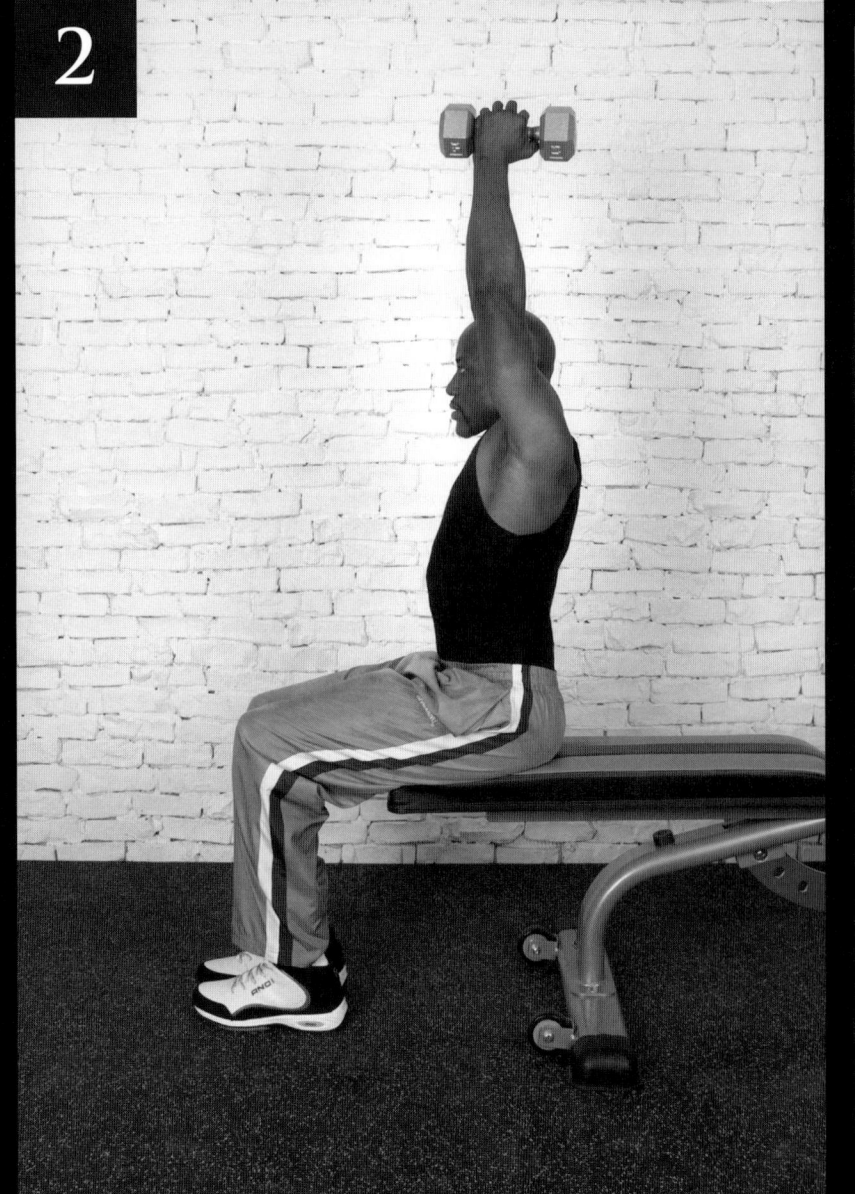
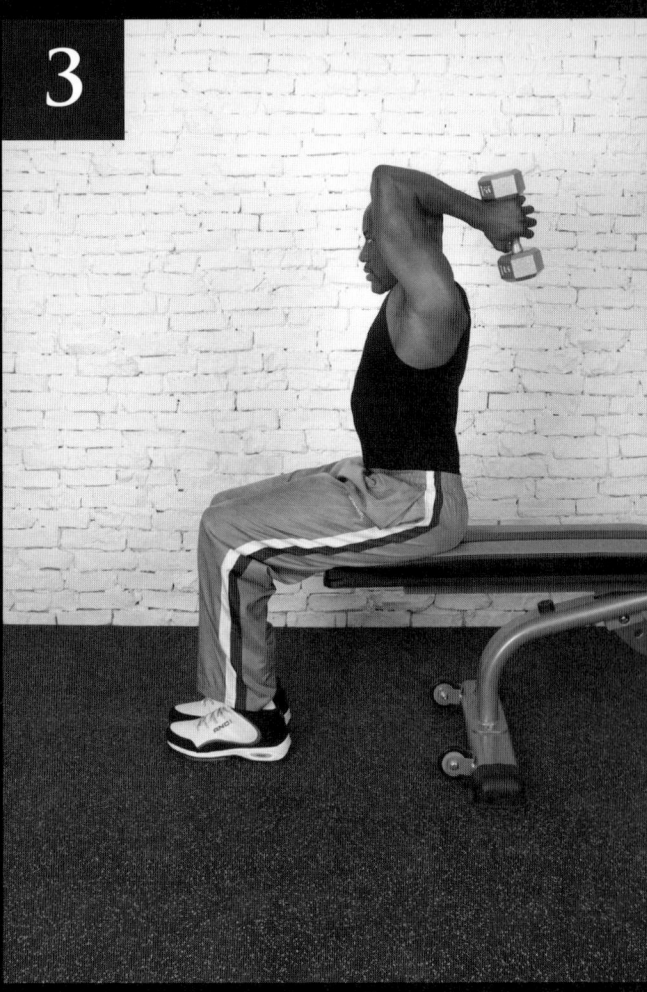

Sitting on the edge of the bench with the weight in a hammer-type position, the weight is elevated above the head. The elbows are then flexed allowing the weight to come to at least 90 degrees or the weight can be allowed to go further past 90 degrees. It is then elevated again overhead and then brought back down safely to the lap. You may have the flexibility to bring the weight to touch your shirt or back. This should be done very gently.

FIT TIP:

Inhale when placing weight behind your head and exhale when lifting weight above the head.

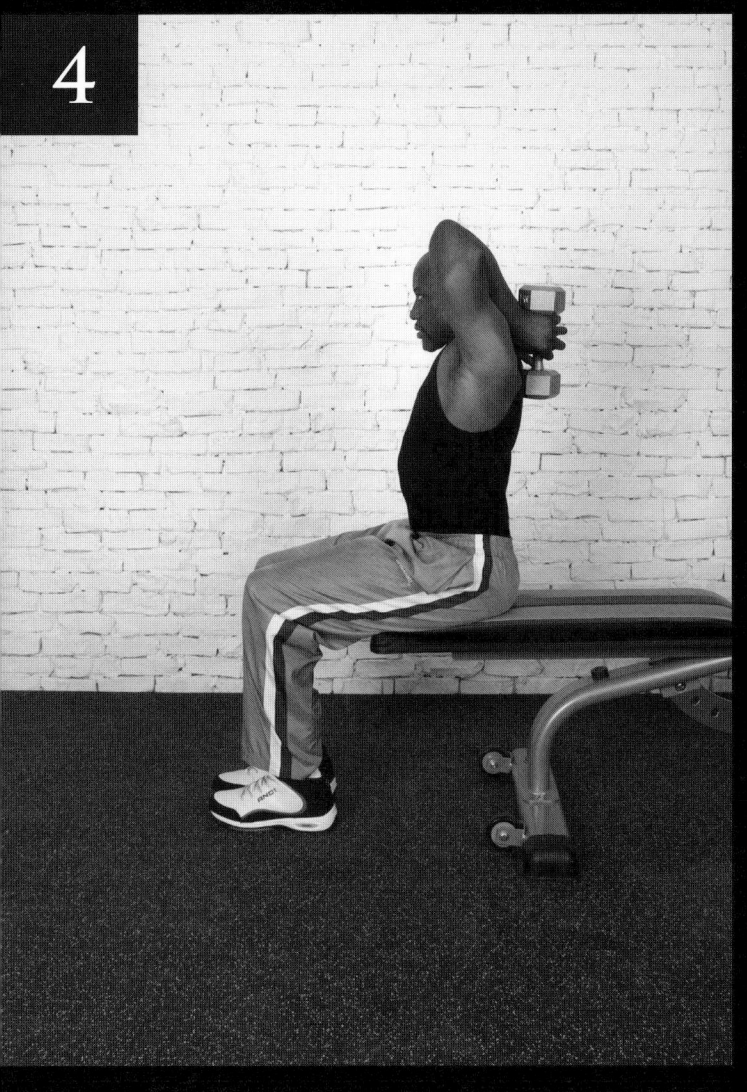

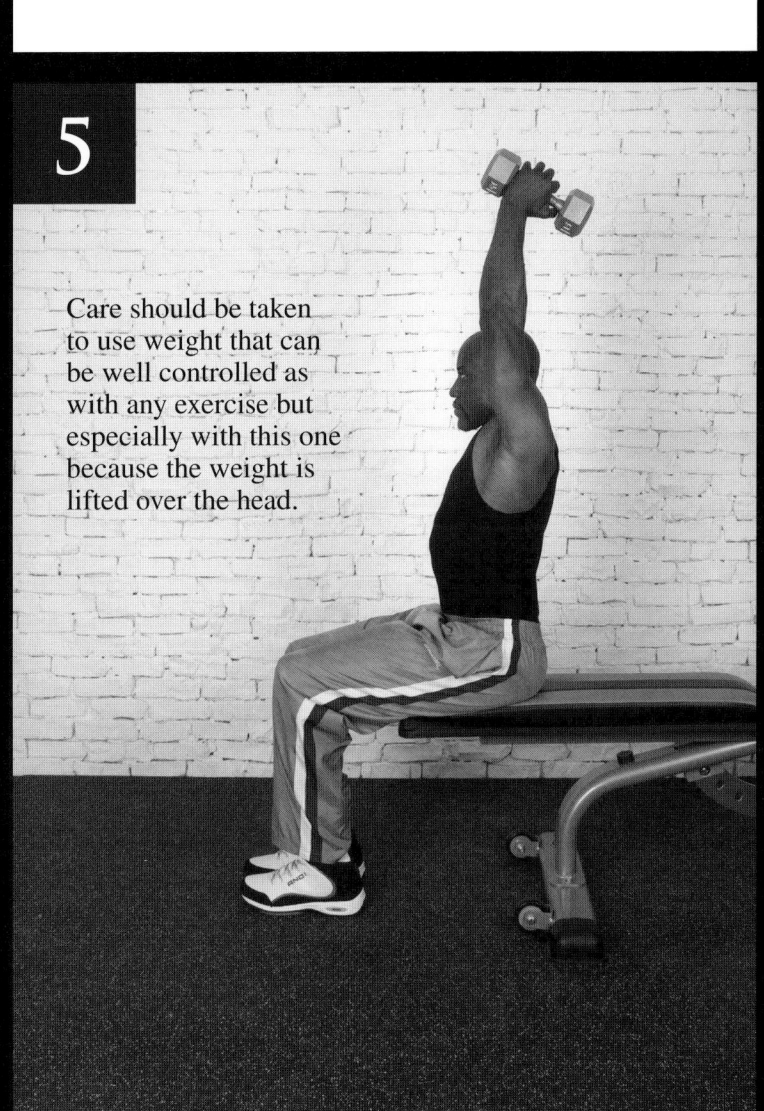

Care should be taken to use weight that can be well controlled as with any exercise but especially with this one because the weight is lifted over the head.

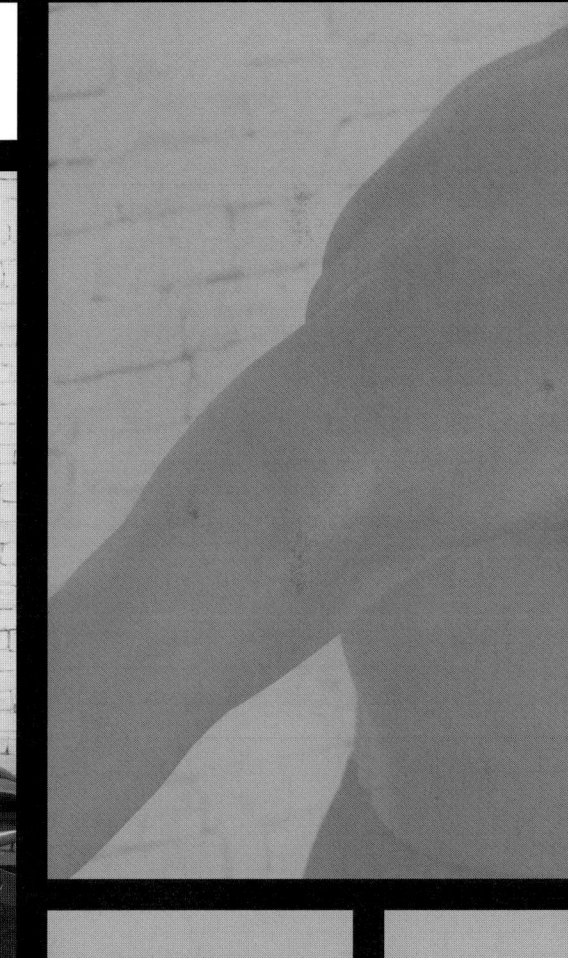

Recommended: 3 to 5 sets of 8 to 10 repetitions.

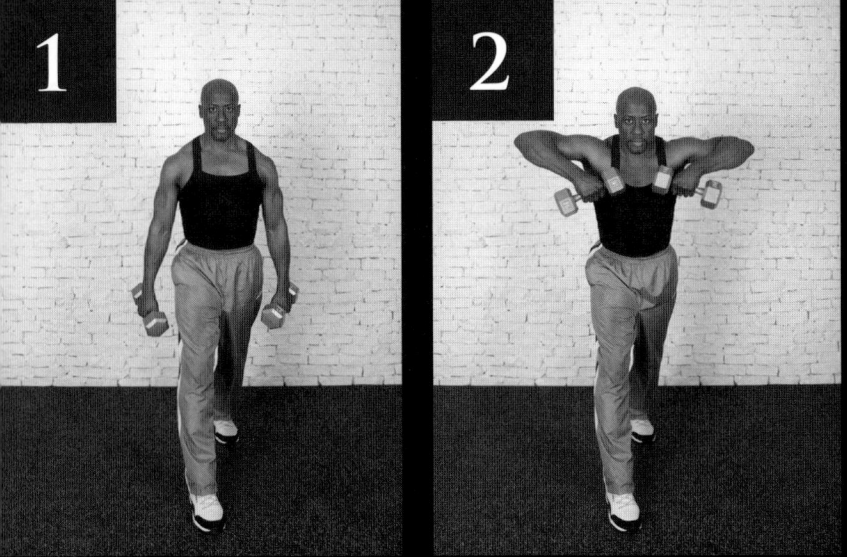

Combined Front Deltoid Rows & Lateral Triceps Extensions

The exercise is done by placing dumbbells in each hand in front of you, with one leg behind you. The weights are brought evenly and symmetrically up to the chest. Care is then taken to extend the elbows laterally with the weights, which is a triceps extension. The weights are then brought back to the chest and then brought downward.

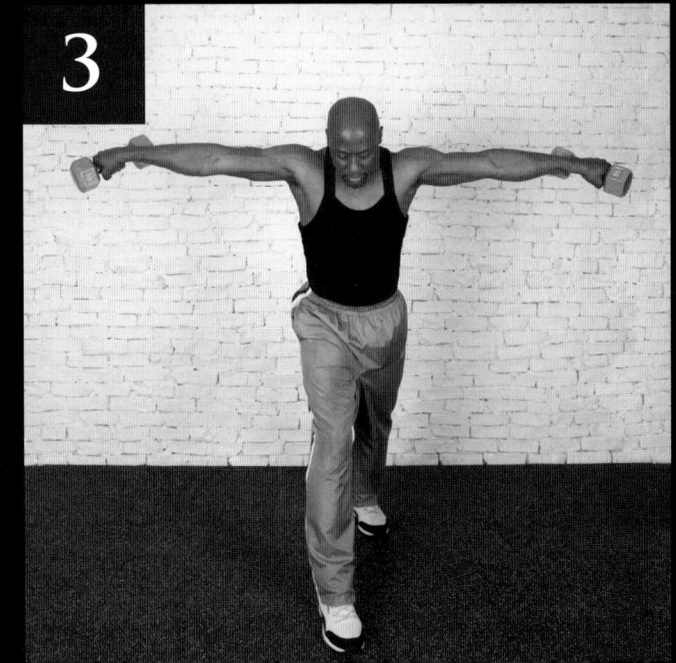

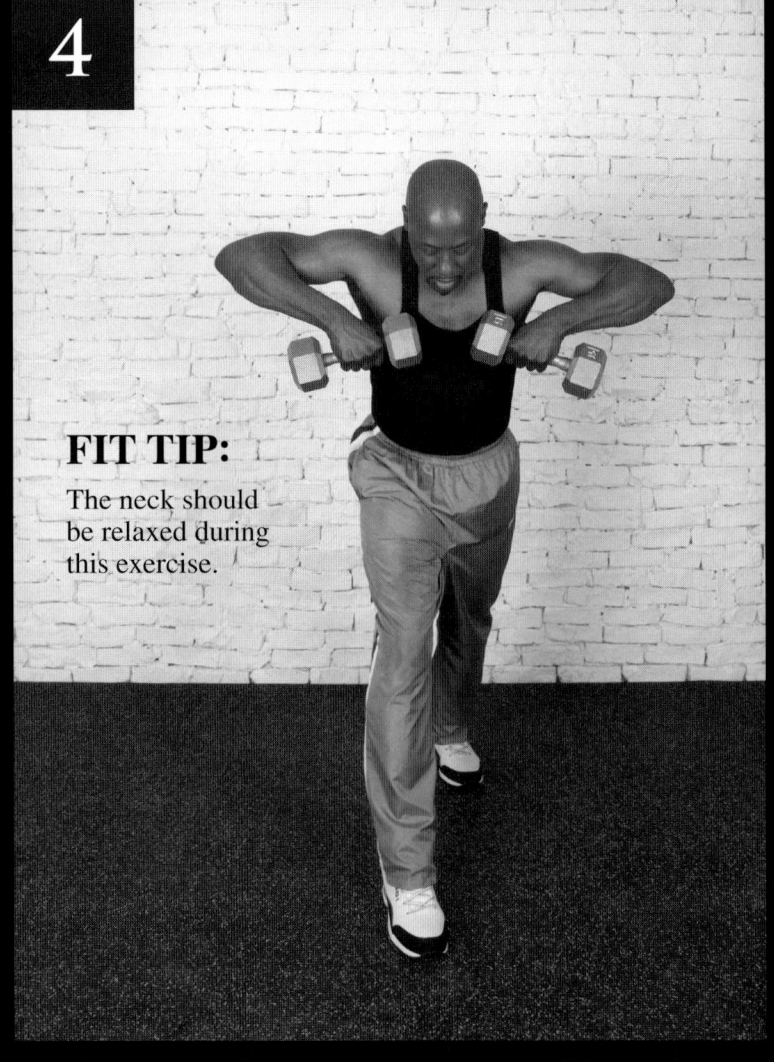

FIT TIP: The neck should be relaxed during this exercise.

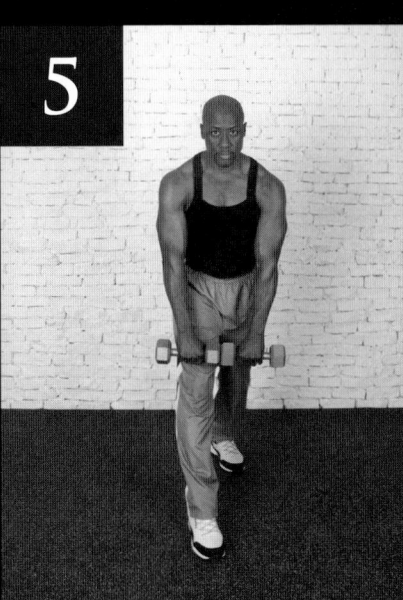

FRONT DUMBBELL DELTOID ROWS

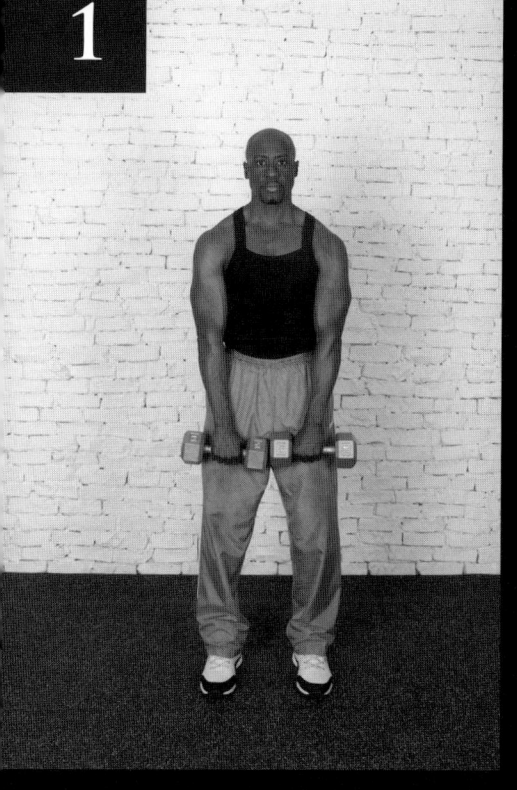

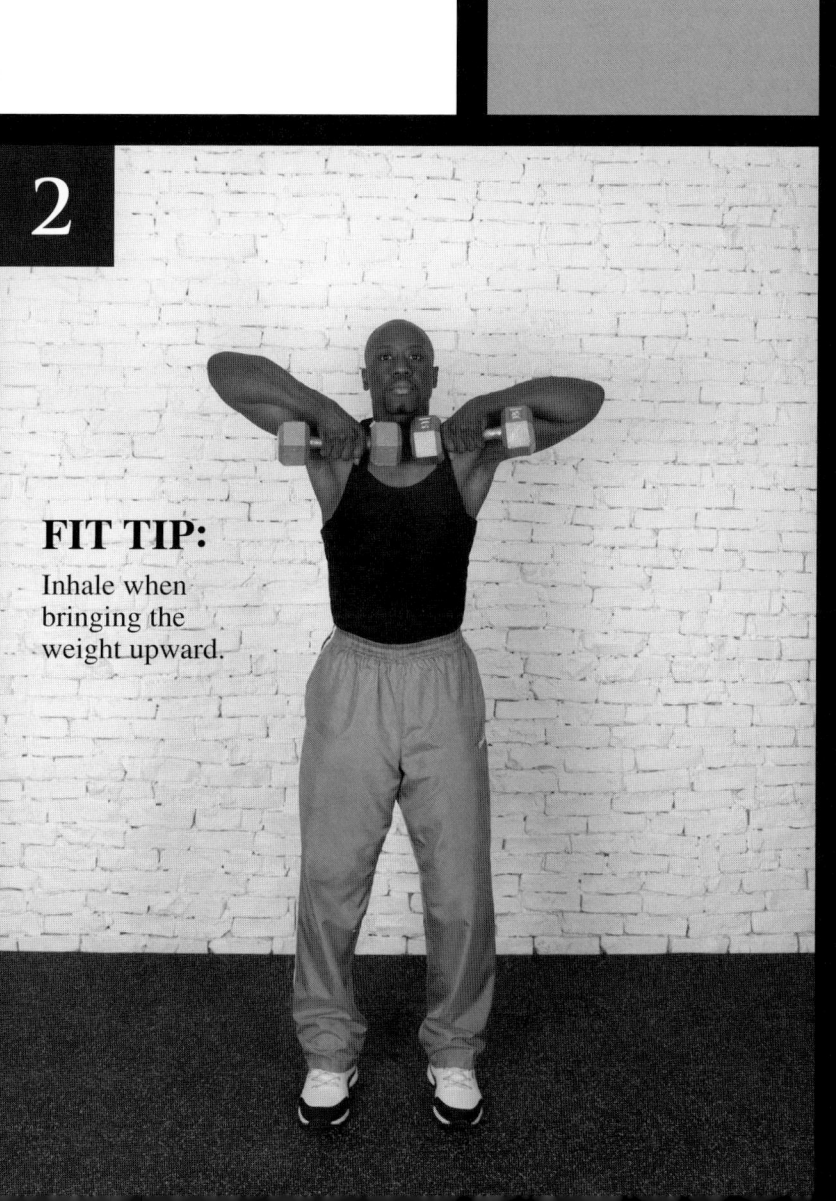

FIT TIP: Inhale when bringing the weight upward.

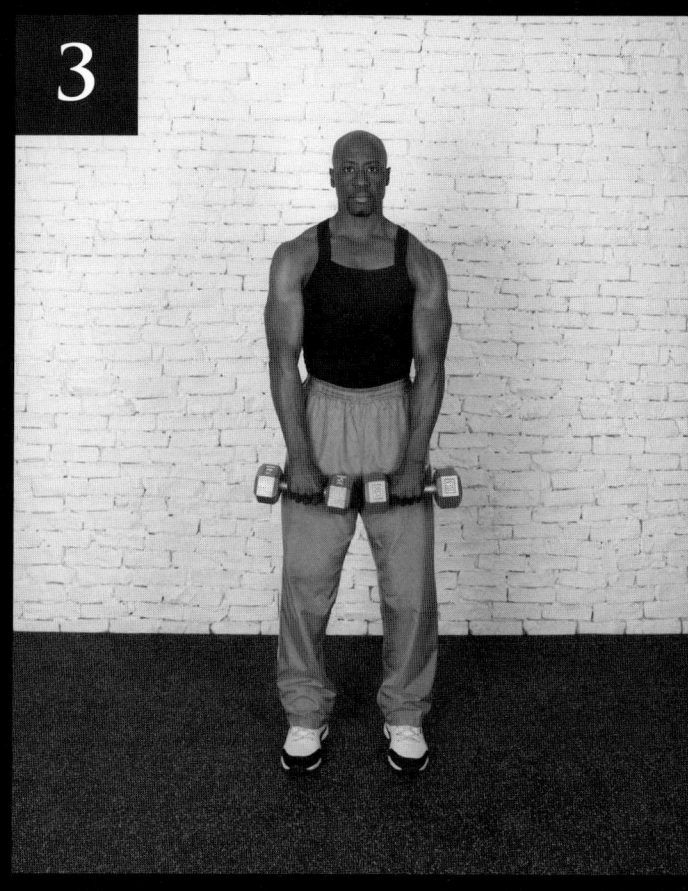

This exercise is done by standing with the feet shoulder-width apart, the dumbbells in front in each hand with the palms facing the thighs. The elbows are then bent and lifted upward, bringing the weight upward toward the neck and then slowly brought downward in a controlled fashion.

COMBINED RHOMBOID ROWS AND TRICEPS KICKBACKS

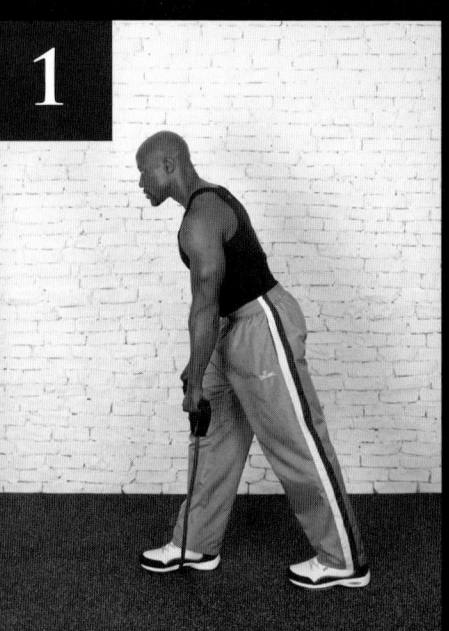

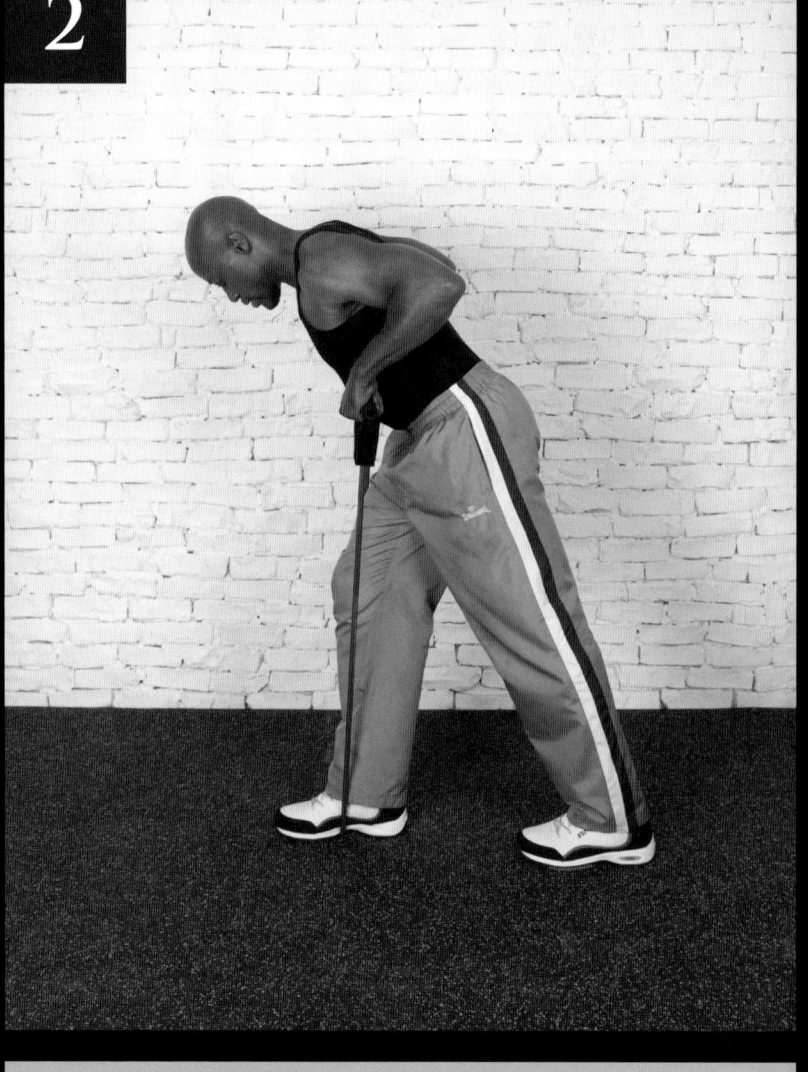

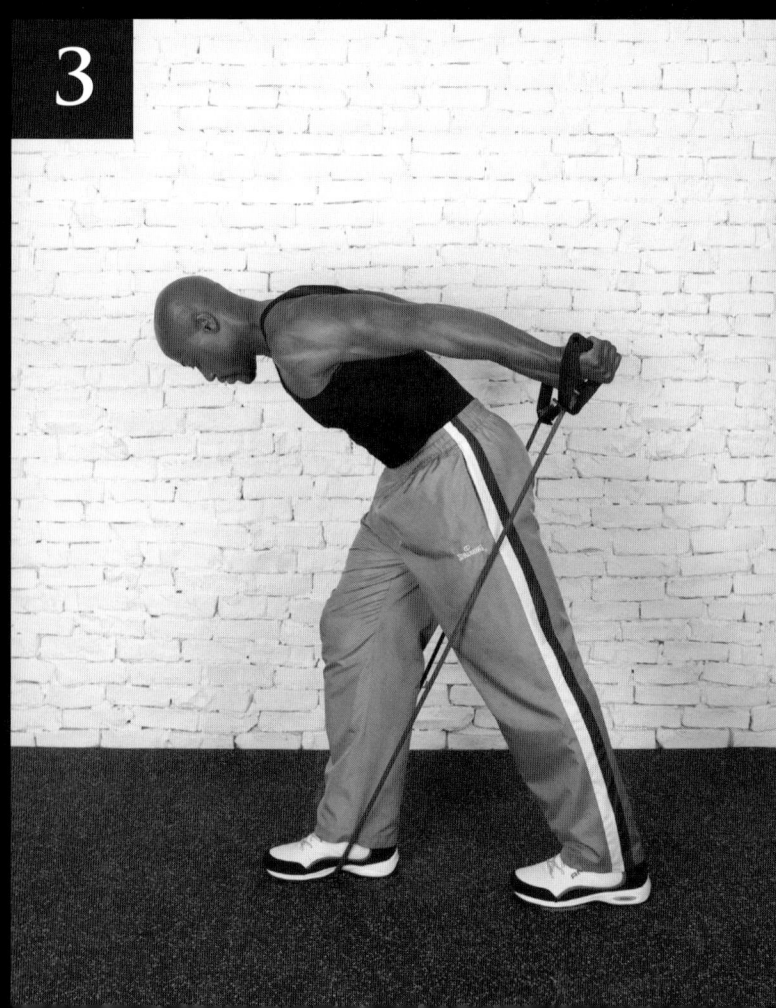

This exercise is done by placing one foot over the mid aspect of the pulley, keeping the front knee over the front ankle and keeping the back leg at least 2 feet behind the front leg.

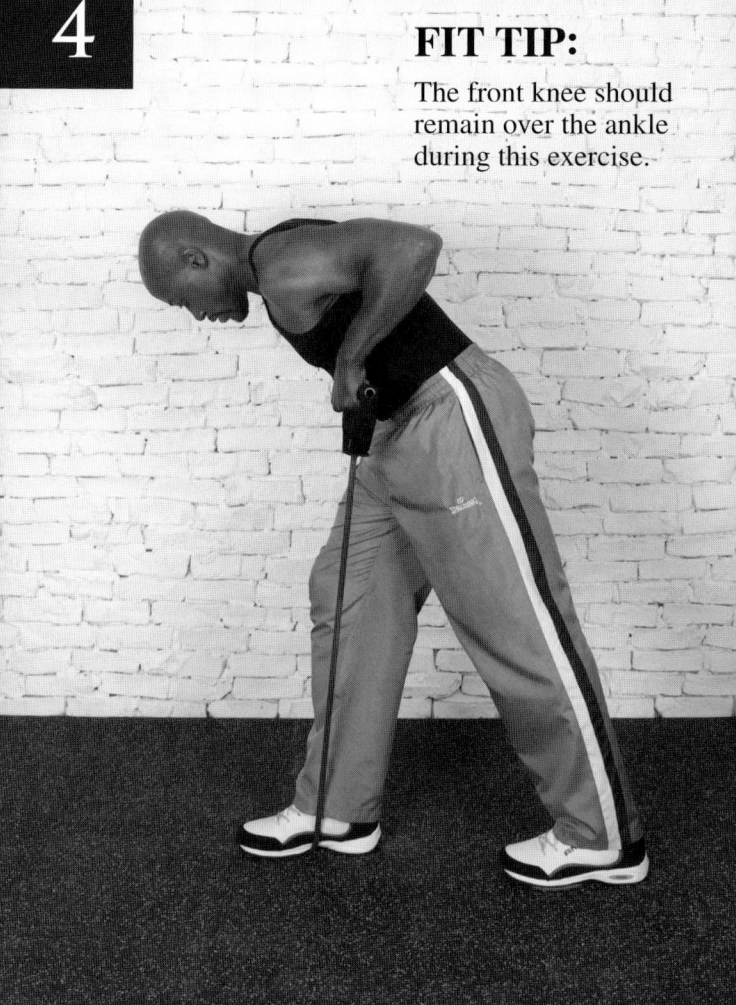

FIT TIP:
The front knee should remain over the ankle during this exercise.

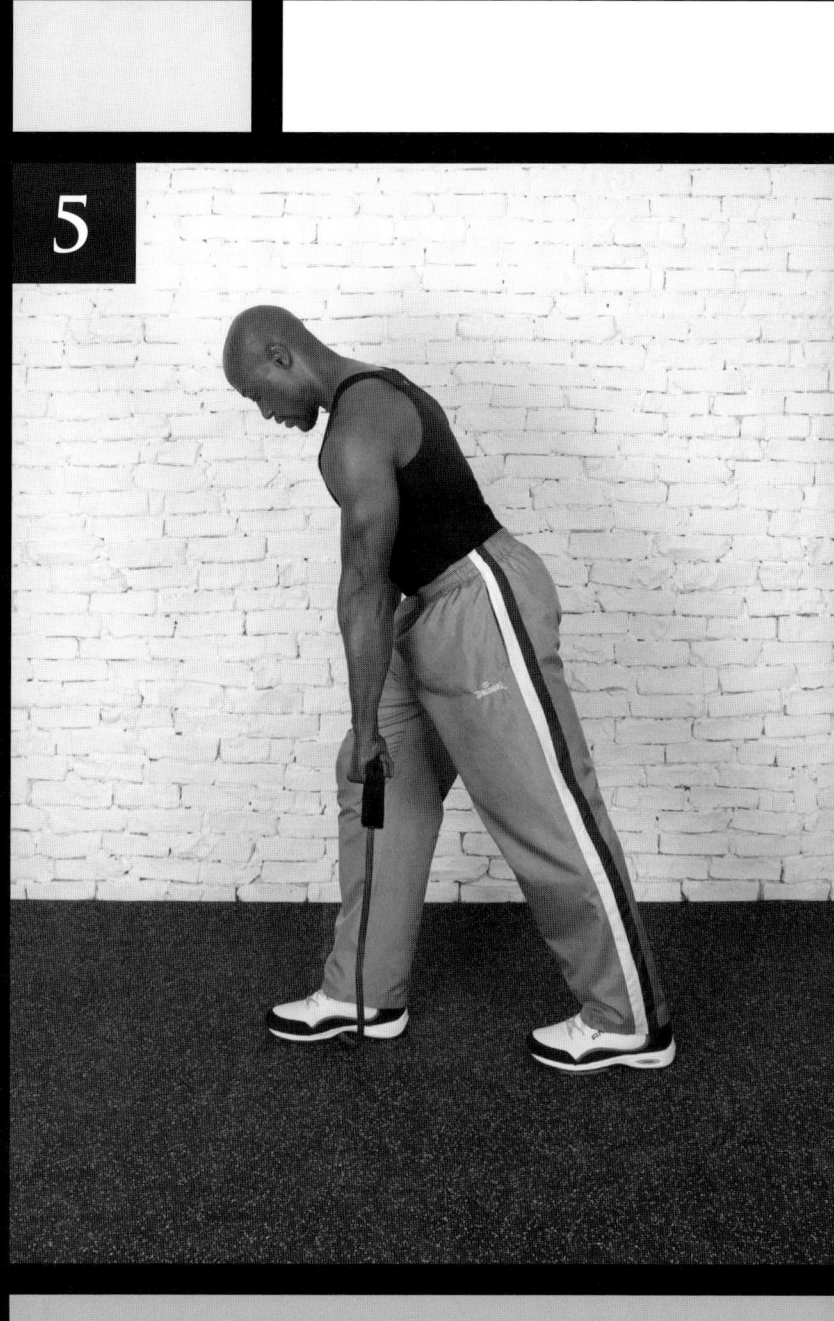

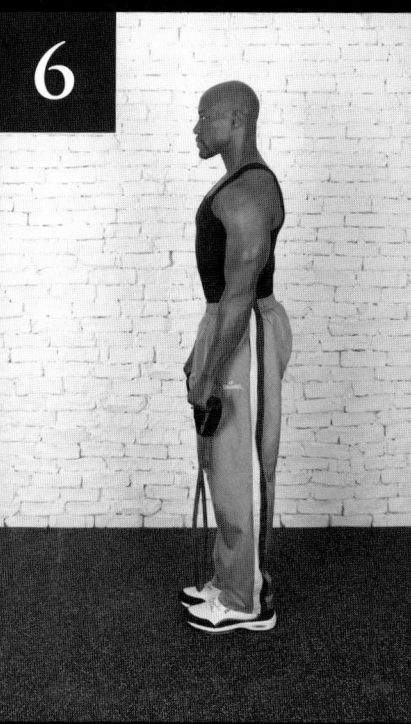

The exercise is executed by leaning slightly forward and lifting both elbows upward while pulling on the rubber band or pulley. Extend the elbows posteriorly, flex the elbows and return to a relaxed neutral position.

Front and Lateral One-Arm Dumbbell Lat (Latissmus Dorsi) Rolls

The exercise is done by placing the right hand on the bench. Allow the left hand to bring the weight downward. Return the weight to the torso.

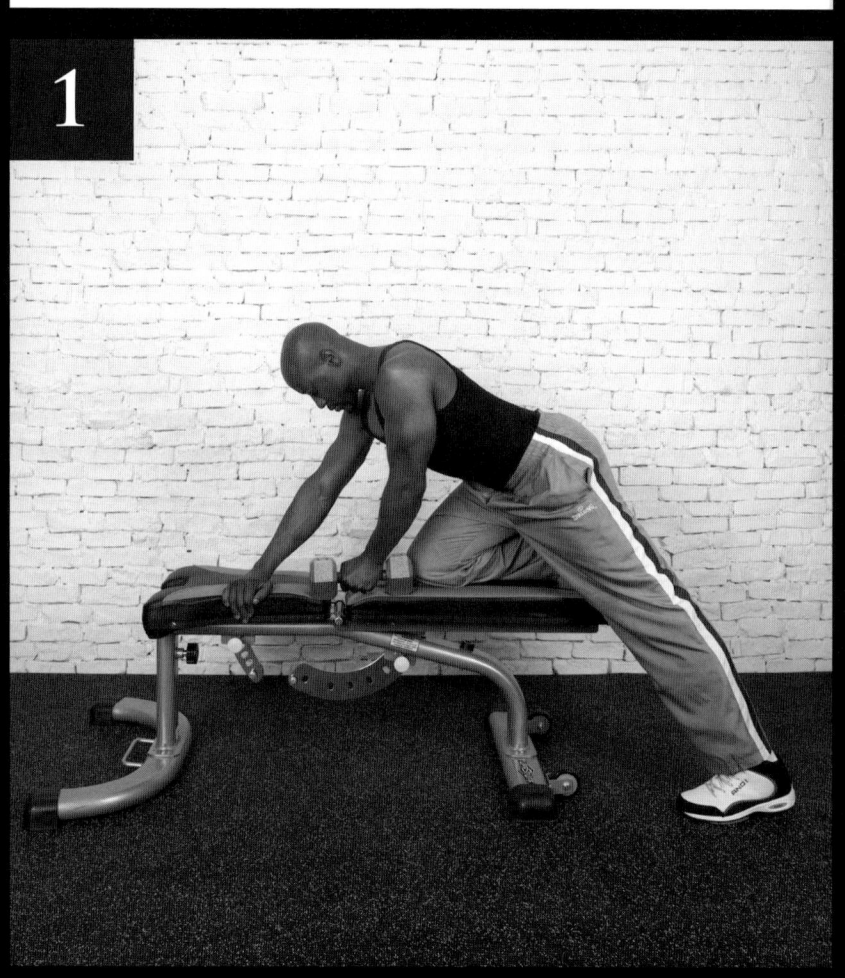

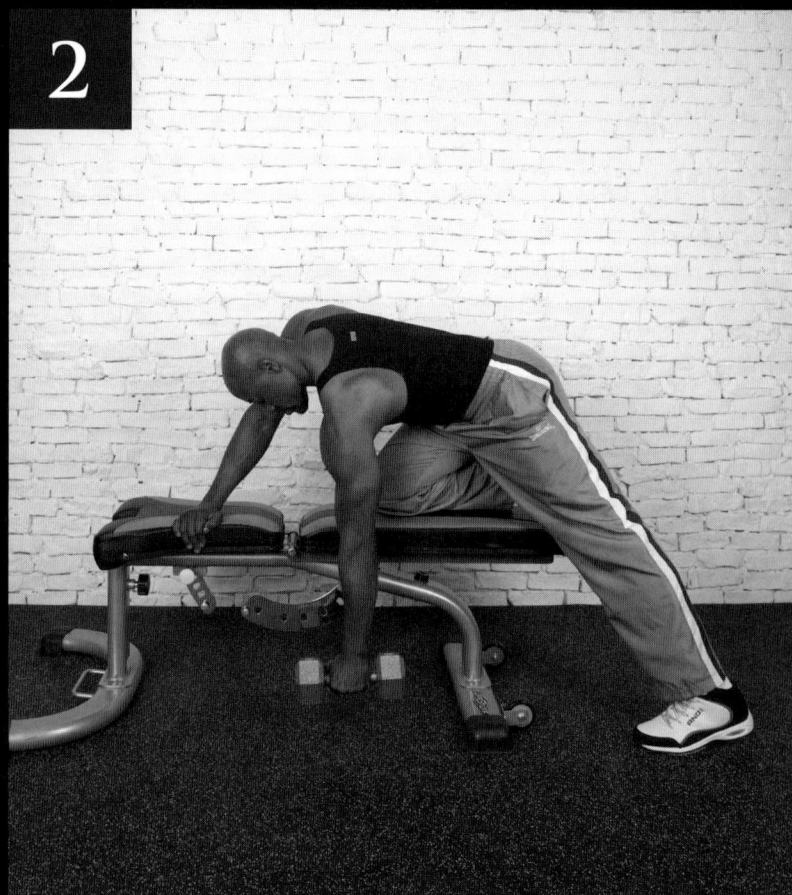

Lift the weight upright and pull upright to the side. Push the weight forward in front of the body and bring the elbow back up to the side to the resting position. The back should remain flat and the left leg should remain safely planted on the floor.

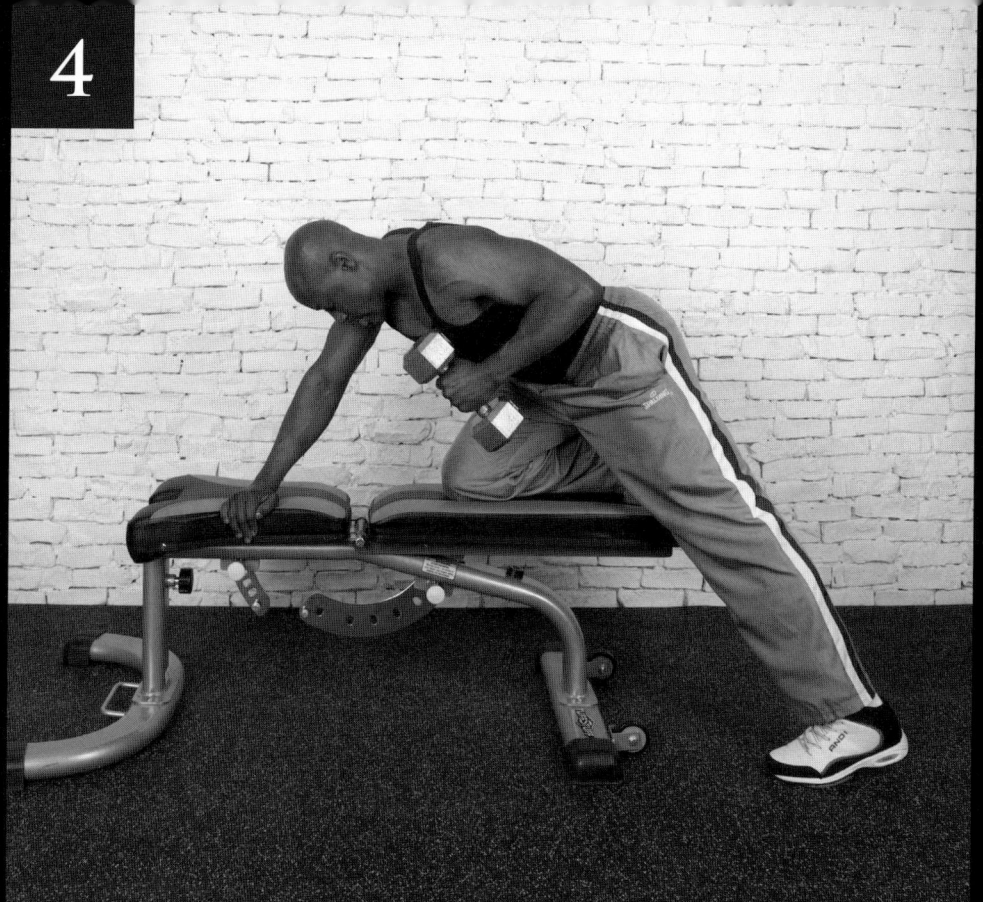

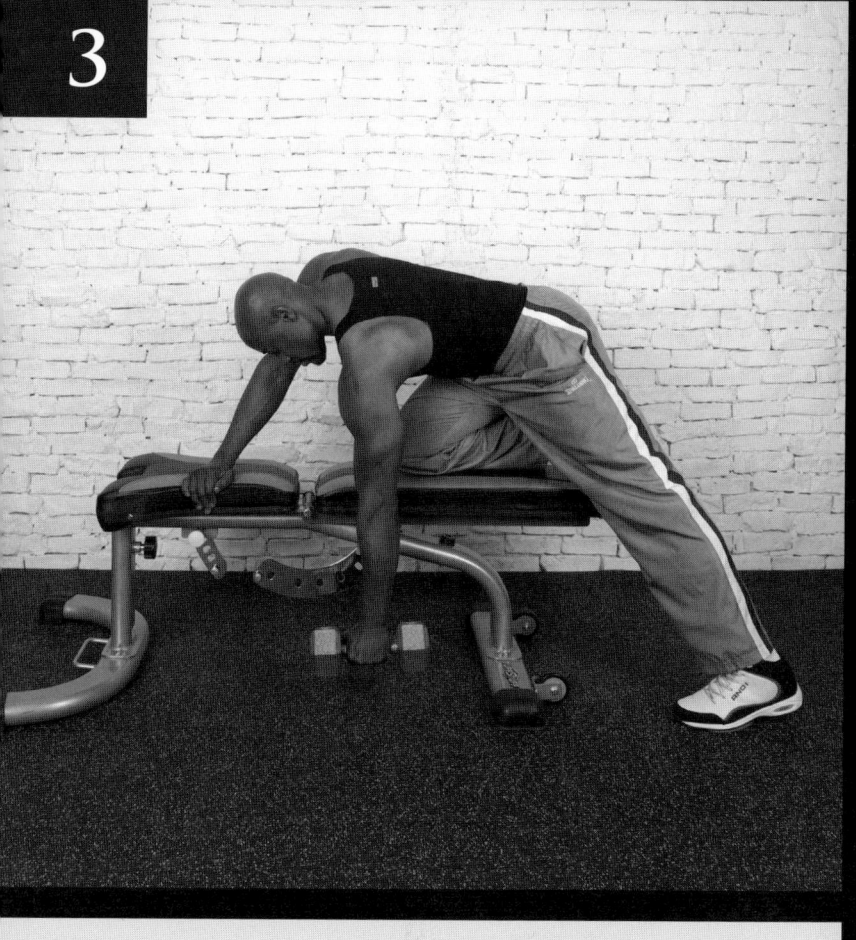

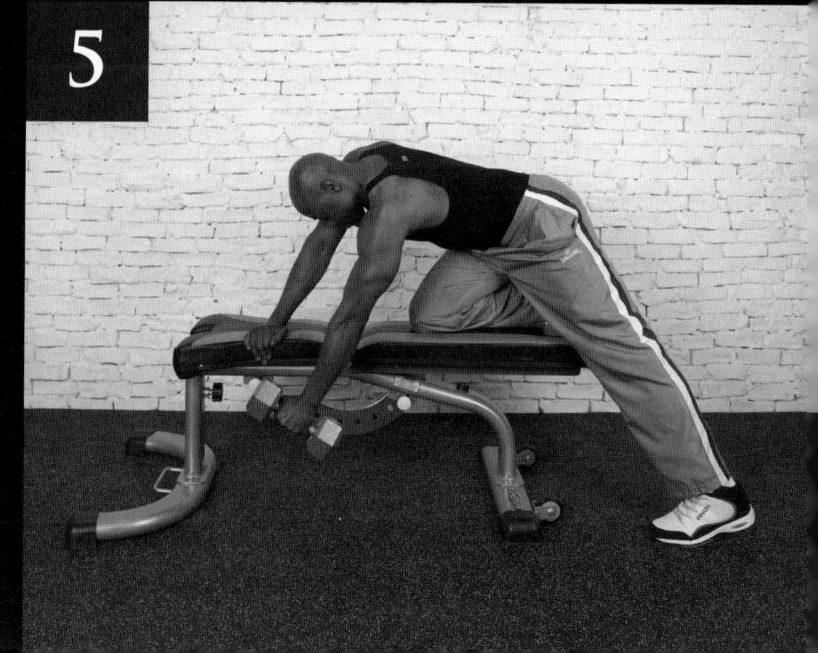

VARIATION OF A LOWER TRICEPS KICKBACK

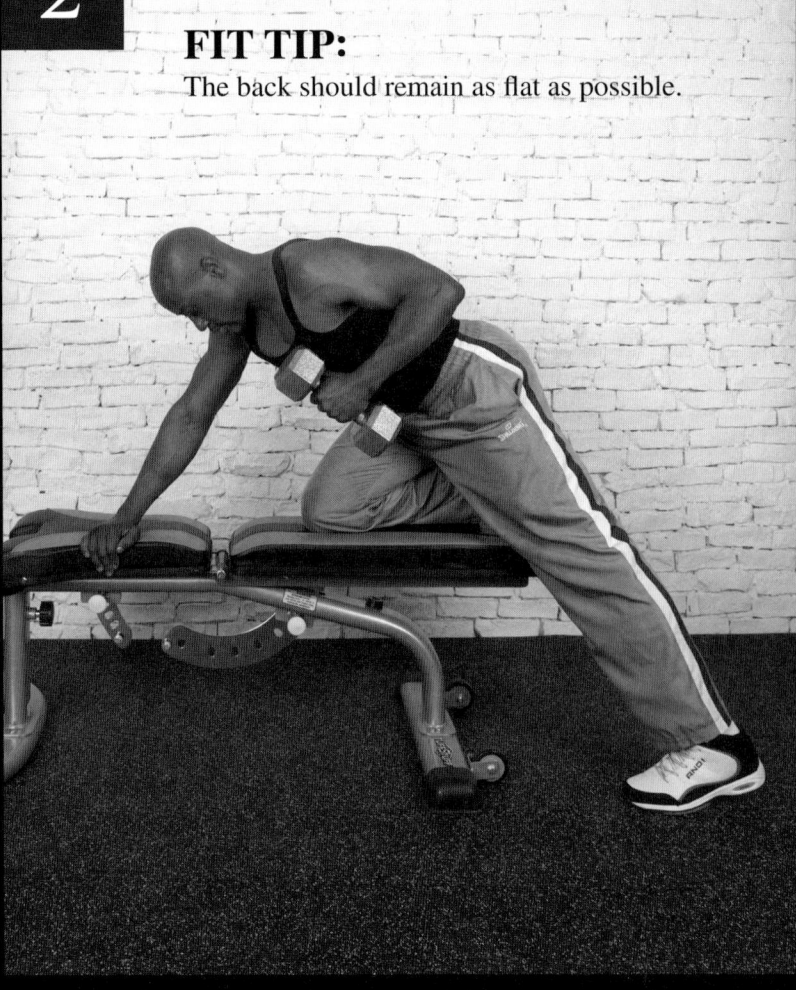

FIT TIP: The back should remain as flat as possible.

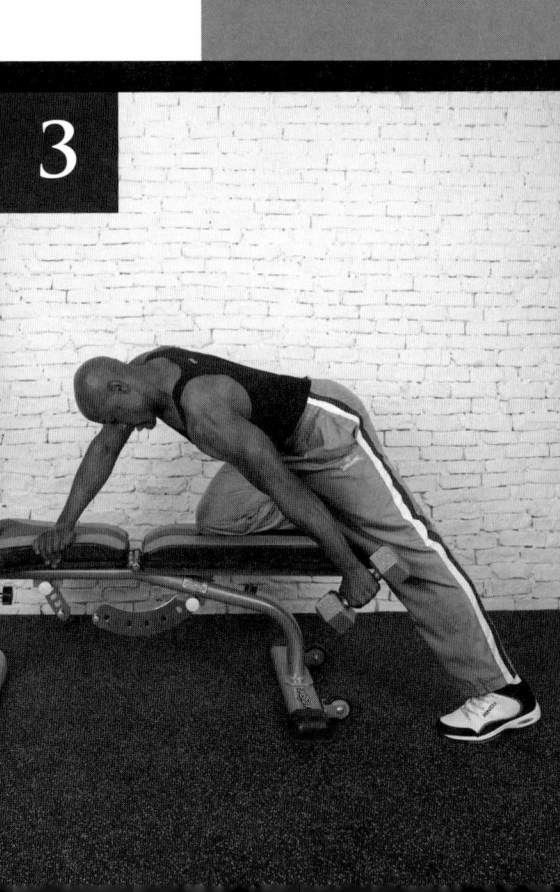

For this exercise, if it is done on the left side, the right knee is on the bench. The right arm is across the body on the bench. The left leg is behind and the foot is firmly planted on the floor. The weight is held in a hammer curl type position. The elbow is elevated and the elbow is then extended with the weight in the hand. The weight is then returned back to the initial position.

Posterior Wrist Curls of the Forearm

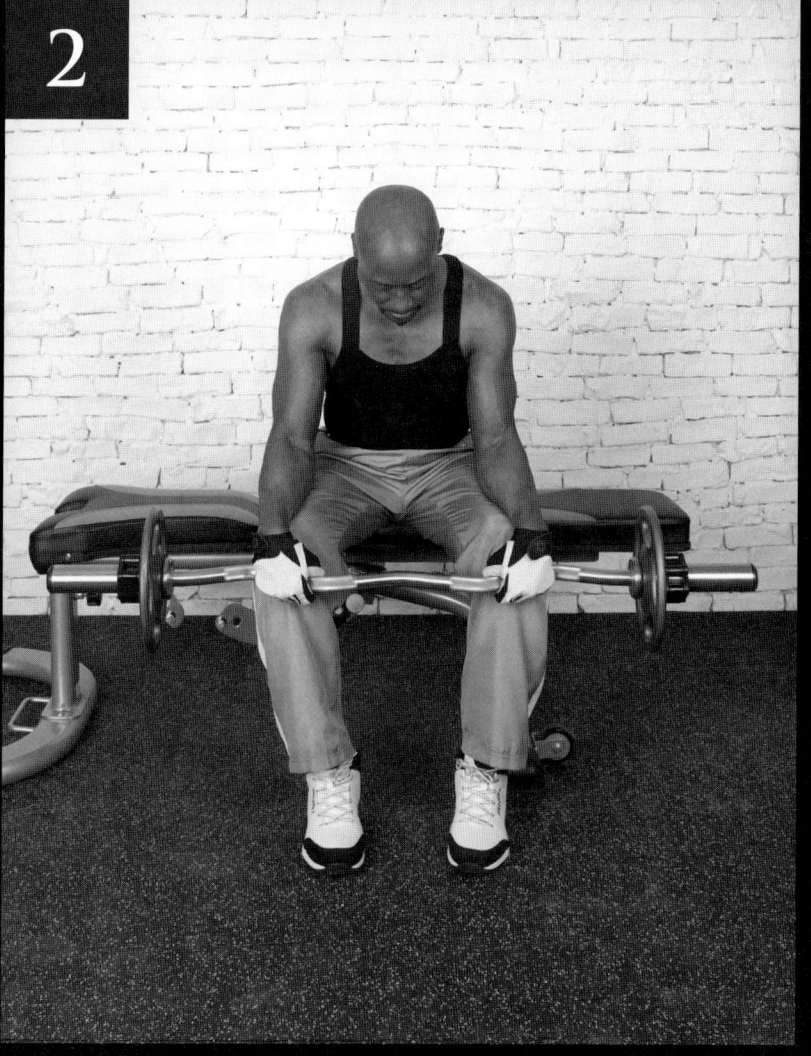

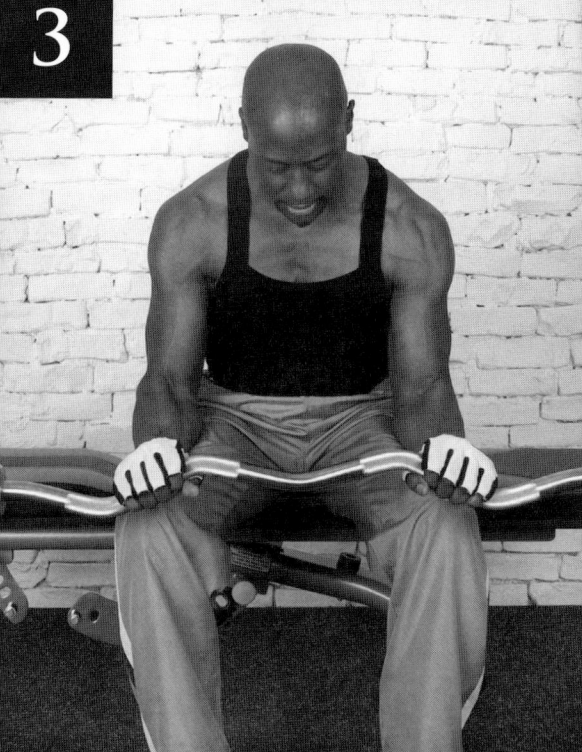

Recommended:
3 to 5 sets of
10 to 15 repetitions.

Sit upright on the bench with the weight bar on your thighs with the palms downward, grasping the bar. Lift the weights by extending your wrists.

ANTERIOR WRIST CURL

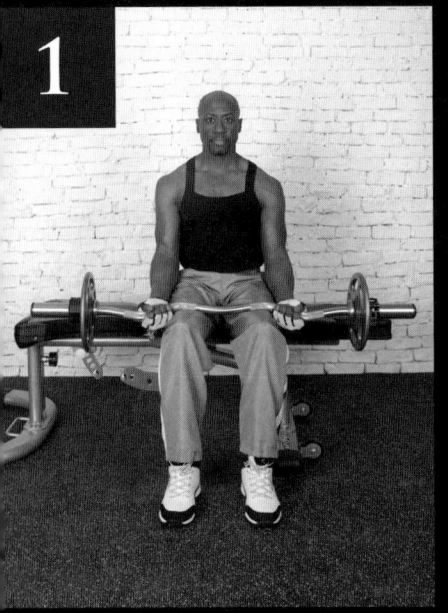

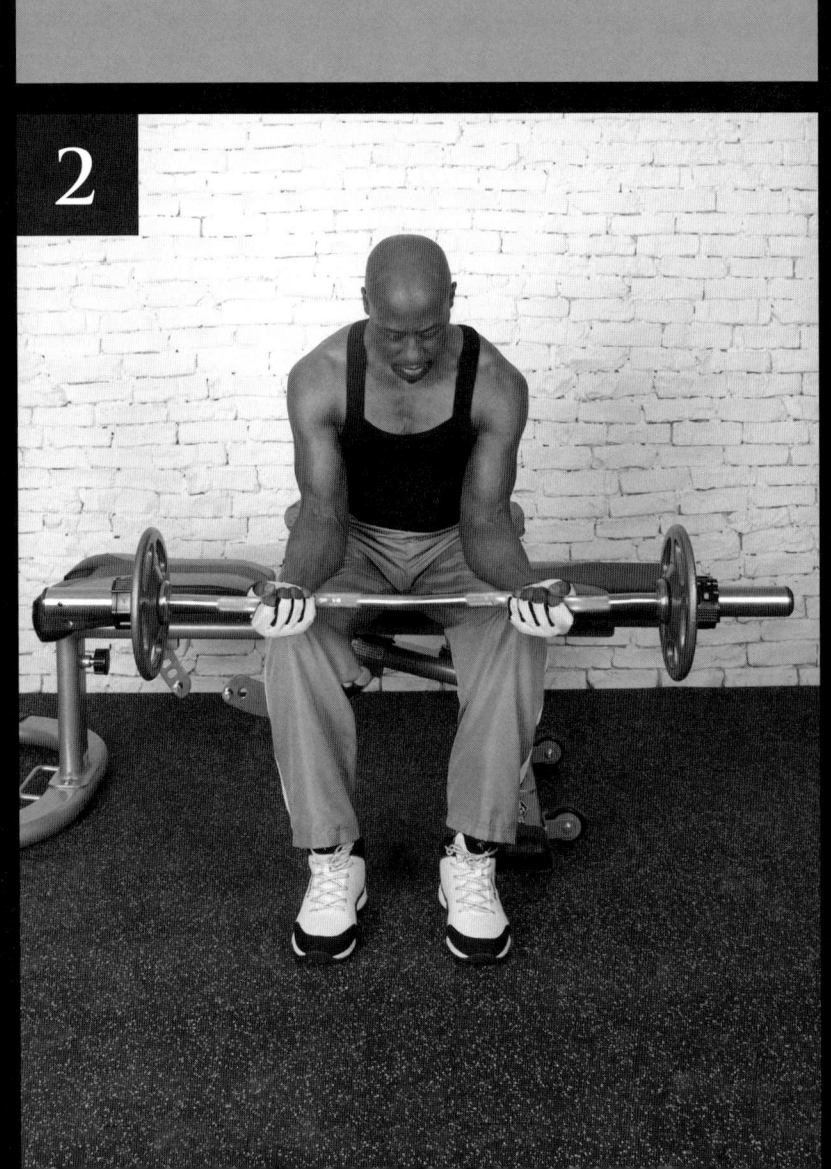

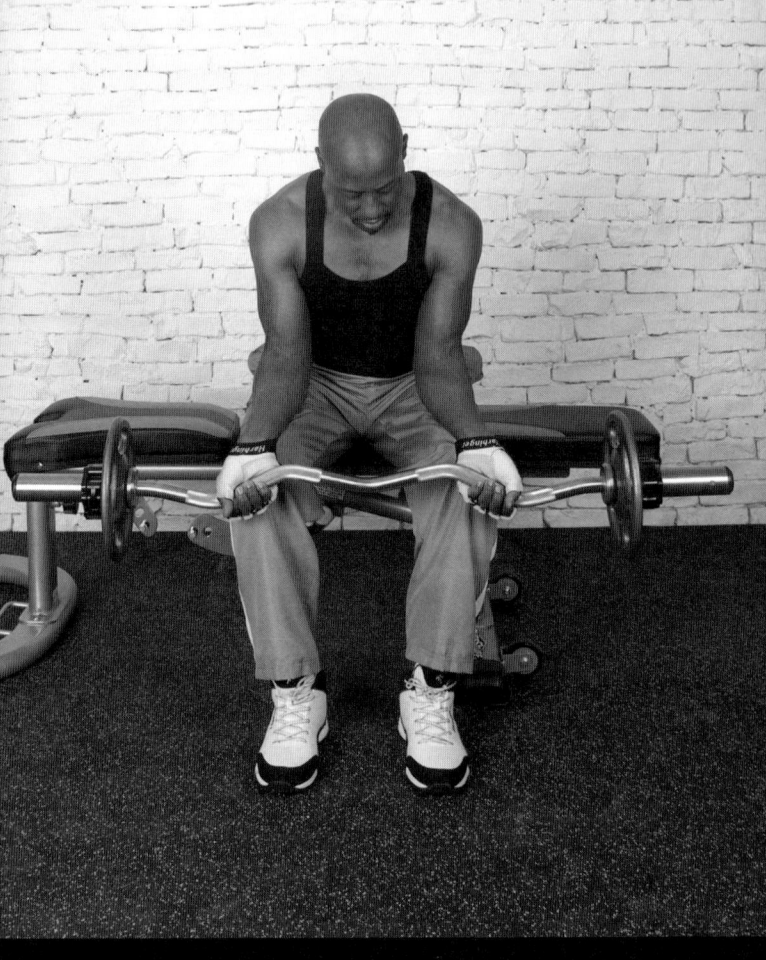

With the T-bar or long bar across the thighs, the bar should be grasped and centered with the forearms on the thighs. The wrists should be extended synchronously while holding the weight and then the wrists are flexed upward. This exercise should be done with the palms facing upward.

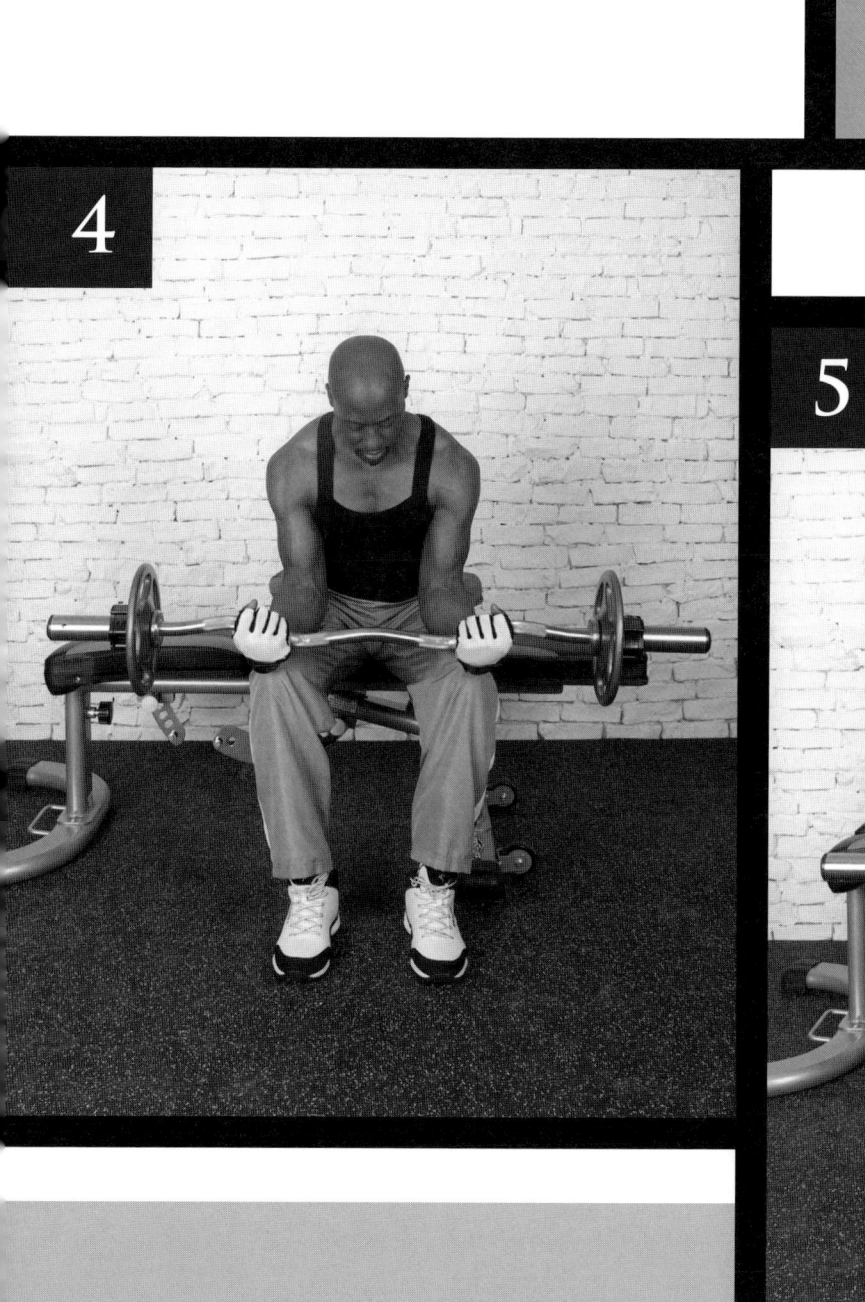
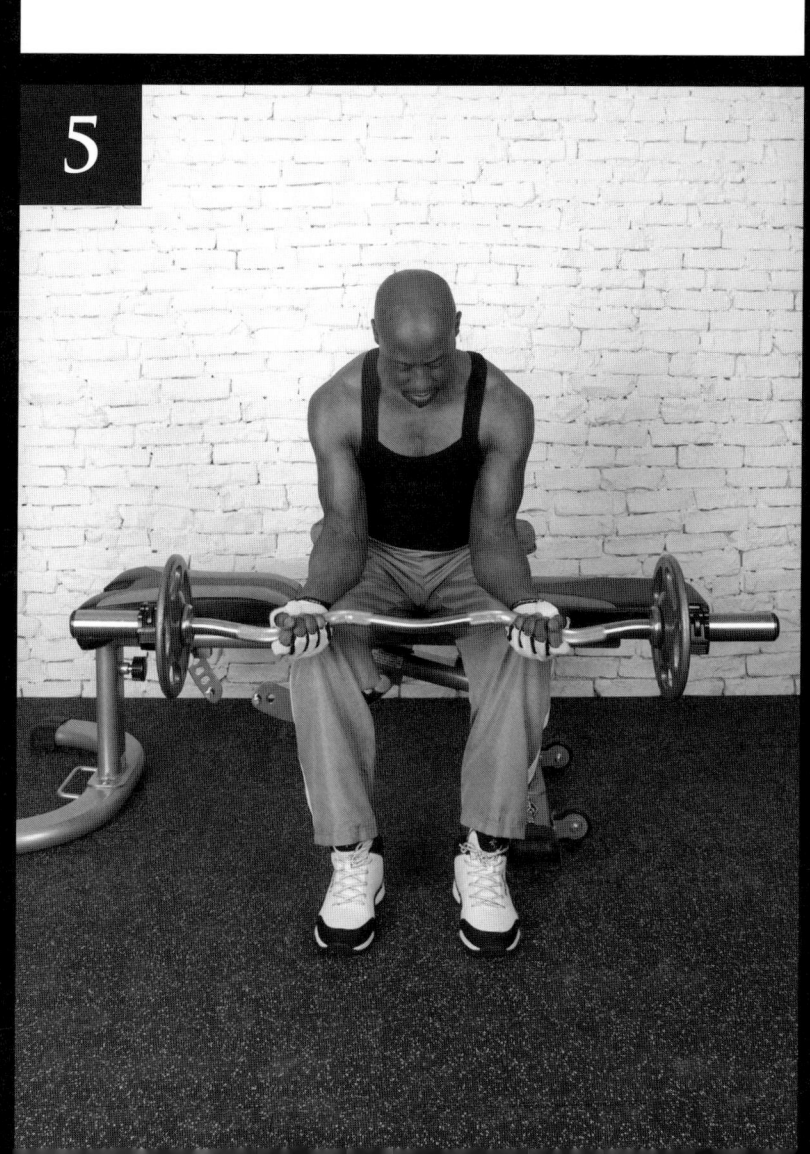
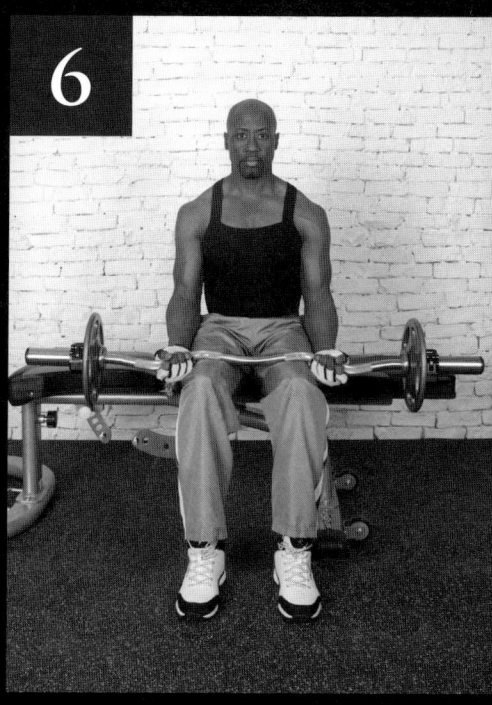

81

Short Curl Bar Upright Row

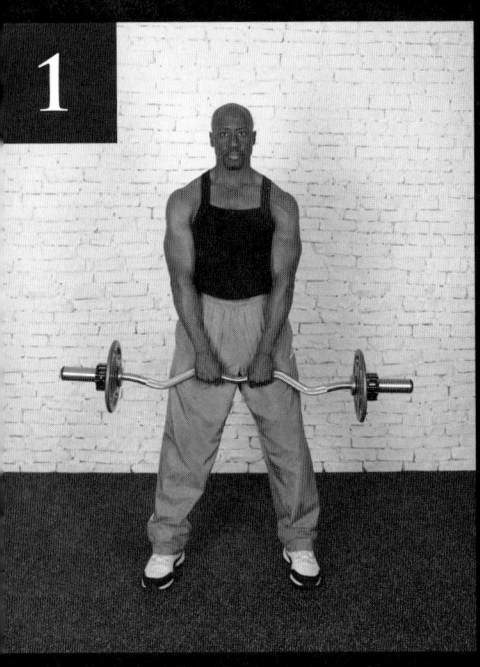

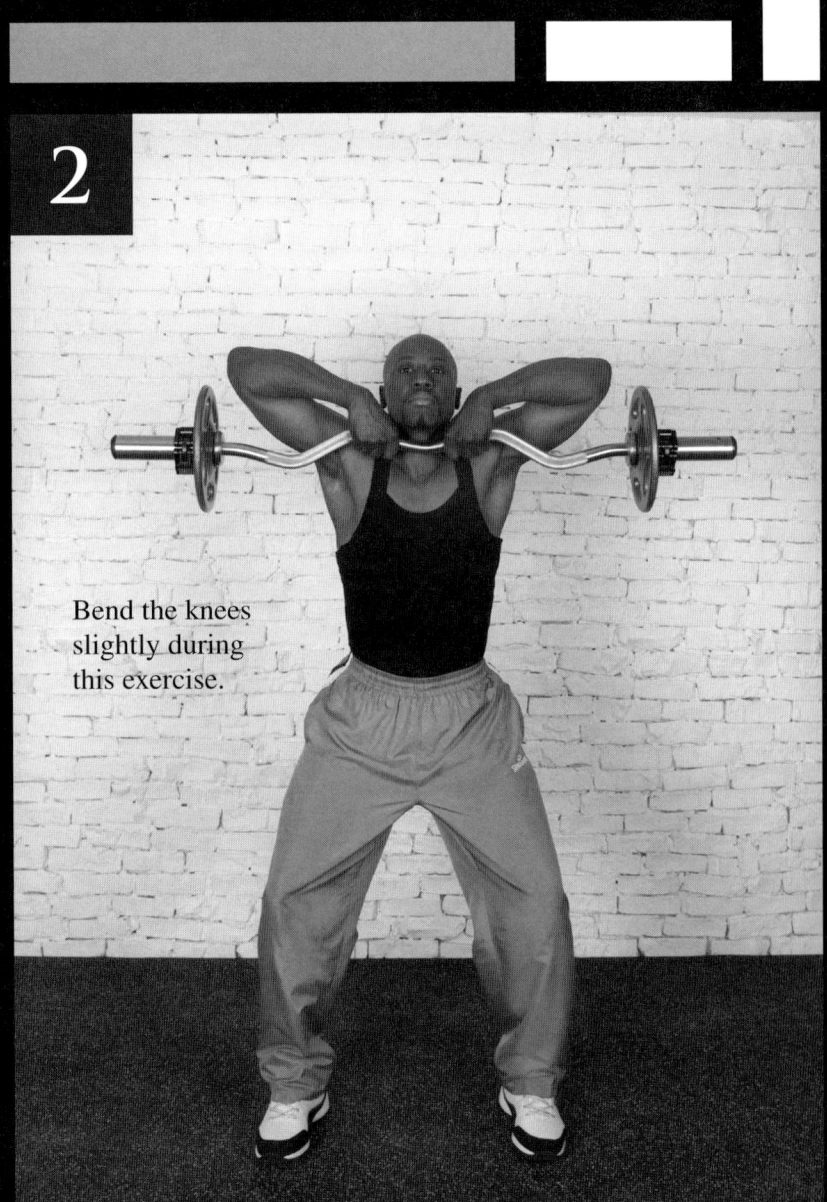

Bend the knees slightly during this exercise.

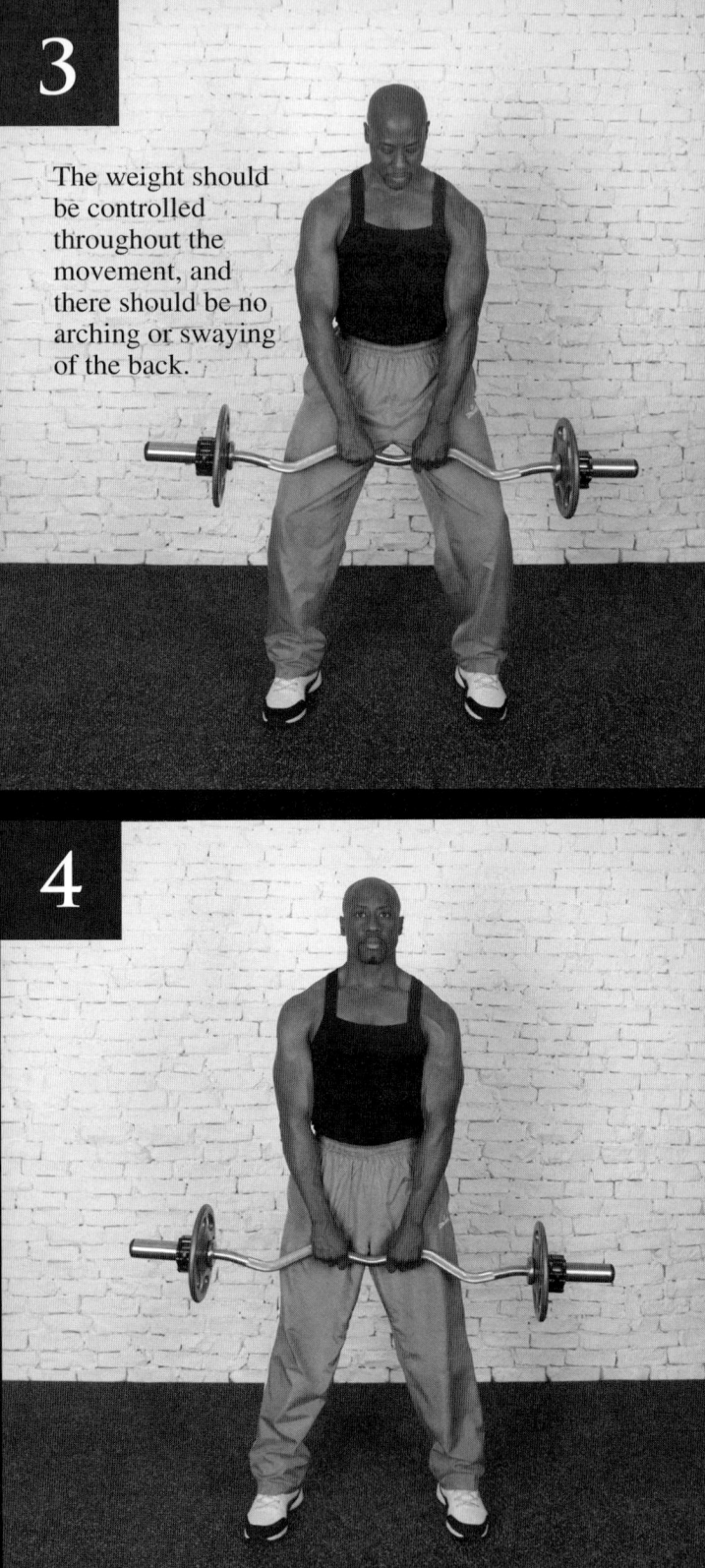

The weight should be controlled throughout the movement, and there should be no arching or swaying of the back.

This exercise is done by either a wide grip, medium grip, or tight grip of the bar. The arms are straight initially. The bar is then lifted up to the level of the chin. It is held and then released downward.

COMBINED UPRIGHT ROW AND SQUATS

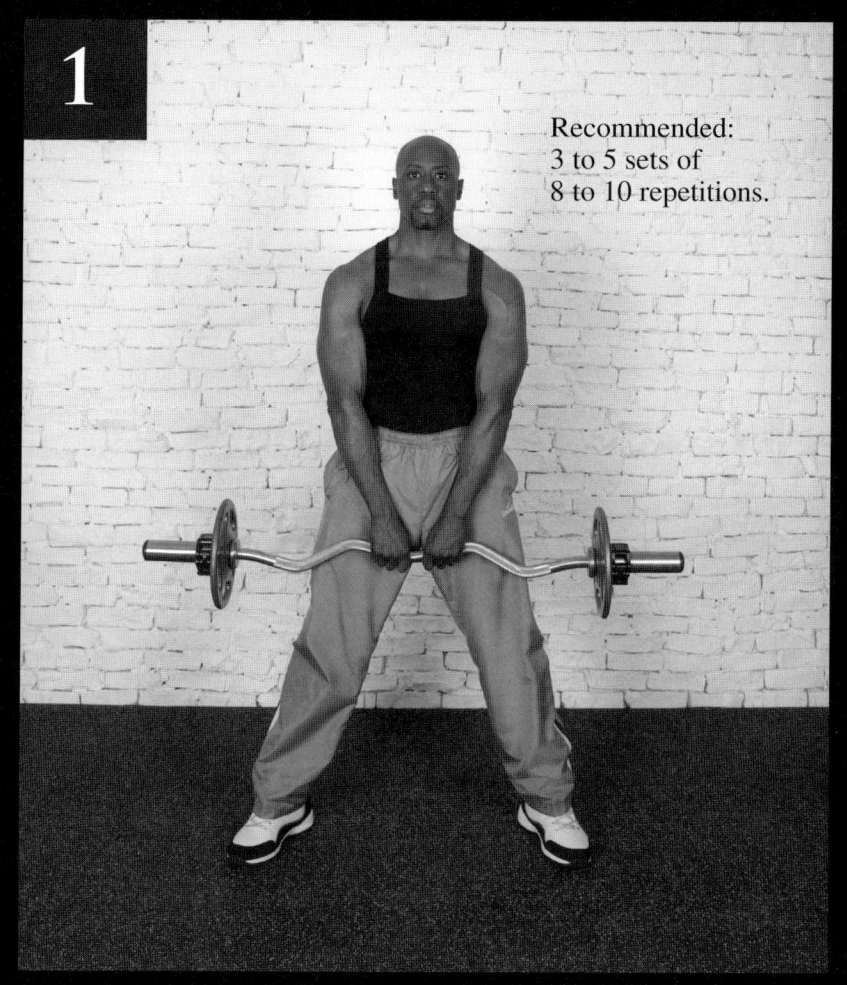

1 Recommended: 3 to 5 sets of 8 to 10 repetitions.

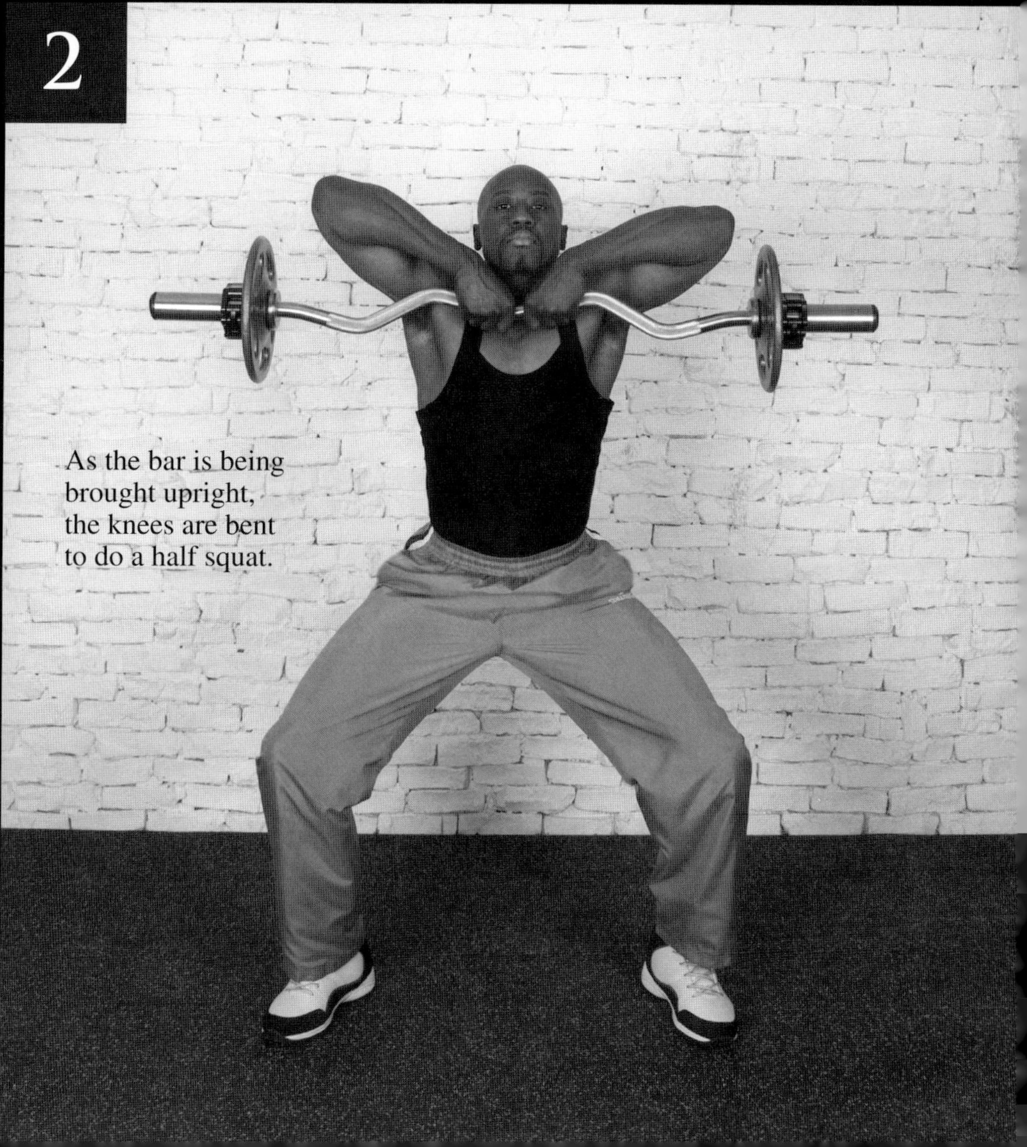

2 As the bar is being brought upright, the knees are bent to do a half squat.

This exercise is done by using a short curl bar with a tight grip. The feet are wider than shoulder-width apart. The back is straight. The shoulders are back. The bar is then brought up to shoulder level.

Posterior Deltoid Row

2 The key here is to bring the elbow up and posteriorly in a synchronized manner without causing any sway or dip in the back or pelvis.

3 Recommended: 3 to 5 sets of 8 to 10 repetitions.

The legs are separated in a runner's type position. The weight is held with the palm facing backwards. The arm is just adjacent to the leg that is forward. The elbow is then elevated to 90 degrees and posteriorly directed and brought back forward and down. The weight should be controlled throughout the movement.

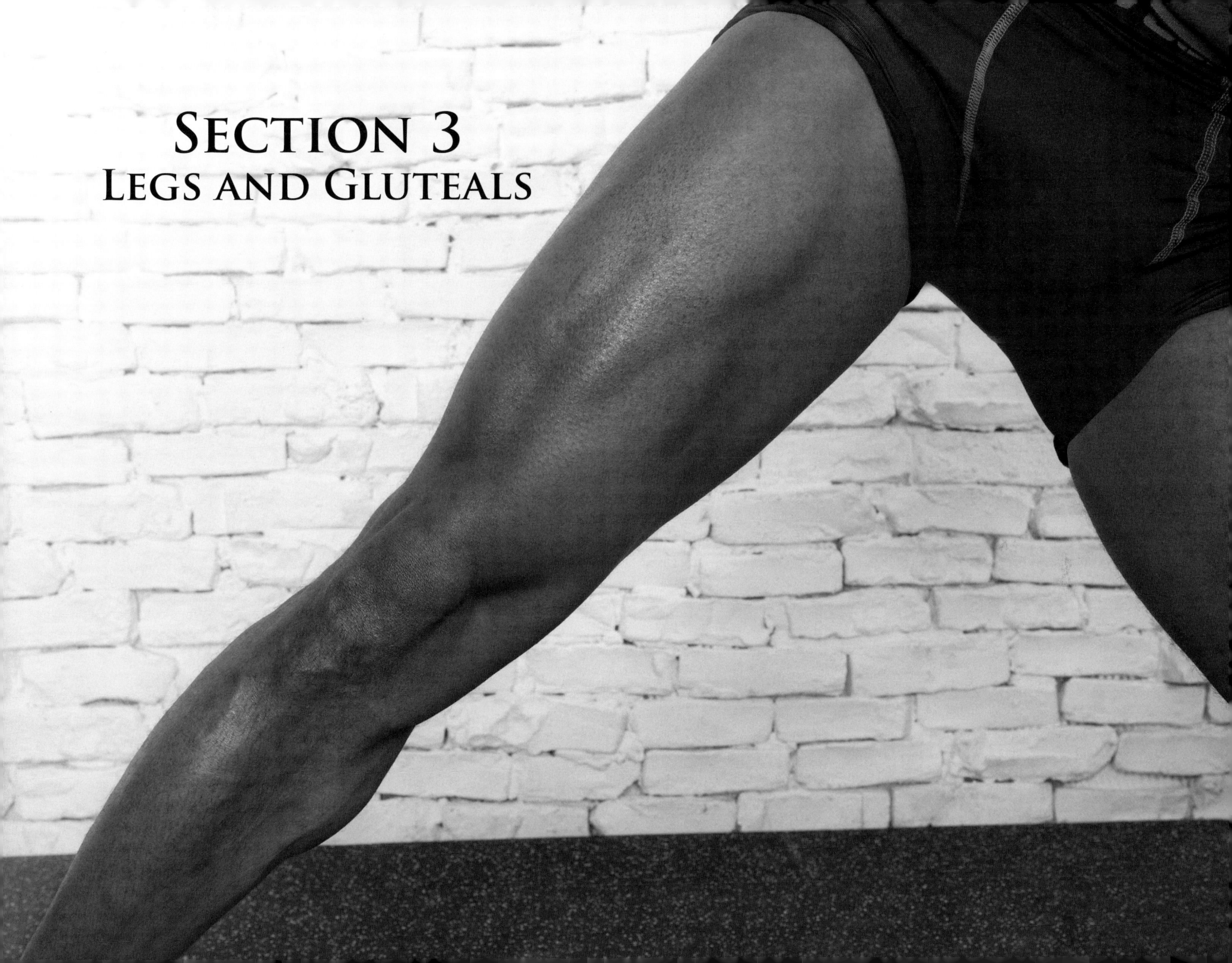

SECTION 3
LEGS AND GLUTEALS

LEG EXTENSION

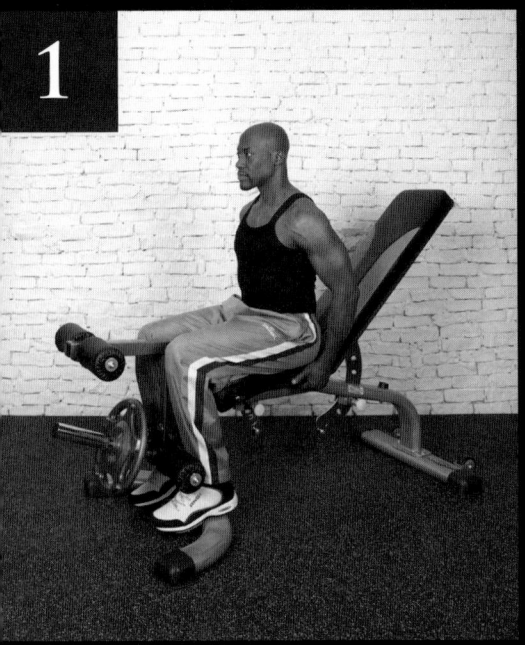

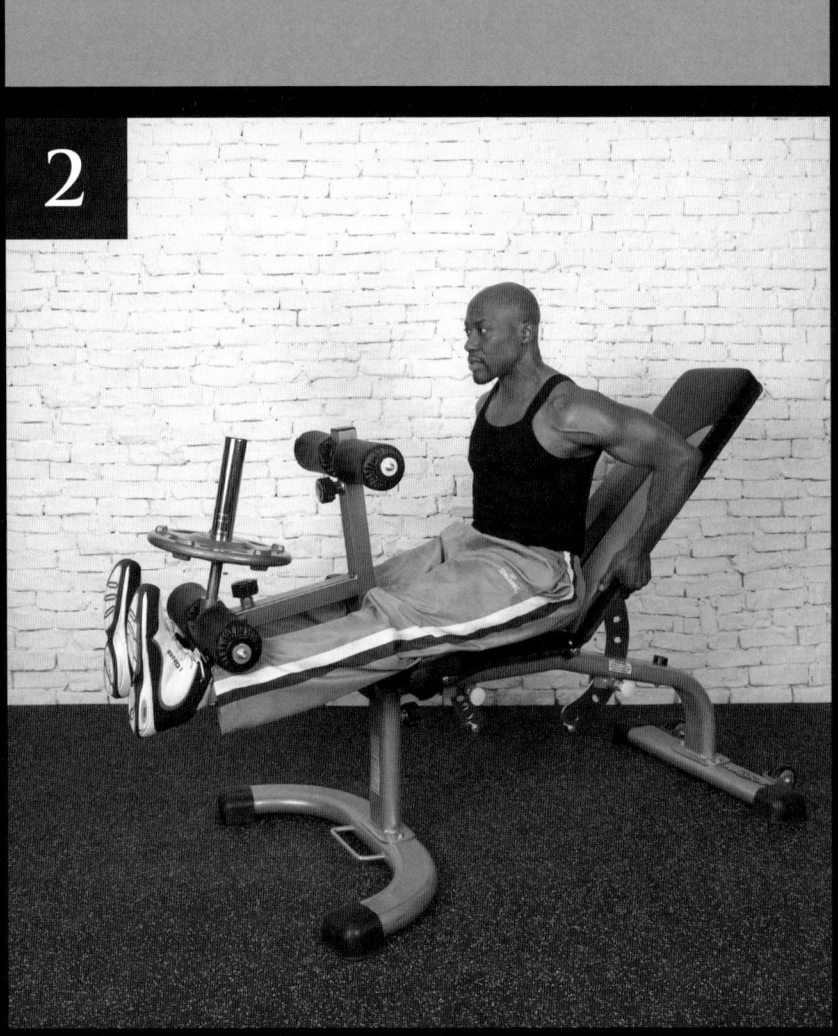

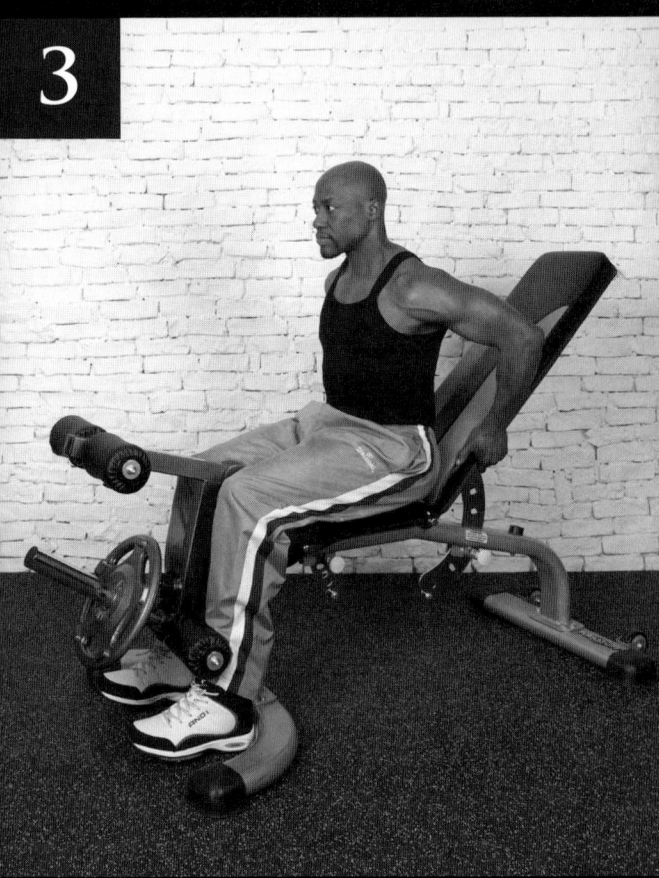

FIT TIP:

Inhale when lifting the weight upward. Exhale when lowering the weight.

This should be done at the seated leg extension machine with the knees at 90 degrees, back straight, and extend your legs and your knees. The weight should be lifted forward.

Hamstring Curls

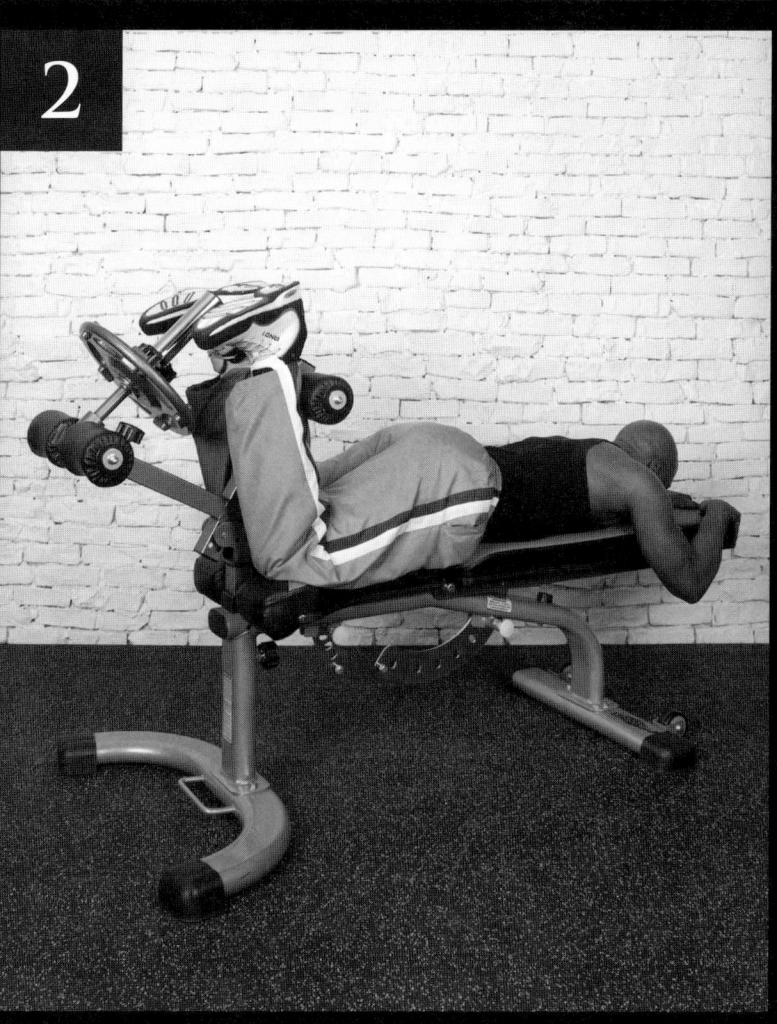

Lie prone on the exercise equipment with the feet tucked behind the heel support. The knees should be bent, bringing up the weight without arching the back. The abdomen should press against the bench. The weight should be lifted and then lowered.

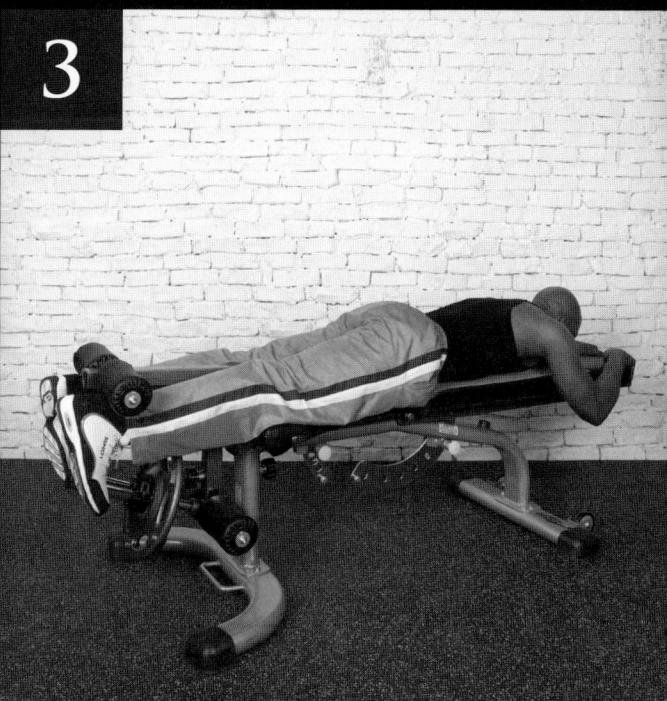

Recommended:
3 to 5 sets of
8 to 10 repetitions.

Bench Assisted Lunge

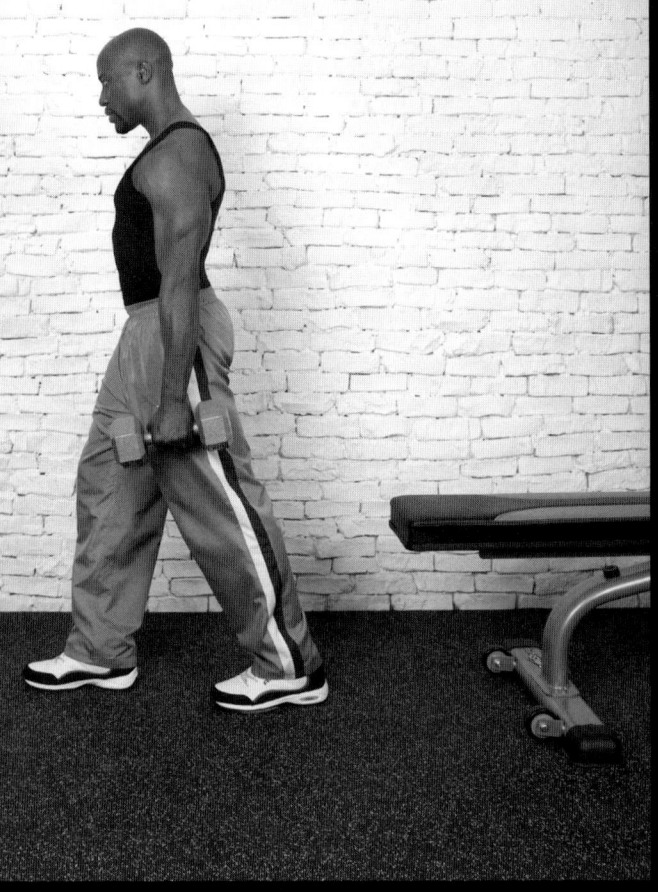

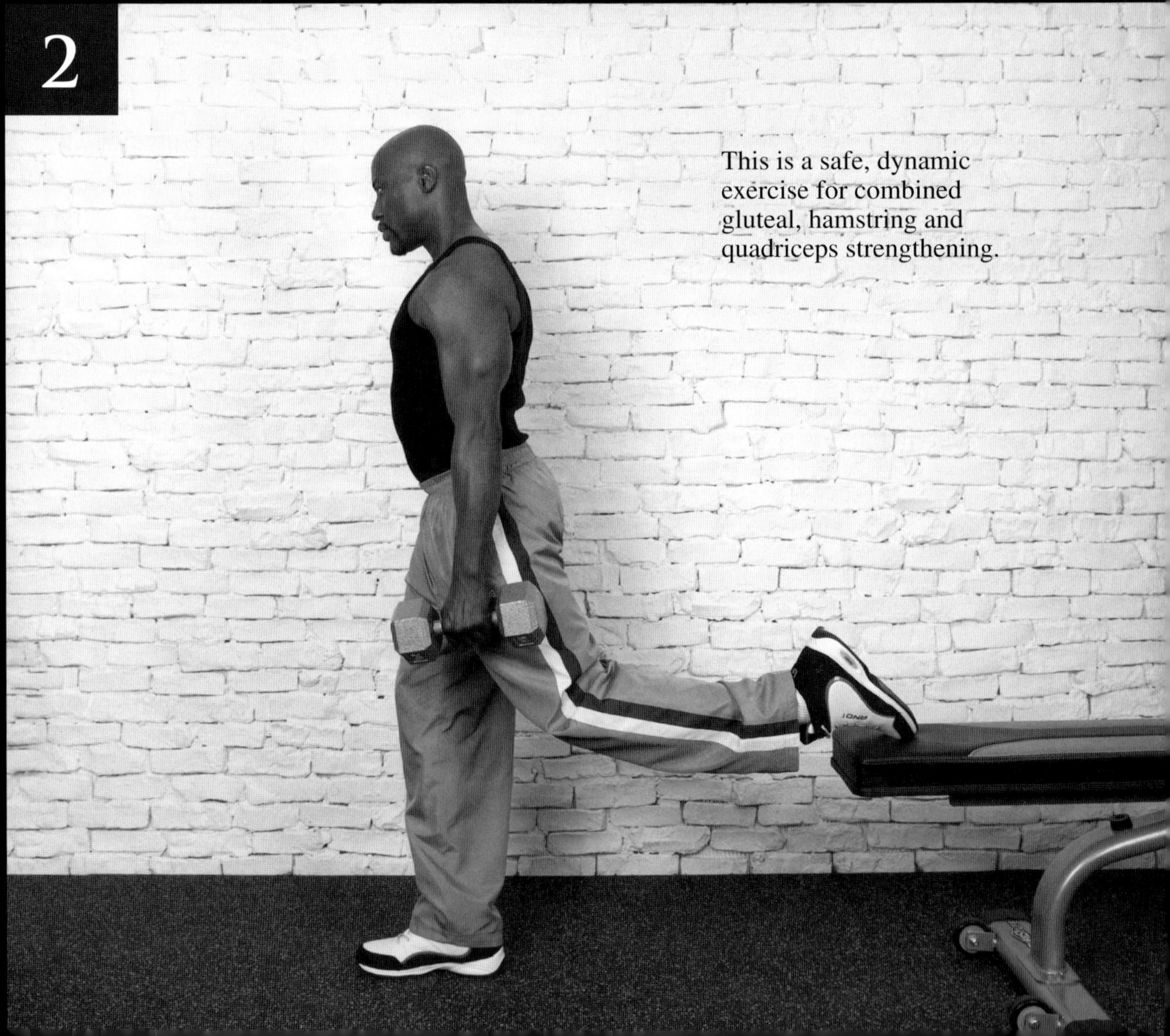

This is a safe, dynamic exercise for combined gluteal, hamstring and quadriceps strengthening.

Start from a neutral standing position with one foot in front of the other, legs apart with the weights in hand, and palms facing the thigh. One foot should be safely placed on the bench, holding both weights in hand. The knees should be bent while holding the weights.

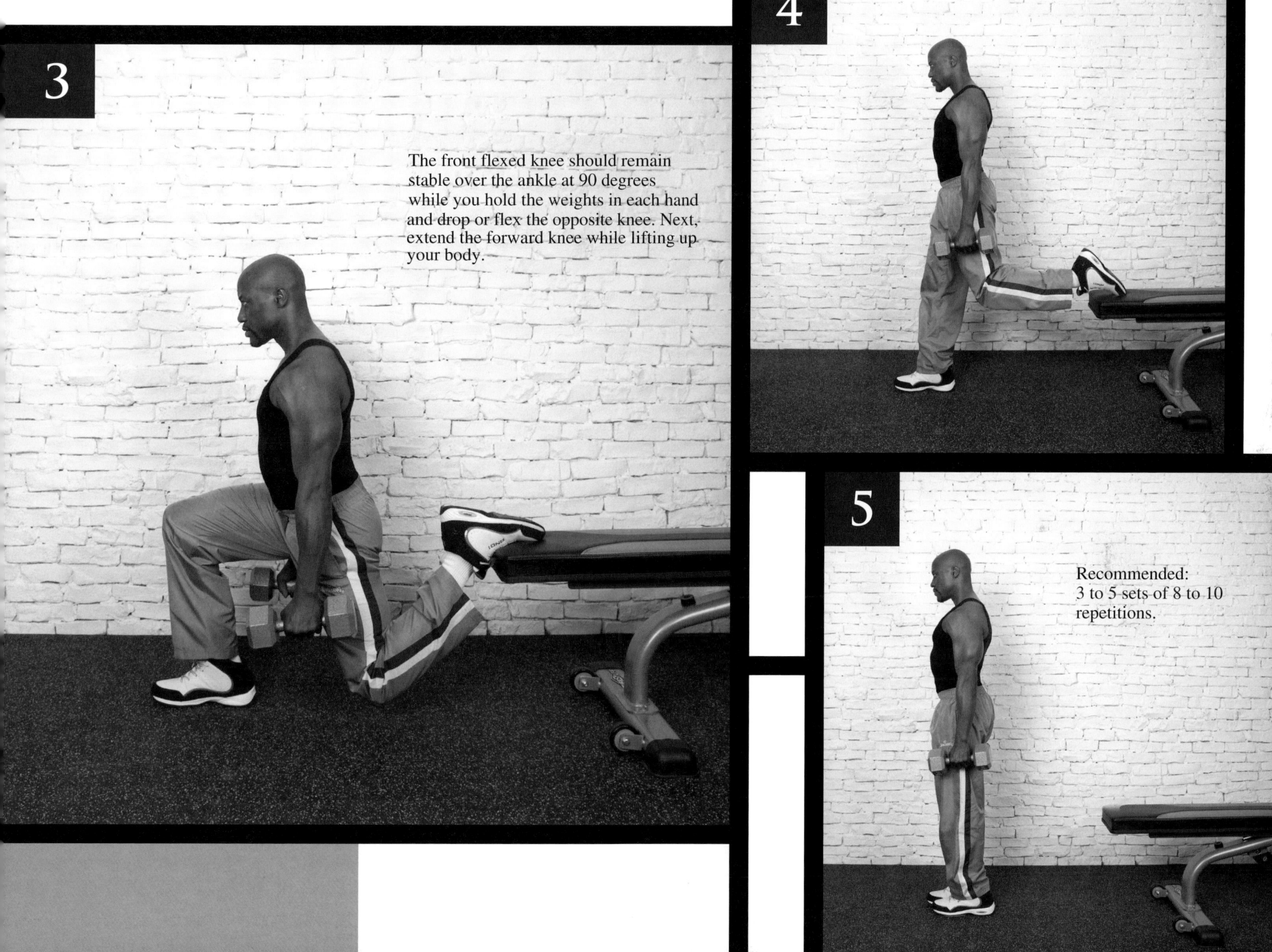

3. The front flexed knee should remain stable over the ankle at 90 degrees while you hold the weights in each hand and drop or flex the opposite knee. Next, extend the forward knee while lifting up your body.

5. Recommended: 3 to 5 sets of 8 to 10 repetitions.

Bench Squat with Weights

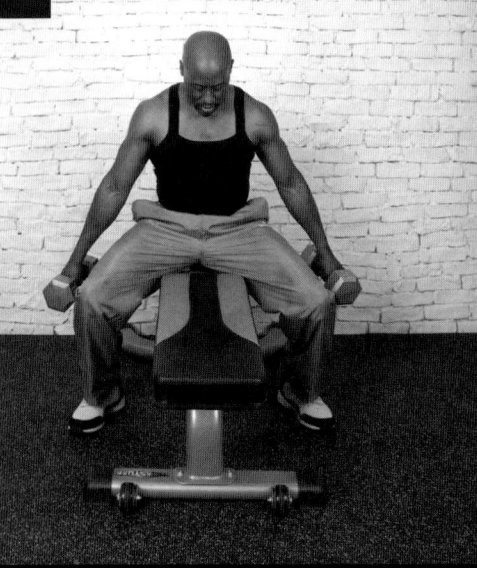

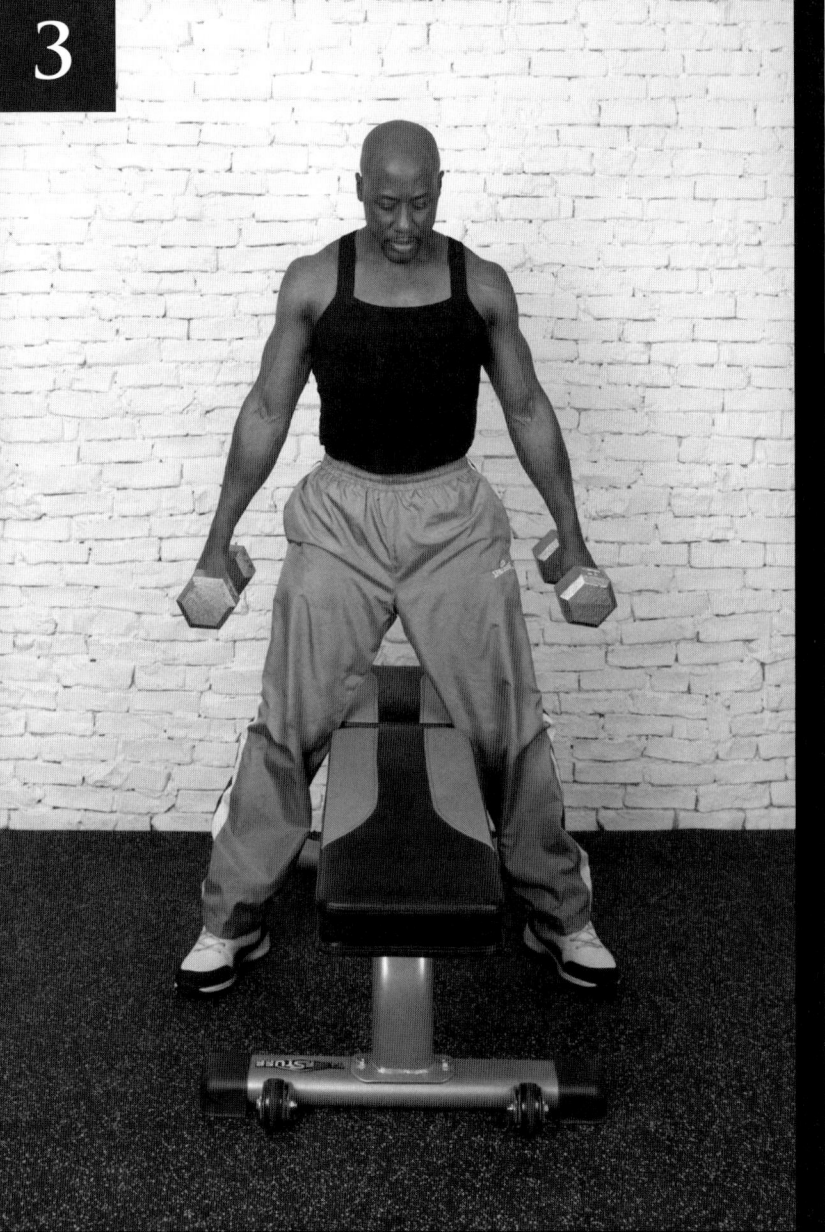

This exercise is executed by straddling a bench with weights in each hand and bending your knees to let your buttocks touch the bench. Squeeze your buttocks after touching the bench. You should slowly come up holding the weights safely.

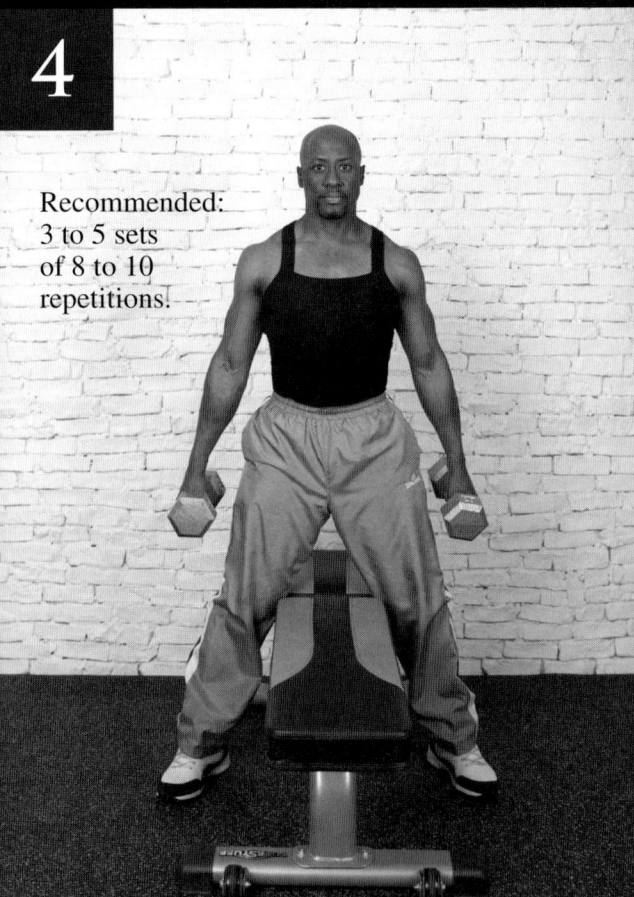

Recommended: 3 to 5 sets of 8 to 10 repetitions.

WIDE SQUAT WITH WEIGHT

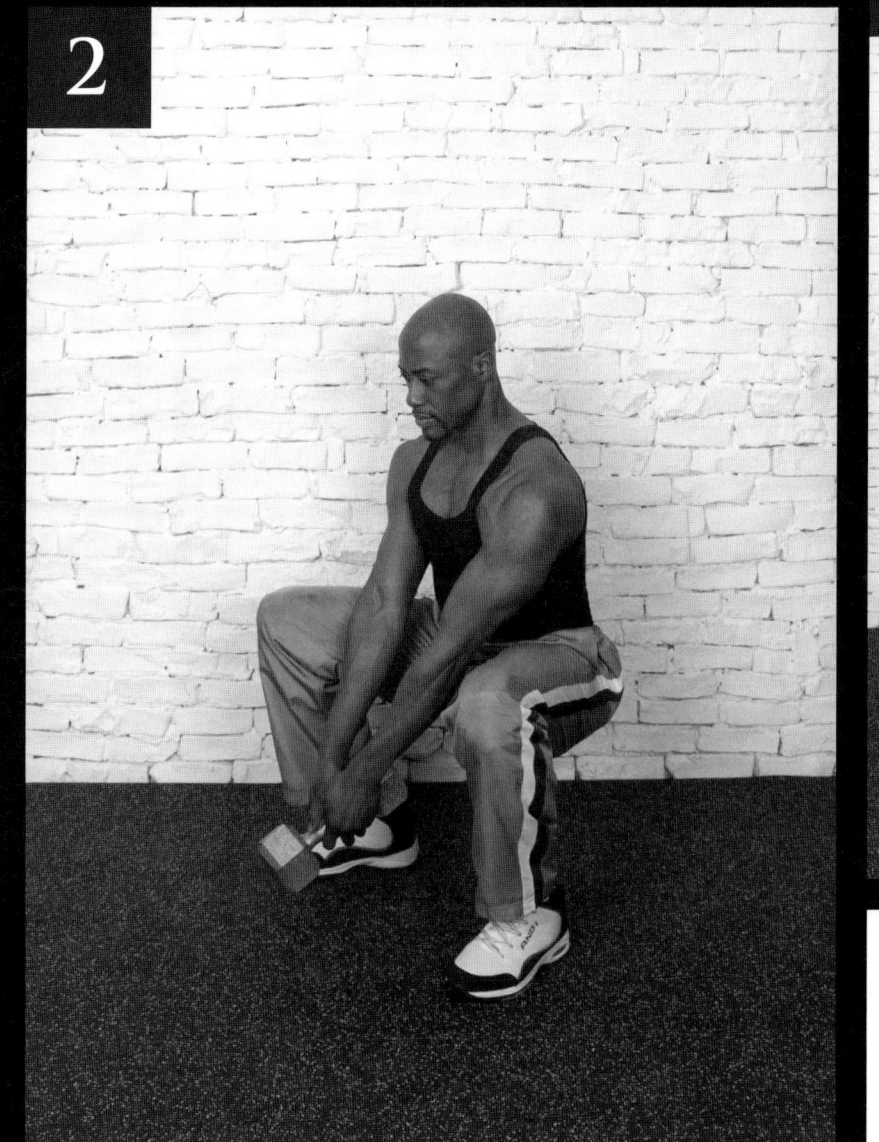

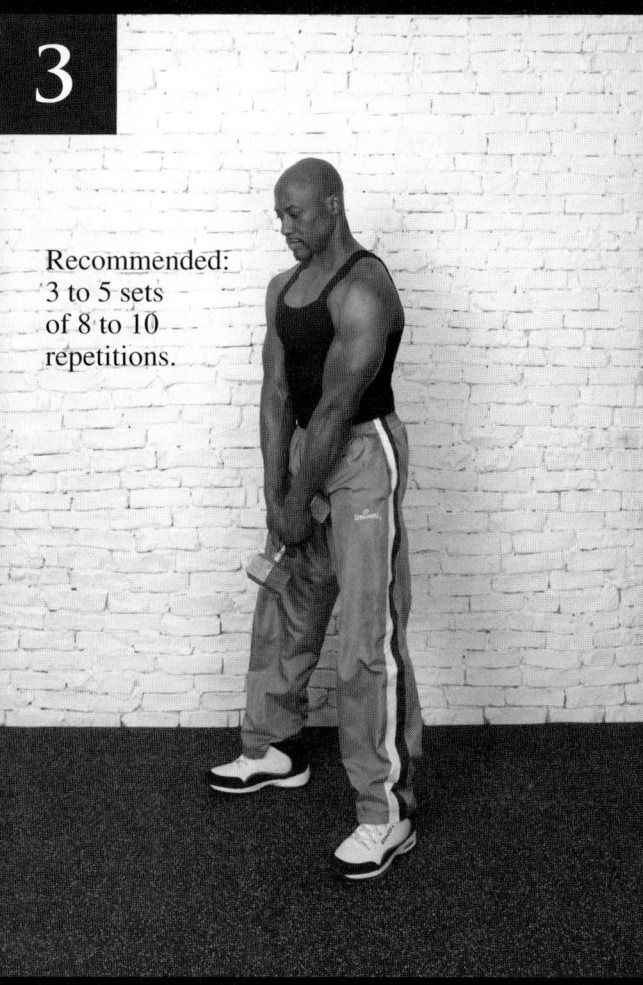

Recommended: 3 to 5 sets of 8 to 10 repetitions.

Start with the feet more than shoulder-width apart, hold the weight in front of you with both hands, squat down with the buttocks even with the knees holding the weight forward, and then lift your body upright holding the weight. The back should be straight, the knees should be kept right above the ankles, and the buttocks should be even with the knees.

Wide Squat with Anterior Deltoid (Shoulder) Raises

1

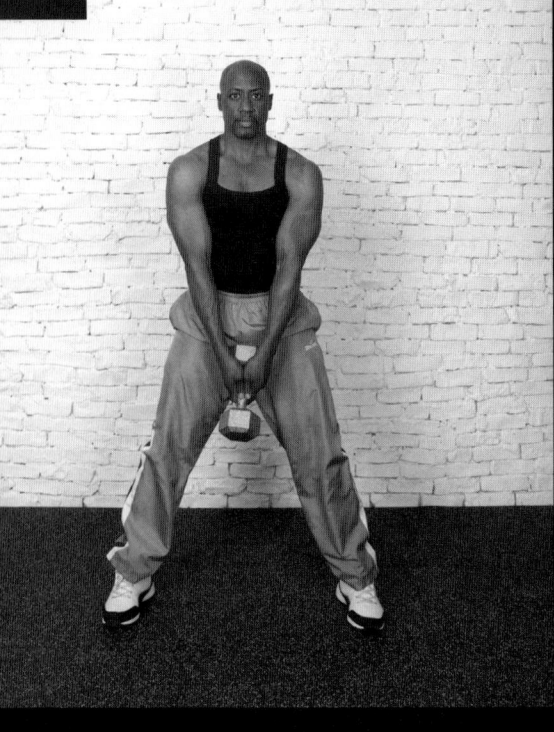

2

FIT TIP: Keep back straight.

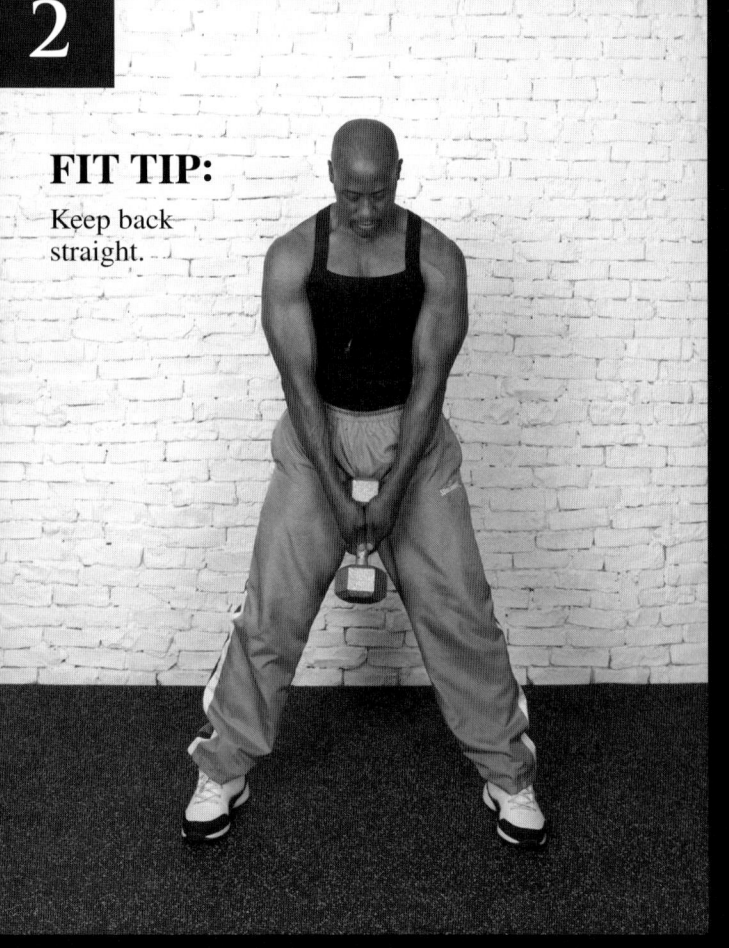

3

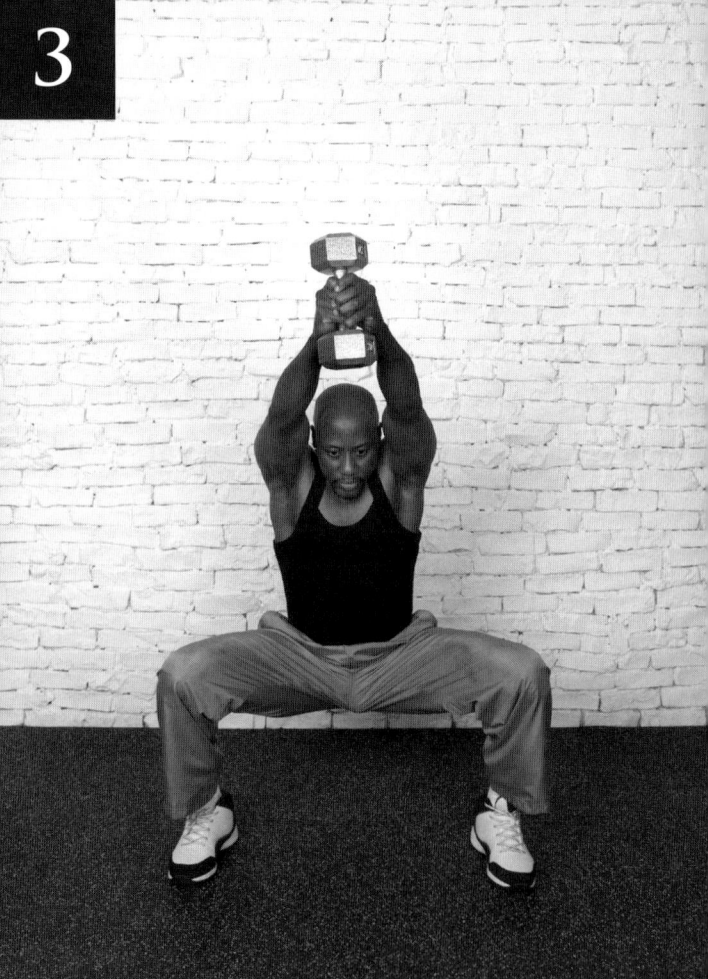

This exercise is done by having the feet wide apart, much wider than shoulder-width apart. Hold one dumbbell in front. Squat down while keeping your feet flat and lift the dumbbell higher than your head, holding your arms straight. The weight should be slowly brought down. As the weight is brought down, stand up out of the squatting position, holding the weight safely in front.

Lateral Side Profile of Wide Squat with Anterior Deltoid (Shoulder) Raises

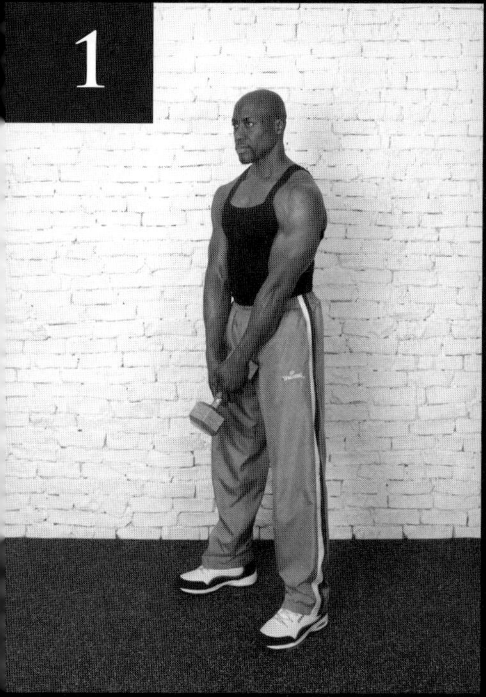

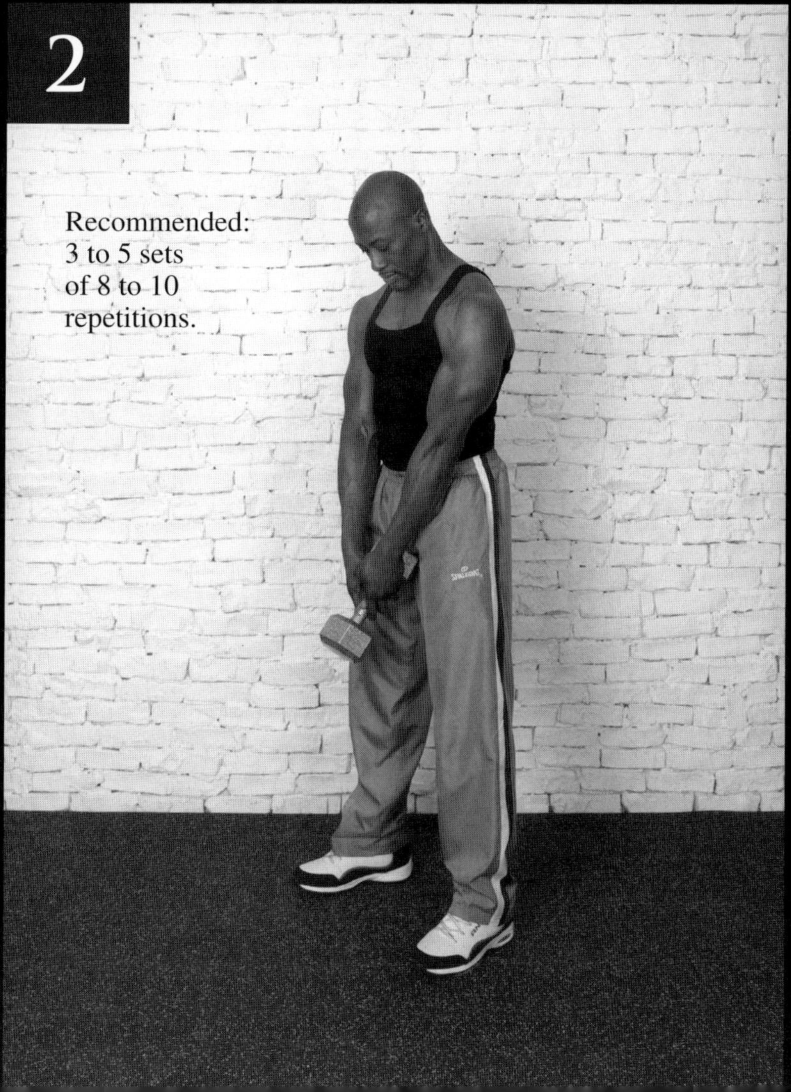

Recommended: 3 to 5 sets of 8 to 10 repetitions.

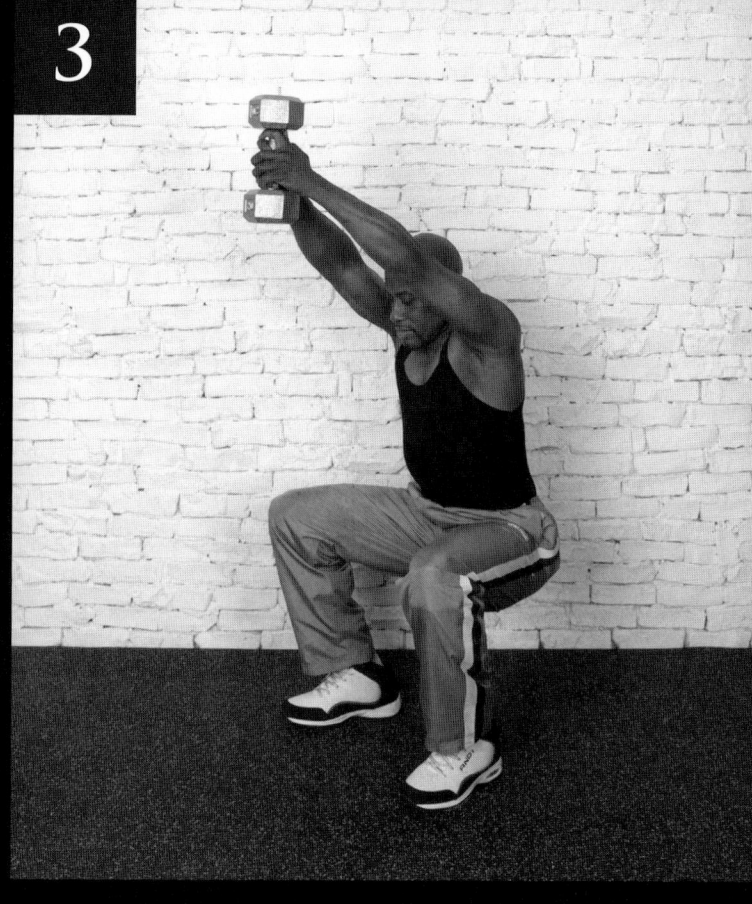
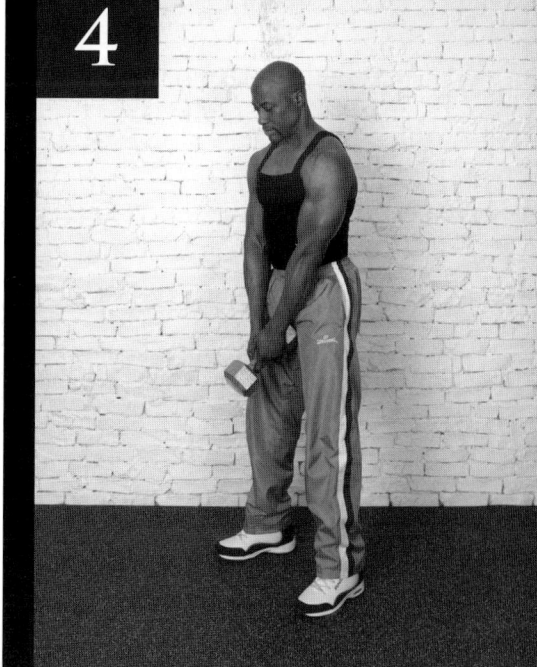

Forward Standard Calf Raises

Using the Captain's Chair

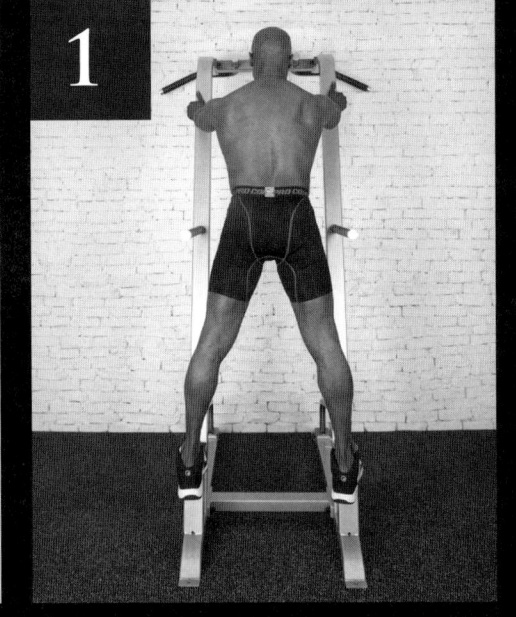

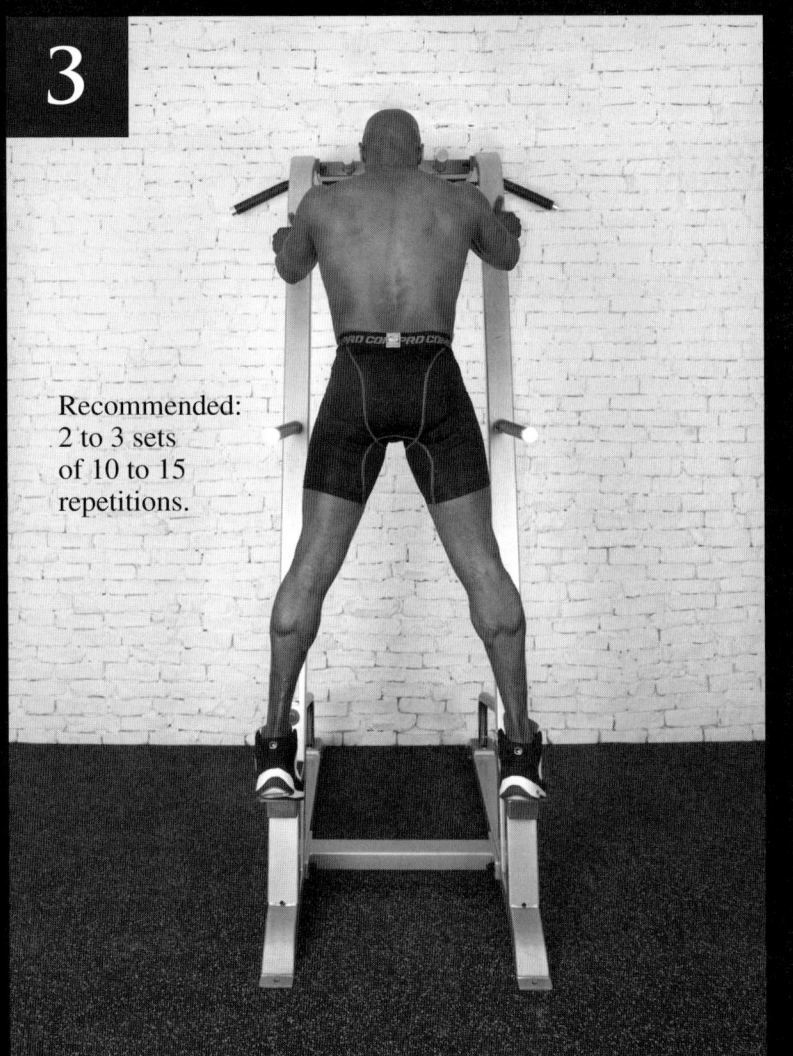

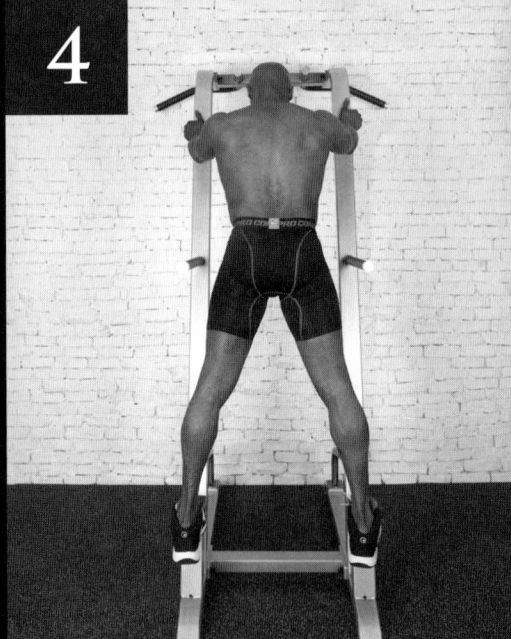

Recommended: 2 to 3 sets of 10 to 15 repetitions.

The Captain's Chair is mounted in the standard position. The feet are on the bottom aspect of the device with just the balls of the feet on the rail. The heels are elevated and then the heels descend toward the floor and then back to neutral position.

EXTERNAL CALF RAISES
Using the Captain's Chair

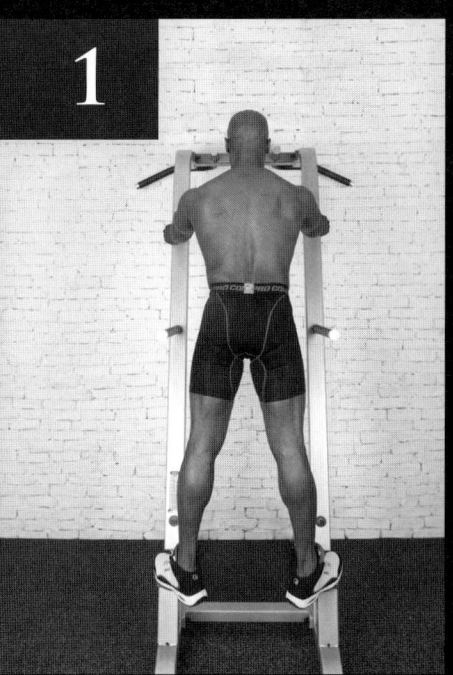

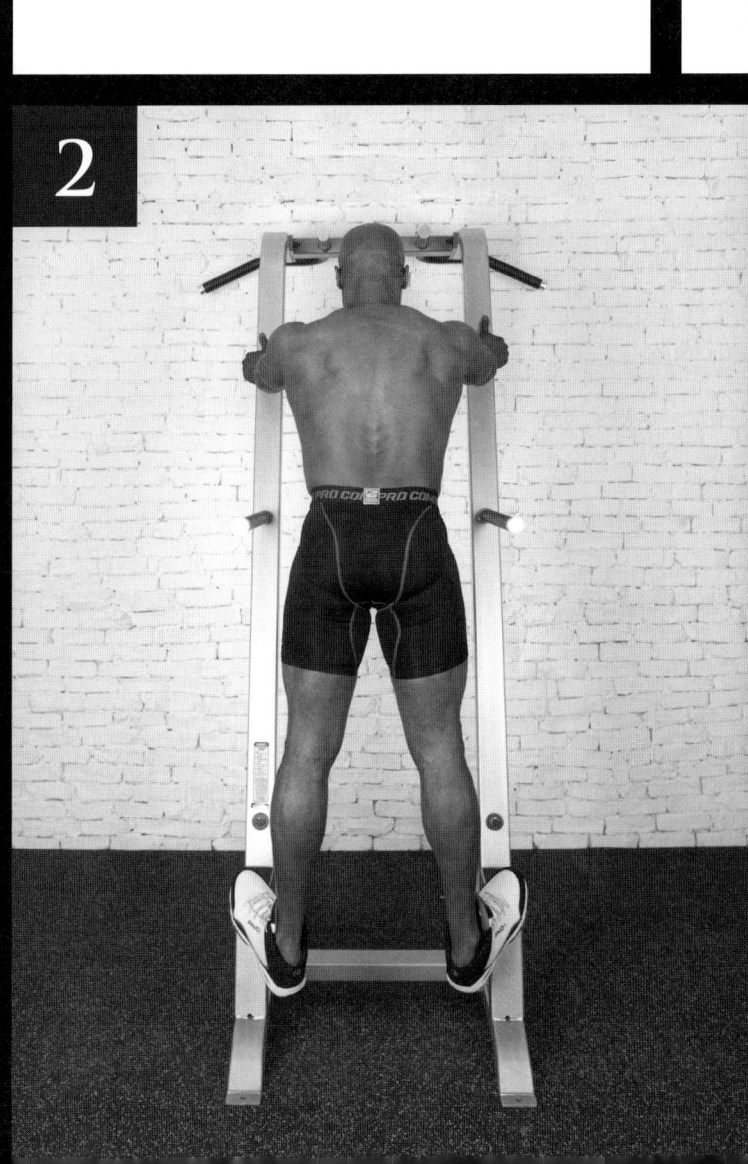

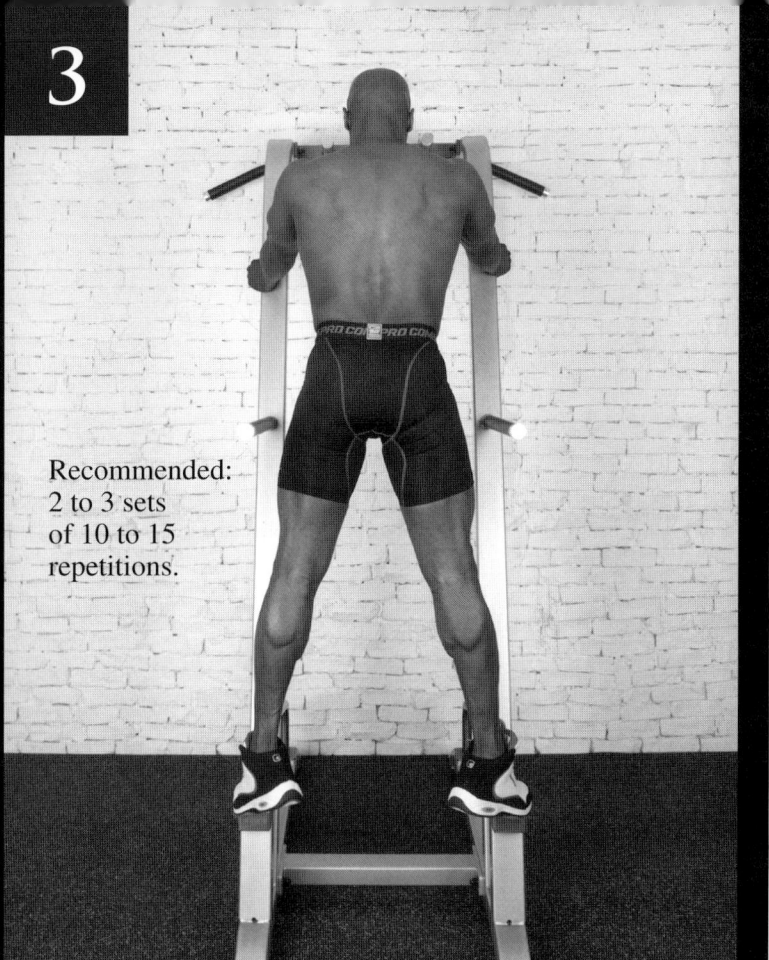

Recommended: 2 to 3 sets of 10 to 15 repetitions.

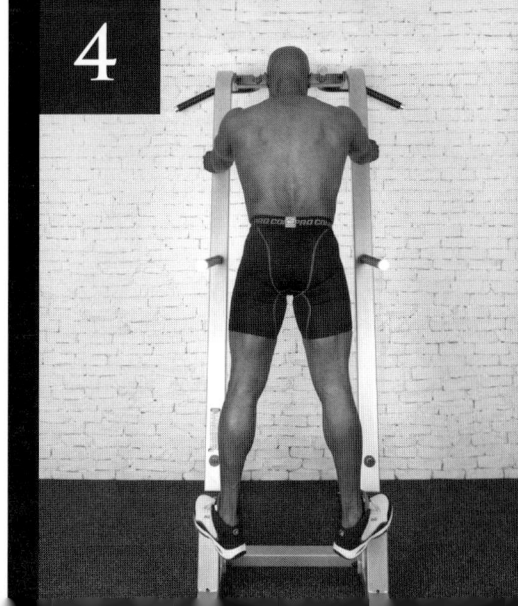

Mounting the Captain's Chair with your toes on the bottom rails with the feet externally rotated, you are to rise up on your toes and then drop your heels toward the floor, then rise back up on your toes.

INTERNAL CALF RAISES
Using the Captain's Chair

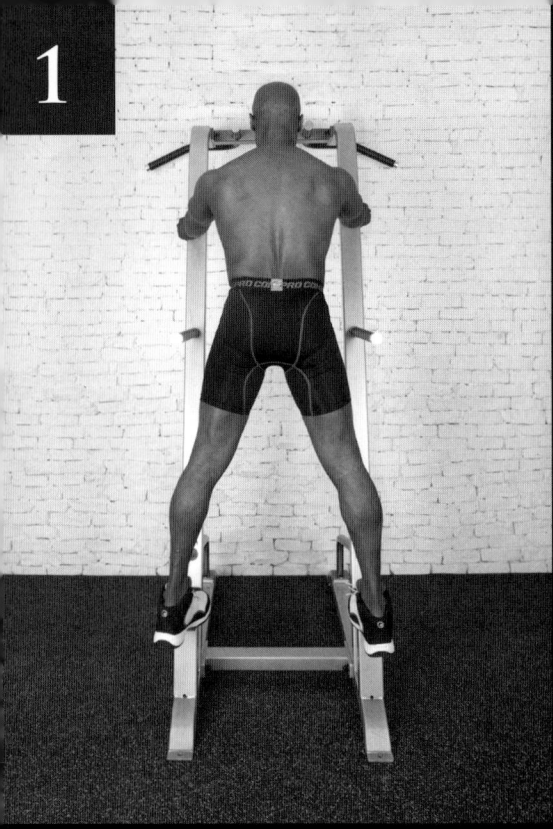

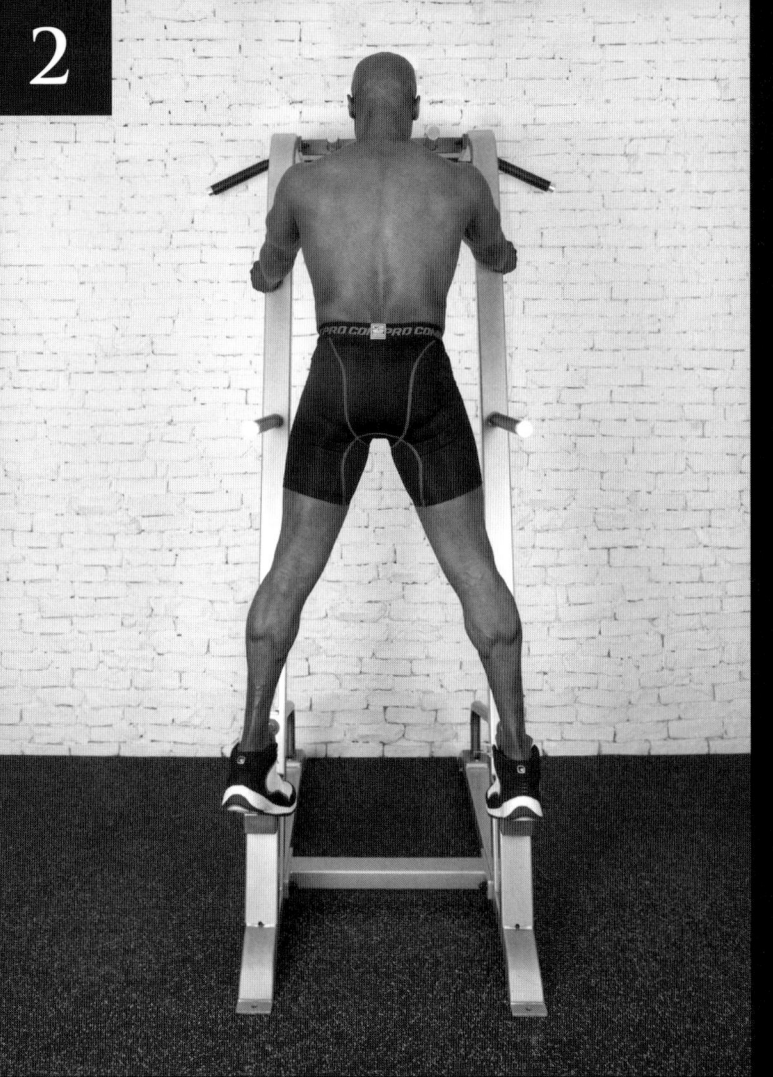

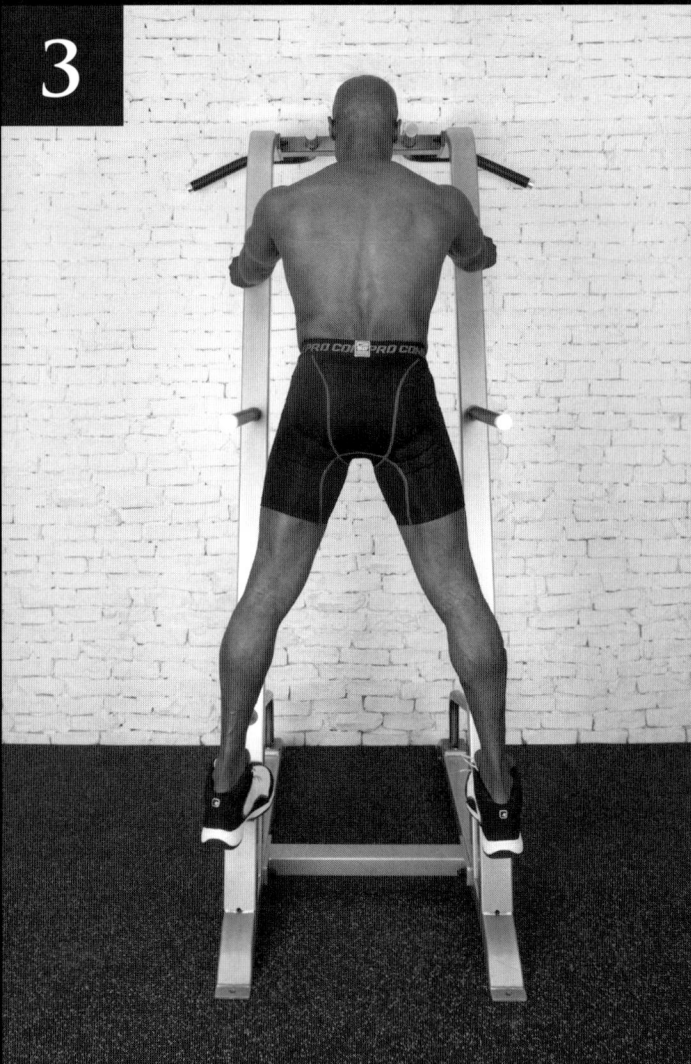

The Captain's Chair is mounted in the standard appropriate position with the toes and balls of the feet on the bottom rail. The toes are internally rotated toward the center line. The exercises are done by raising upward on your calves then letting your heels descend downward and then lifting up again and returning back to the standard mounting position for the Captain's Chair.

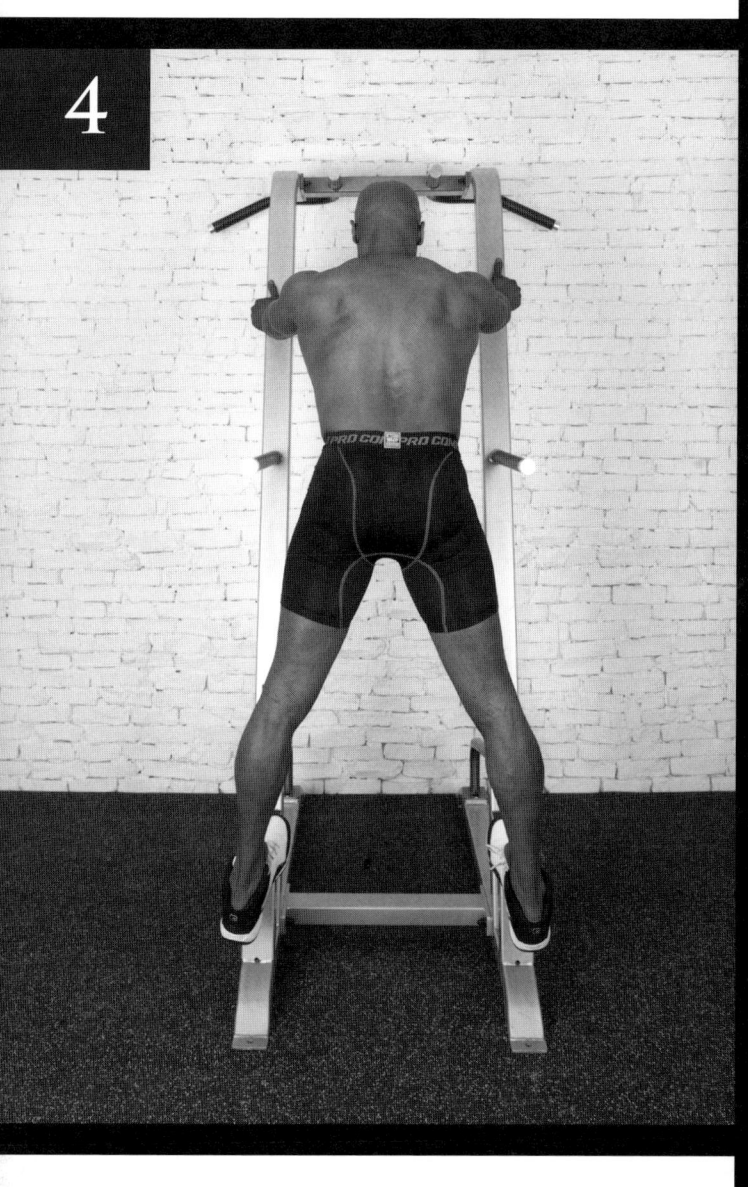

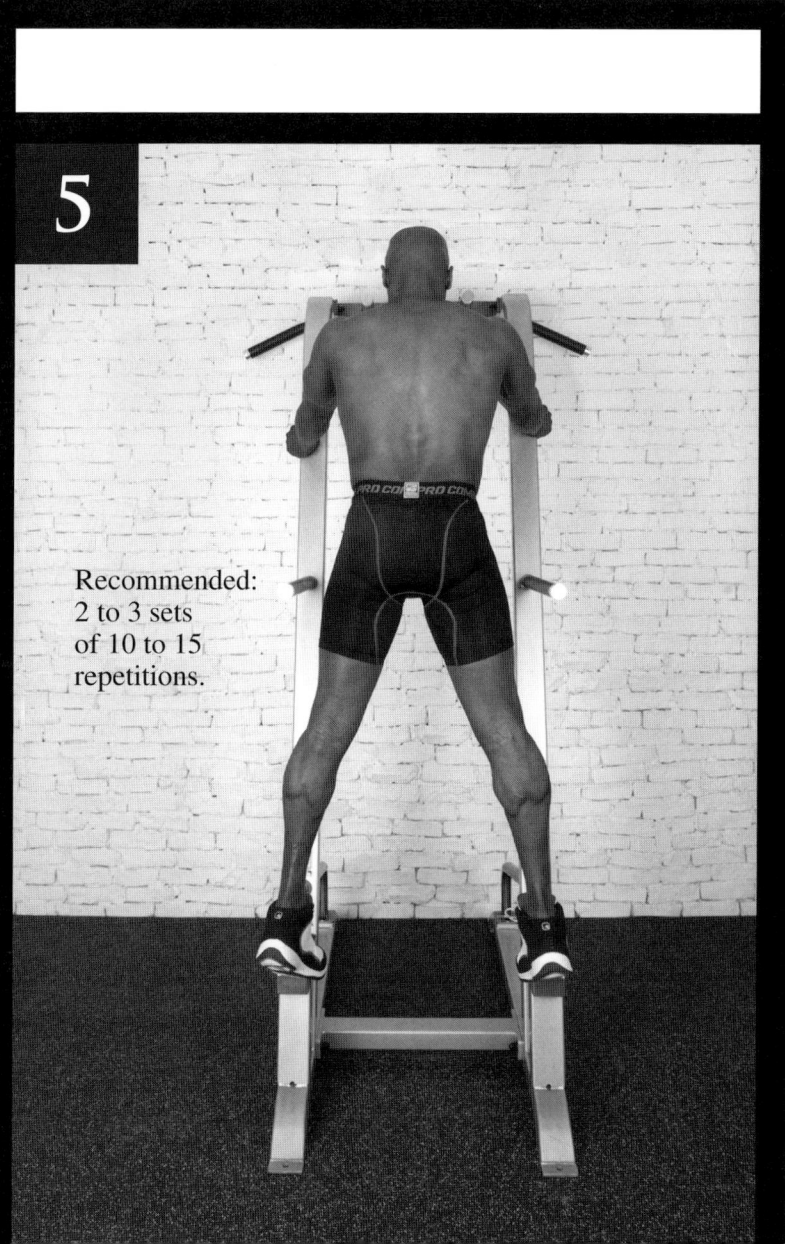

Recommended: 2 to 3 sets of 10 to 15 repetitions.

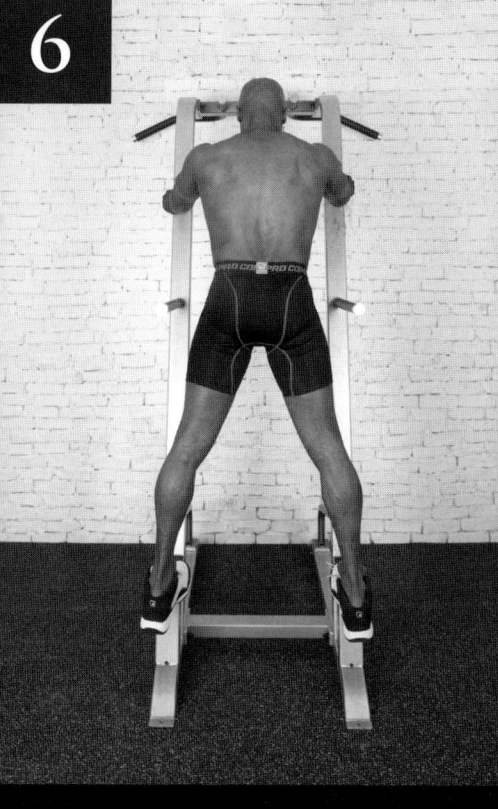

Lateral View of Calf Stretch

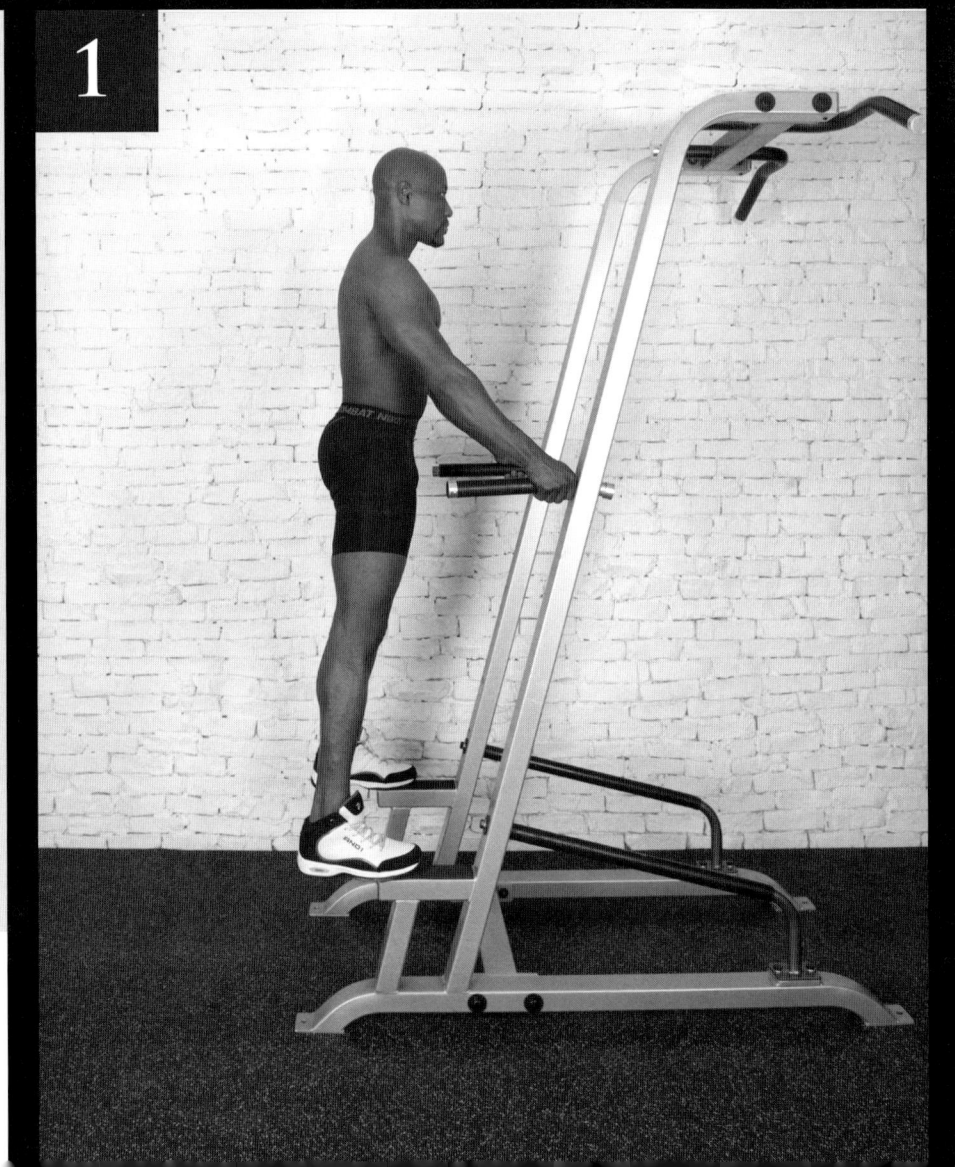

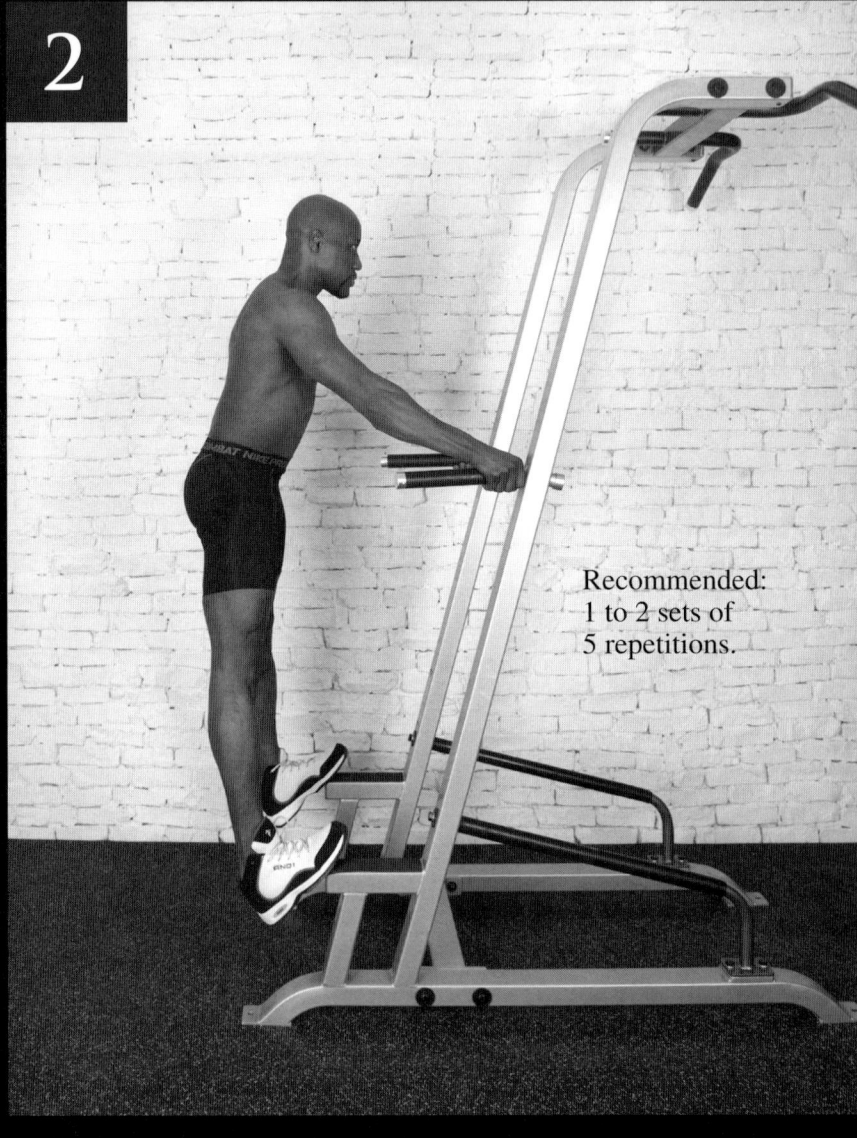

Recommended: 1 to 2 sets of 5 repetitions.

The Captain's Chair is mounted in the standard position as previously discussed. The heels are then pushed toward the floor and the body is stabilized by having the hands hold on to the Captain's Chair handrails. The stretch should be held for 30 seconds to 1 minute. This is a static stretch with no bouncing or swaying during the stretch.

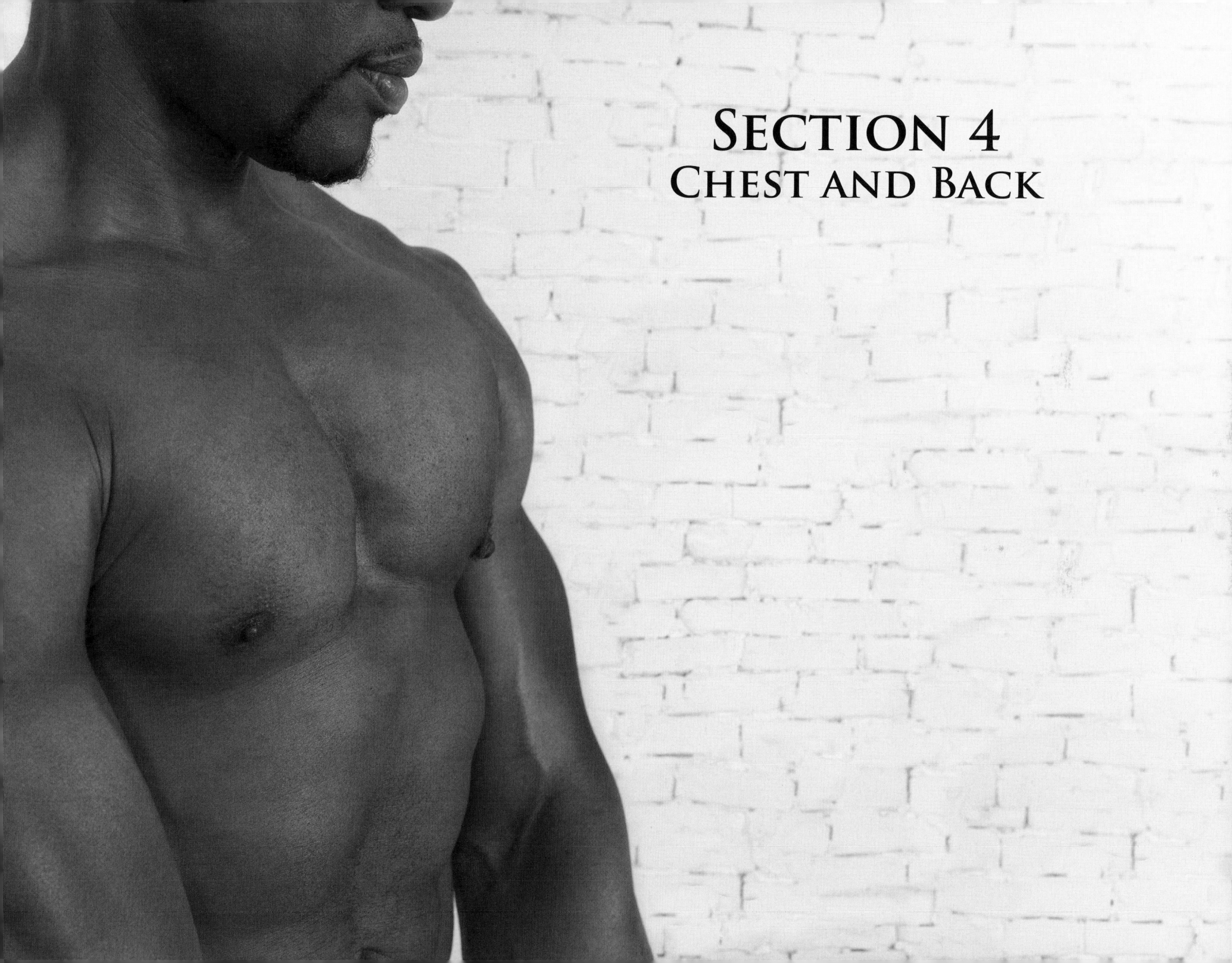

SECTION 4
CHEST AND BACK

Lateral Rhomboid Raises

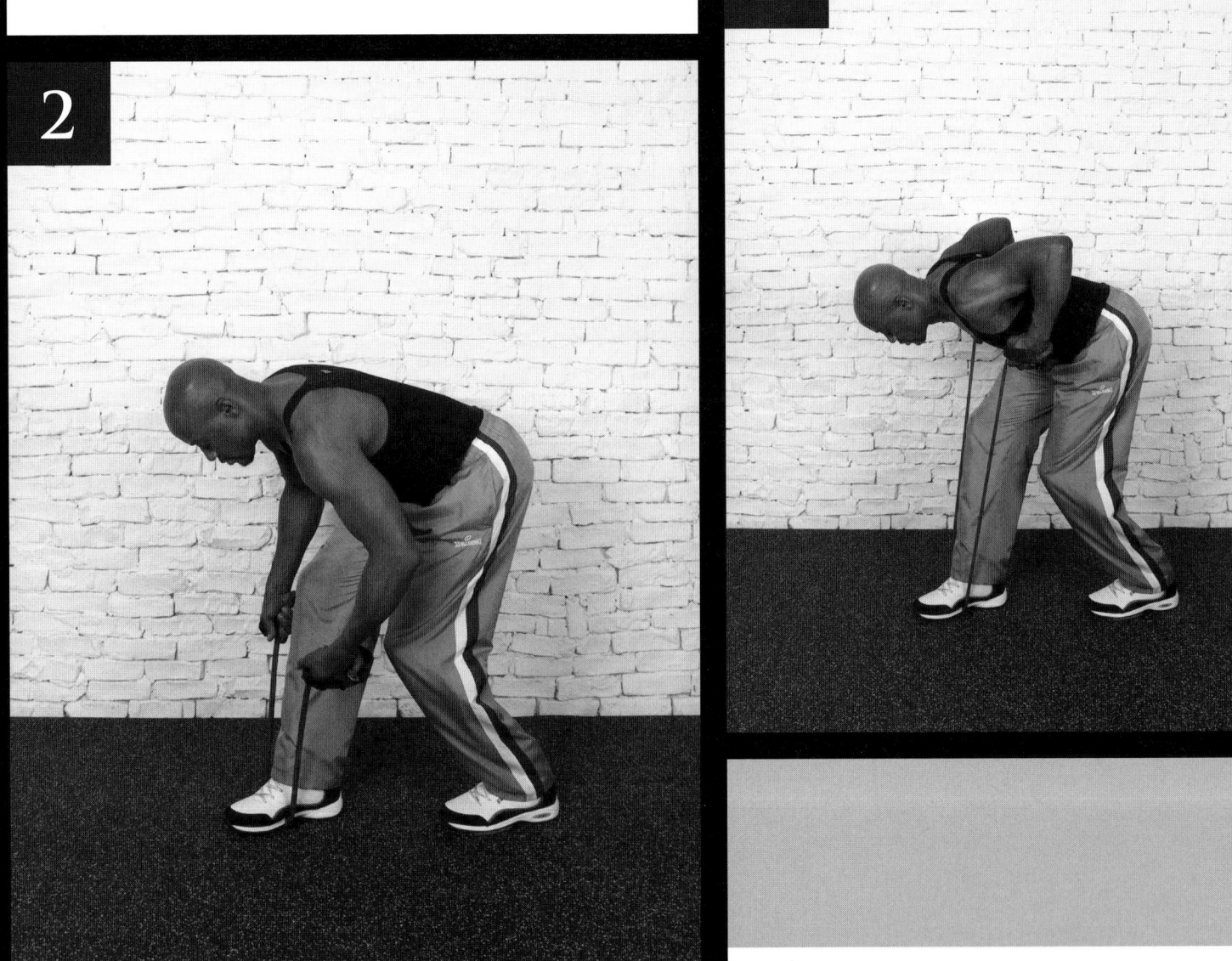

This exercise is done with the pulley, starting from the neutral position. The pulley is placed under one foot. The torso is flexed forward. As you lean forward, pull upward on the pulley while keeping both knees slightly flexed. (Consider doing 3 sets of 15 to 20 repetitions.)

Posterior Pulley Raises

For Rhomboid and Latissimus Dorsi

Recommended:
3 to 5 sets of
8 to 10 repetitions.

The exercise is done by holding the pulley with one foot, bending the torso forward, holding the pulley safely, and lifting the elbows in a coordinated manner, bringing the elbows posteriorly and up.

Regular Bench Press

The standard mount for a bench press is done. The weights are in each hand and balanced. The weights are then extended overhead, evenly and synchronously, and then lowered in a downward position with the elbows slightly past 90 degrees. The weights are then elevated again over the chest.

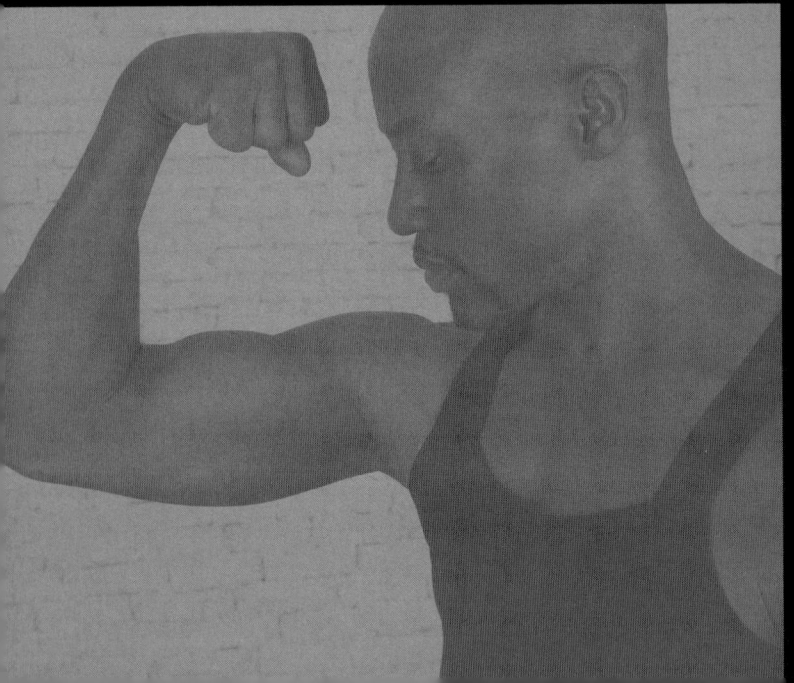

1

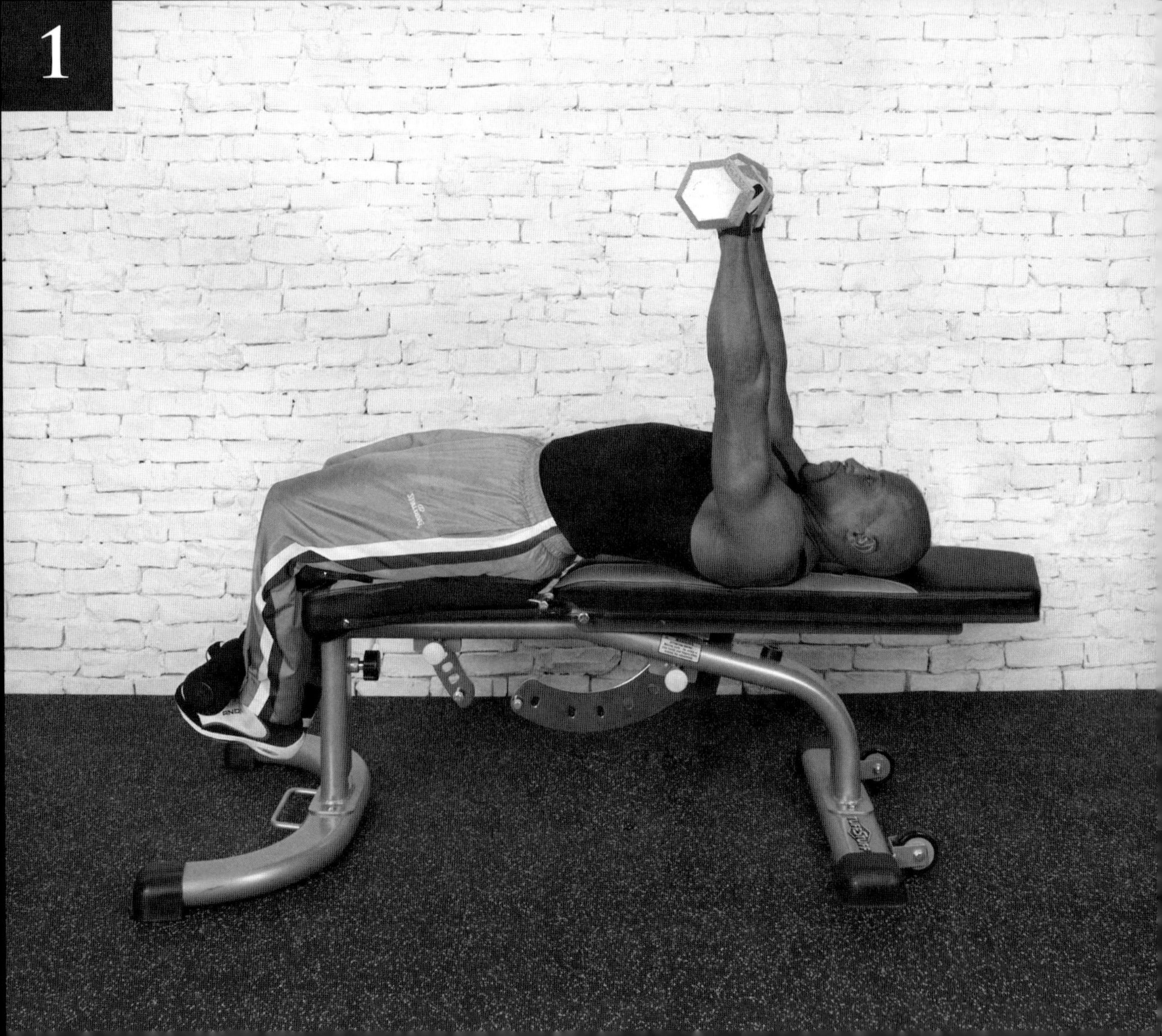

2

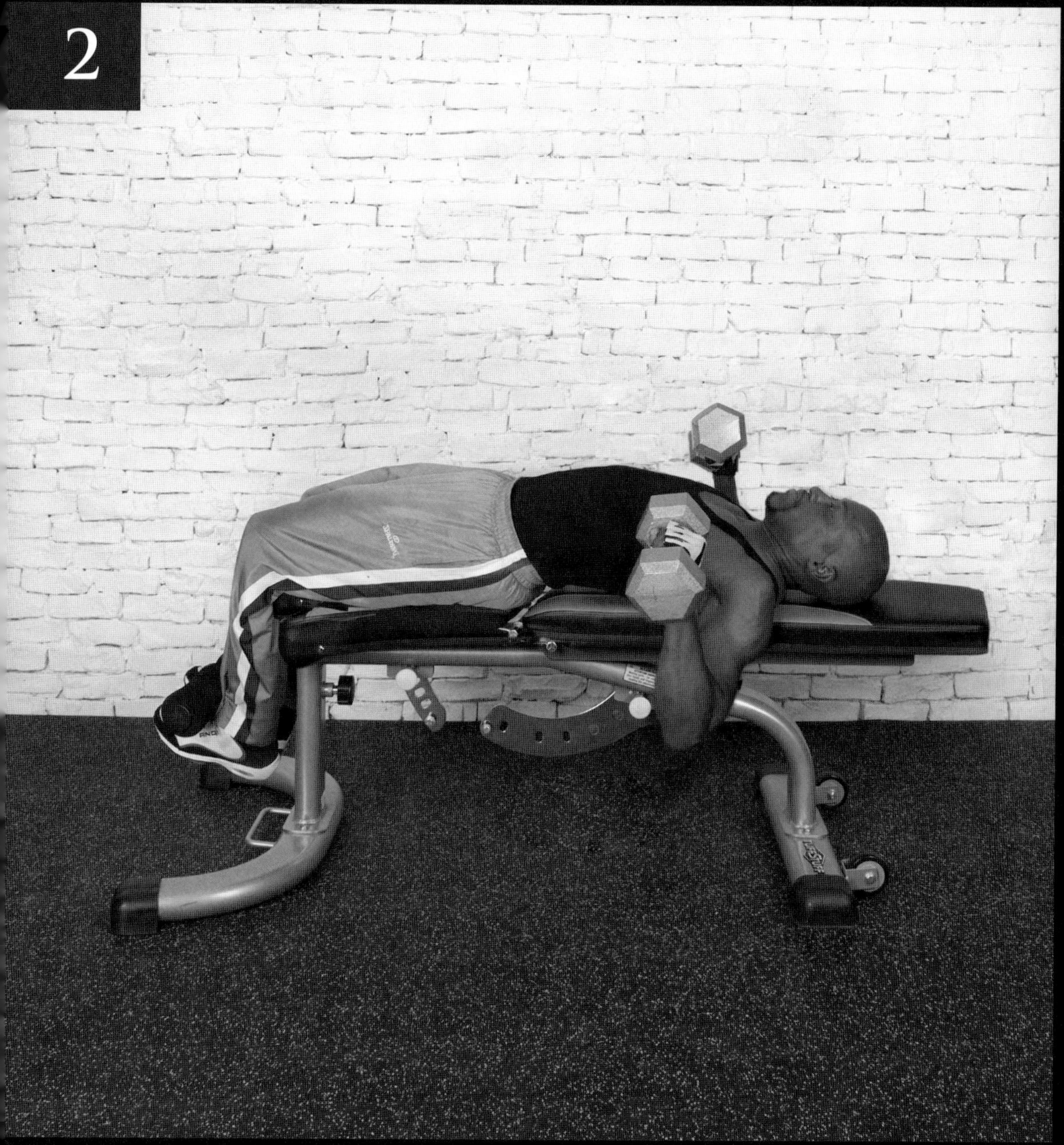

3

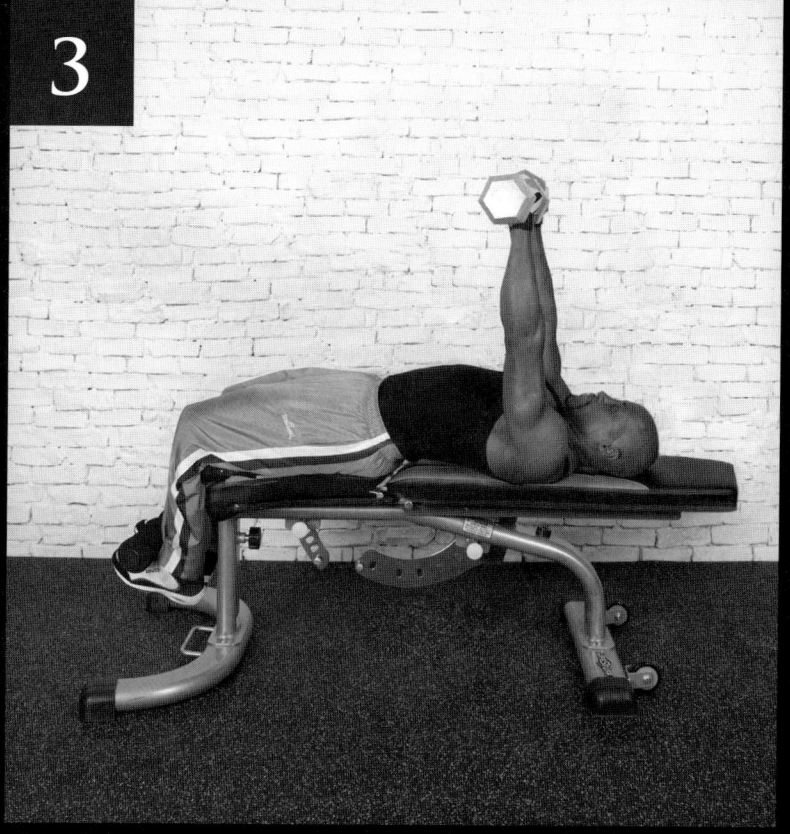

Recommended:
3 to 5 sets of
8 to 10 repetitions.

DECLINED BENCH PRESS
For Lower Pectoral Muscles

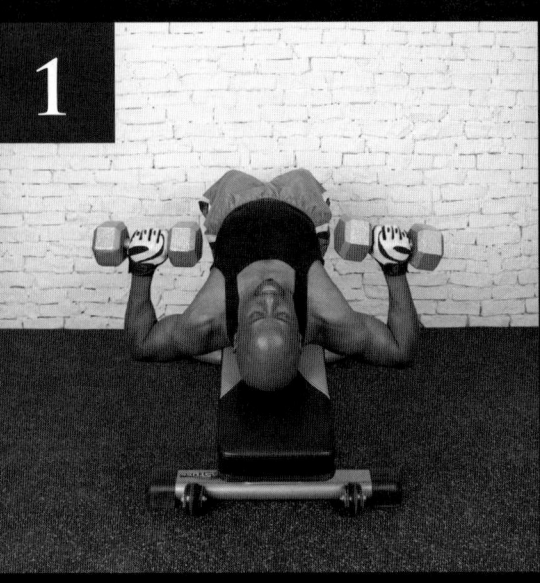

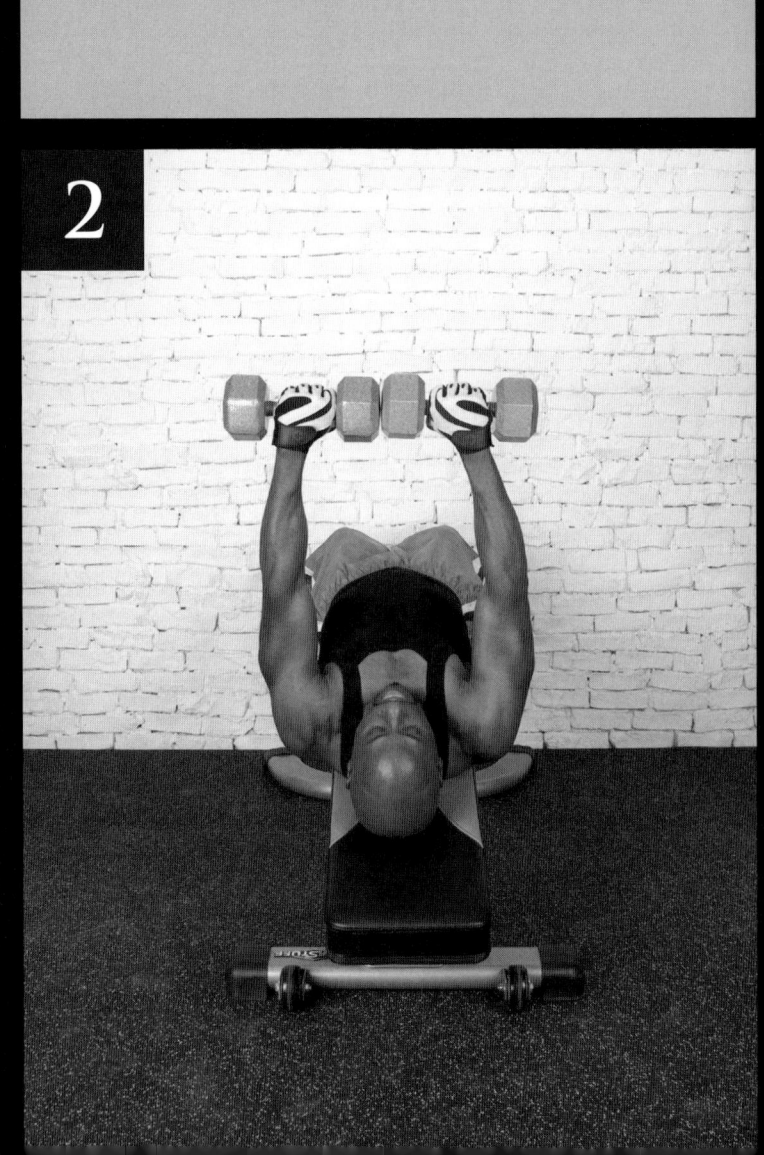

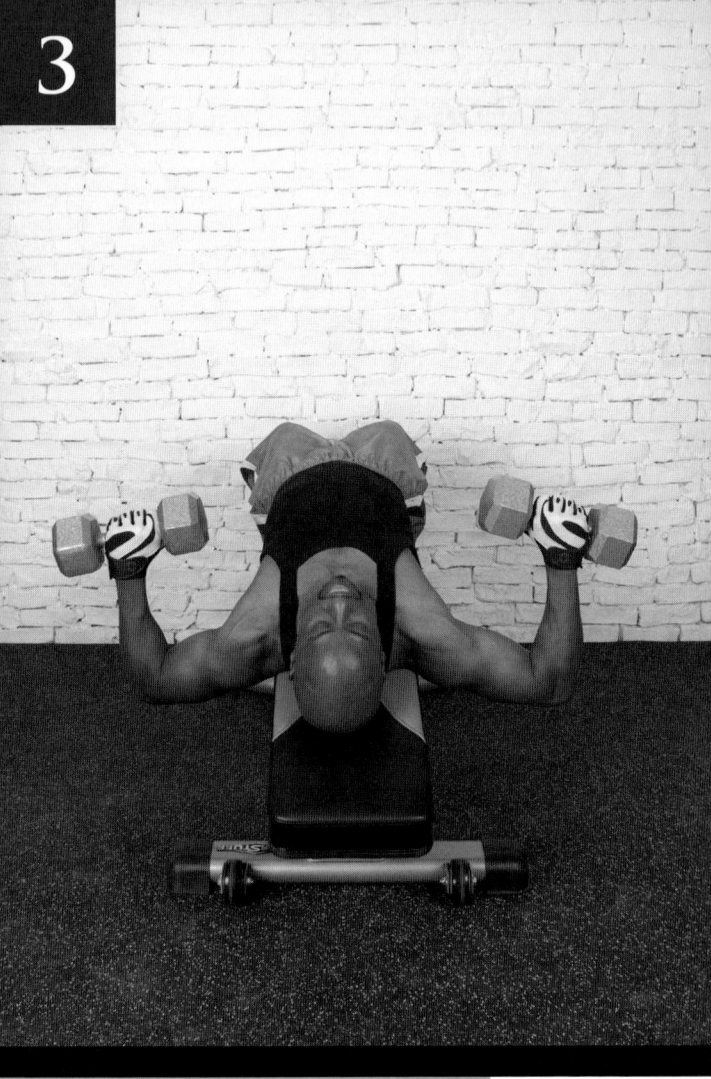

The standard mount for the declined bench is done. The weights are in each hand and balanced. The weights are then extended overhead, evenly and synchronously, and then lowered in a downward position with the elbows slightly past 90 degrees. The weights are then elevated again over the chest.

Side Views of the Declined Bench Press

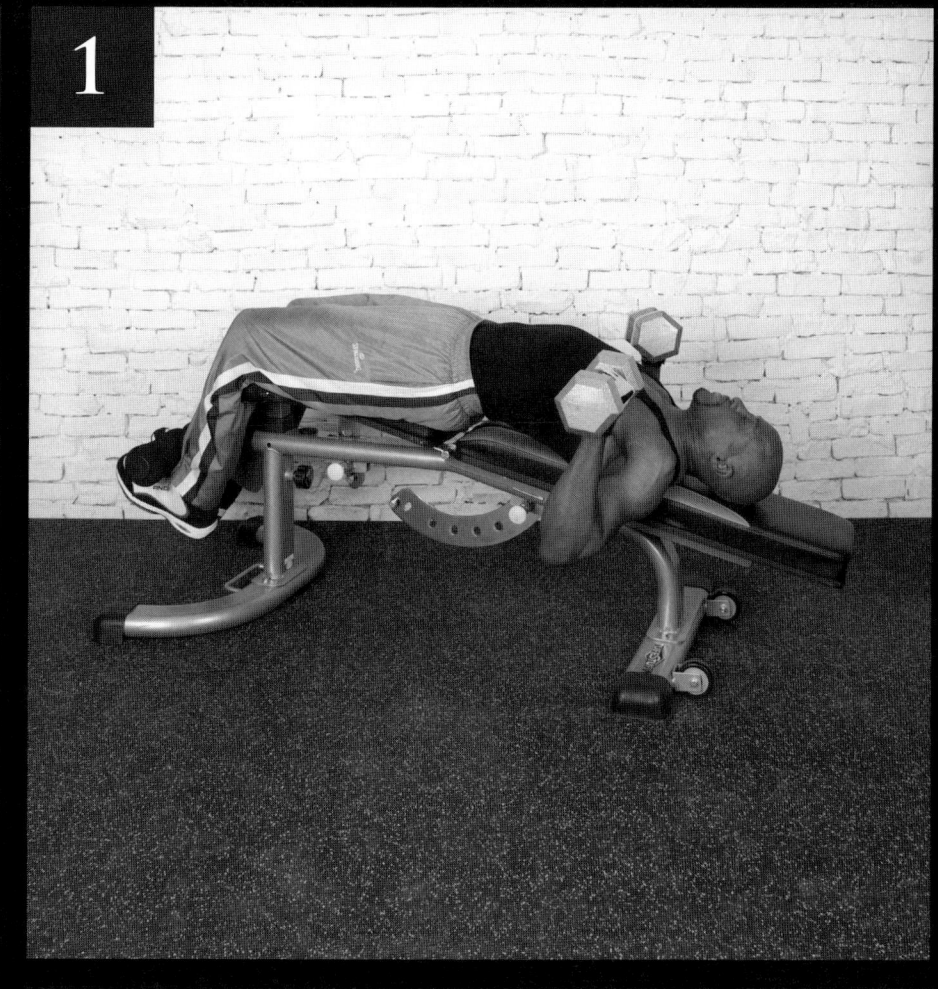

Recommended:
3 to 5 sets of
8 to 10 repetitions.

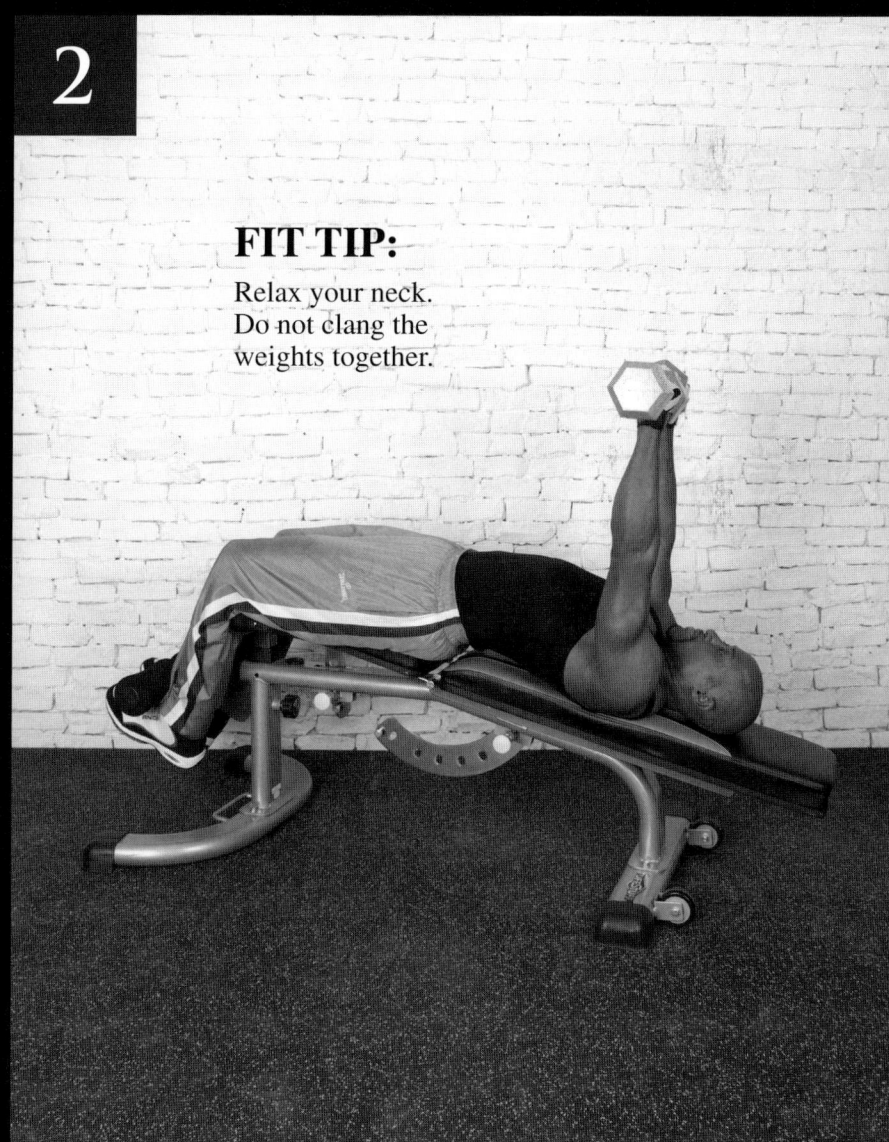

FIT TIP:

Relax your neck. Do not clang the weights together.

Incline Bench Press

For Upper Chest

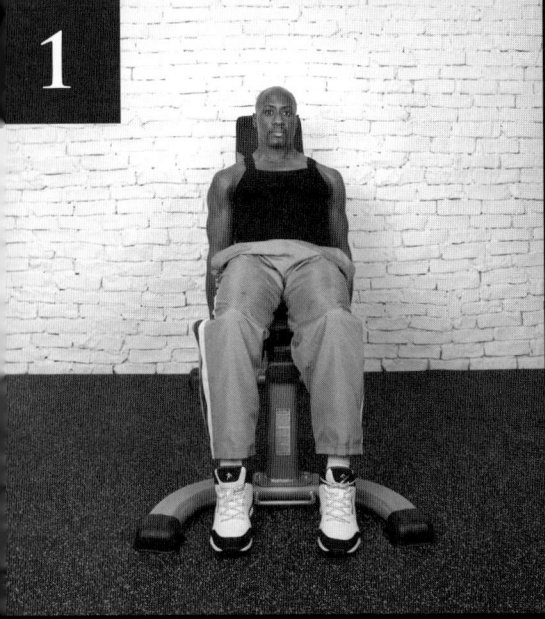

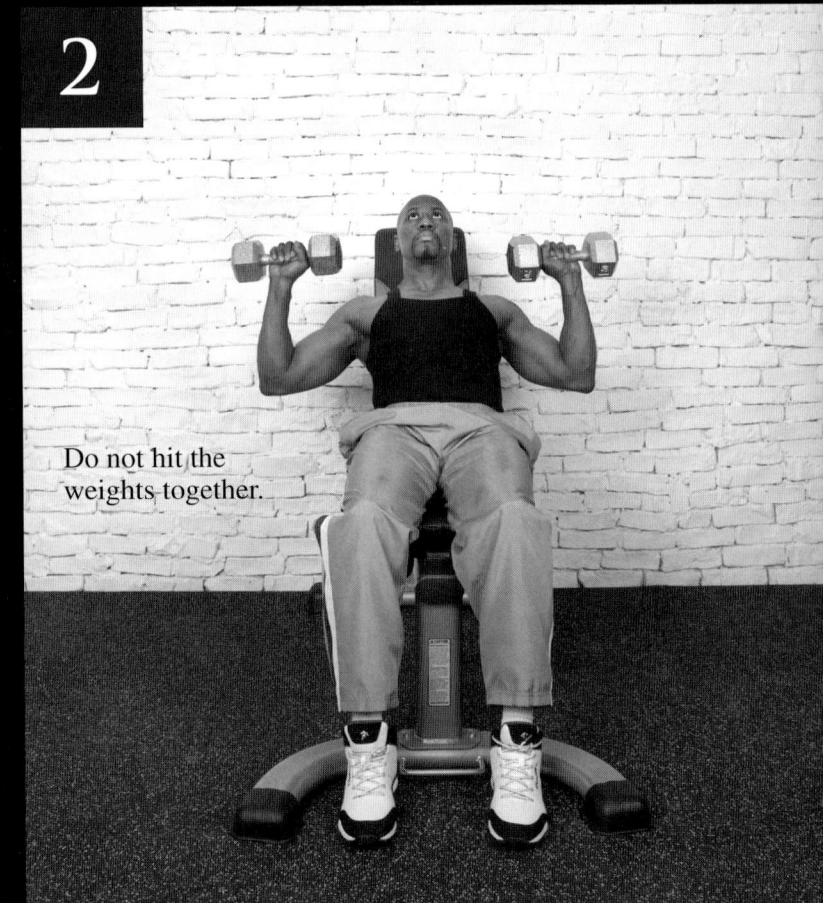

Do not hit the weights together.

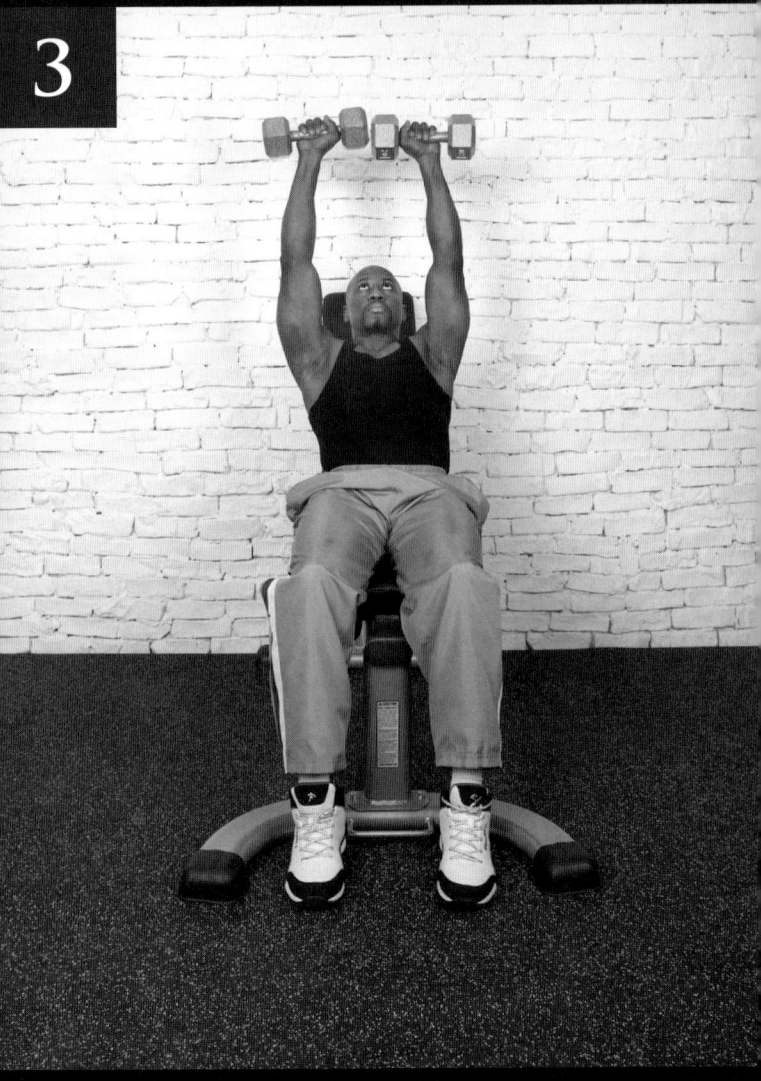

The weights should be positioned as if doing a hammer biceps curl with the weights next to the body. Bring the weights up to shoulder level and then extend the elbows and the arms above the head evenly and smoothly.

4

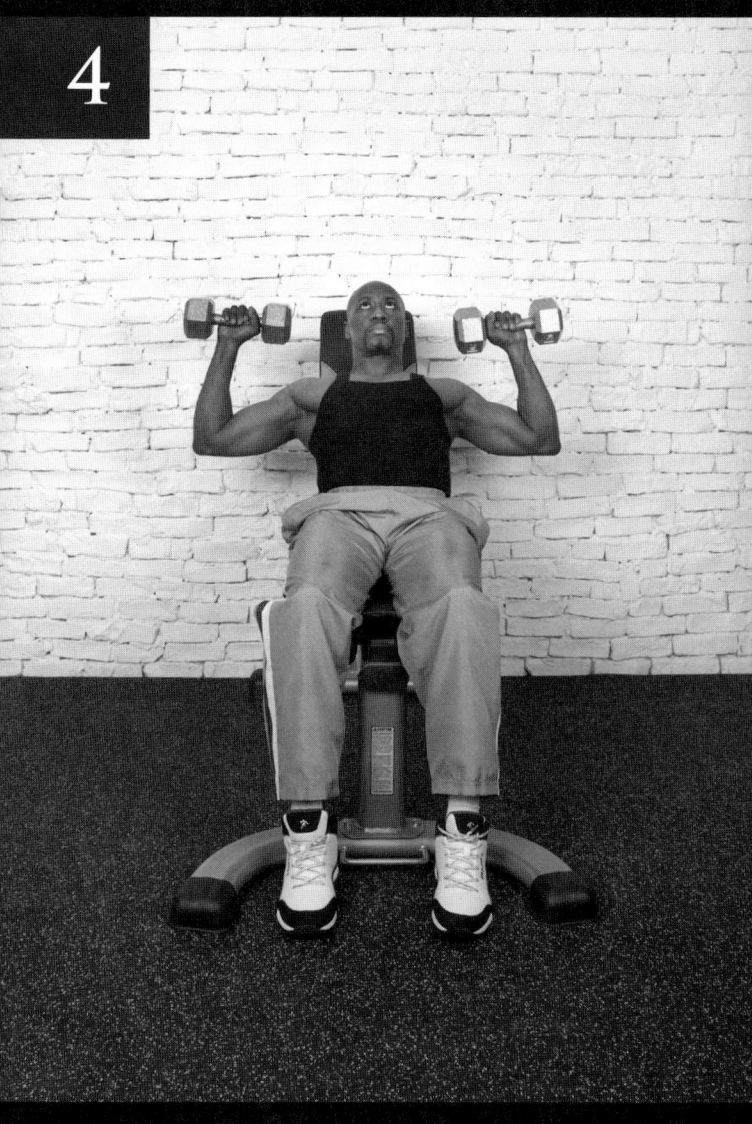

5

The incline of the bench should be 30 degrees, which is the angle from the floor up.

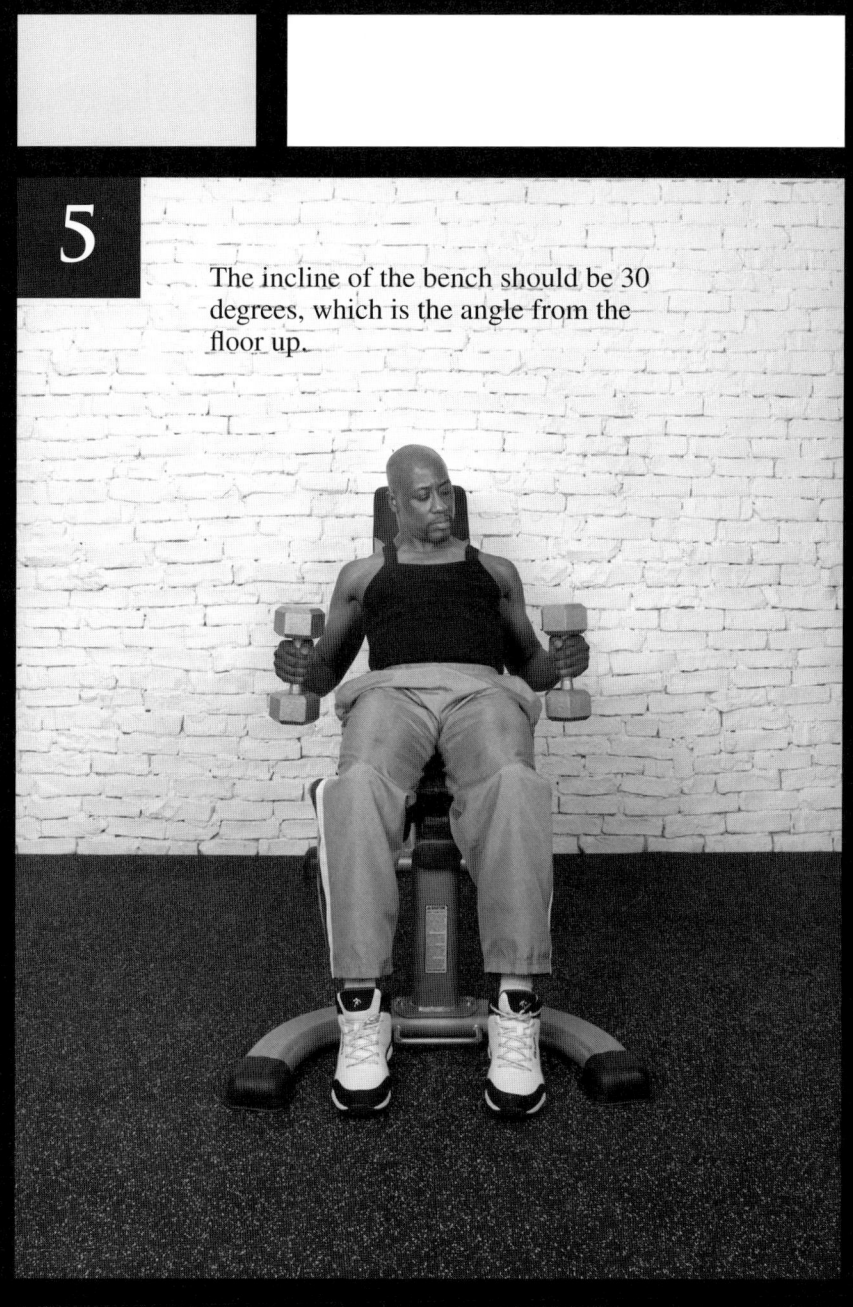

6

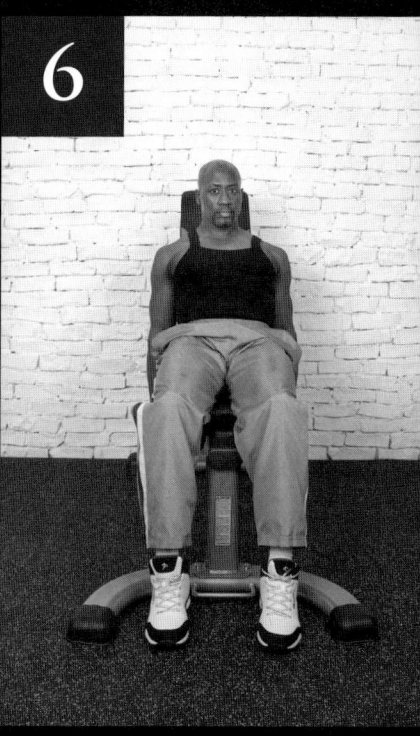

Recommended:
3 to 5 sets of
8 to 10 repetitions.

The exercise should be done with weights that can be handled without taking away from the integrity of the movement. The movement is clean, slow, and focused.

Incline Pectoral Flys

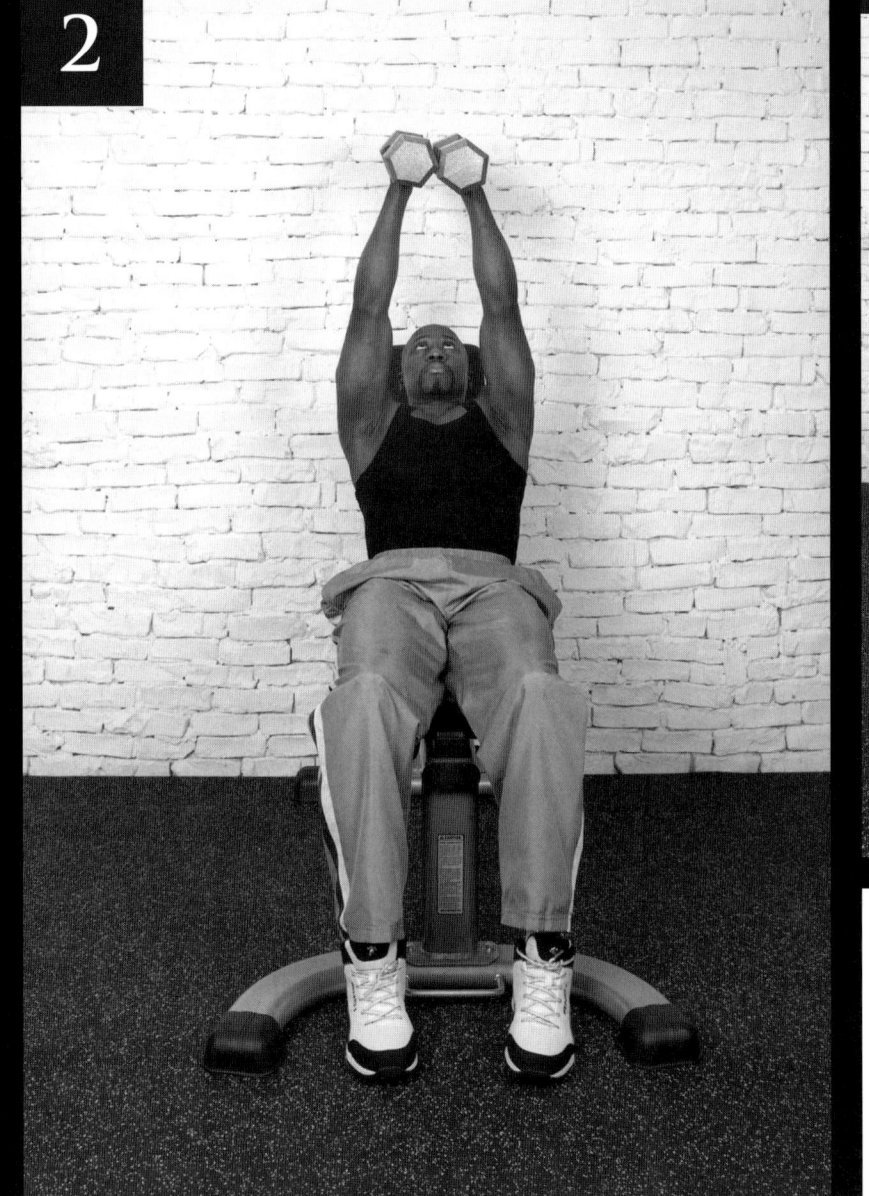

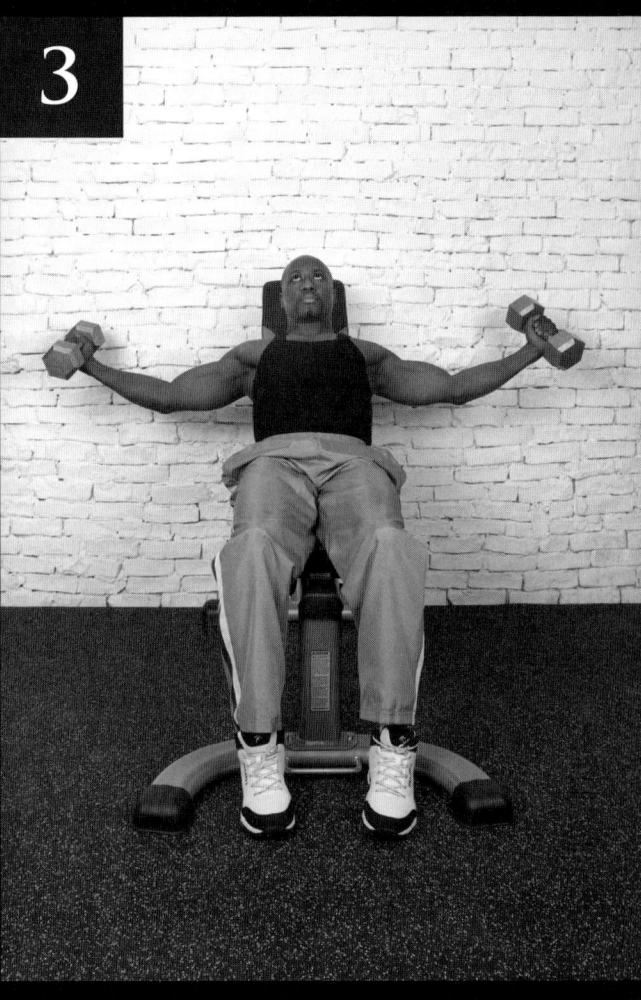

The chair is at a 30 degree incline. The weights should be brought above the head in a synchronized manner with the palms facing each other. The arms should then be opened as if holding a barrel on the chest.

4

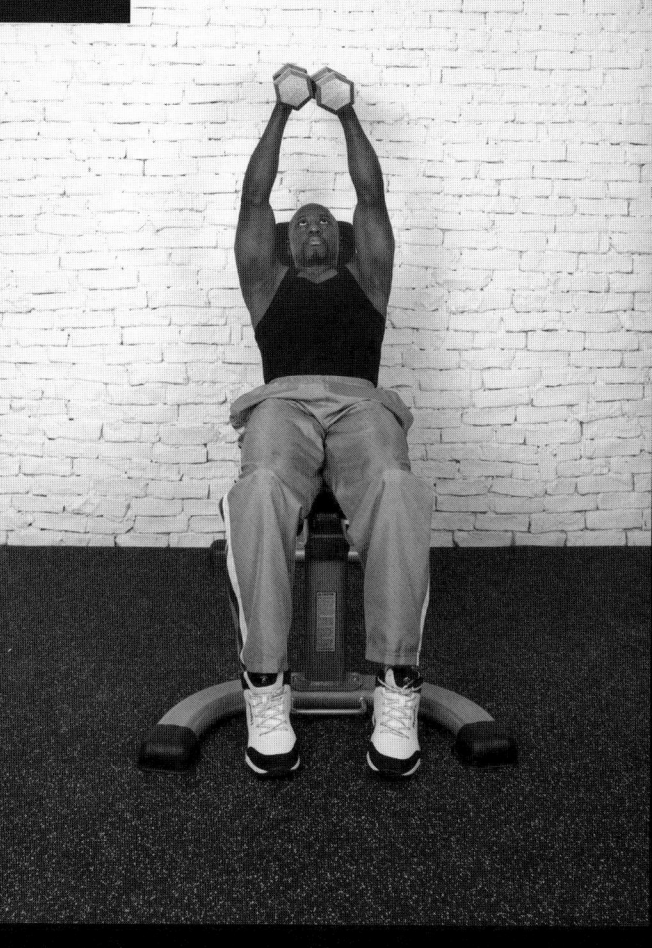

5

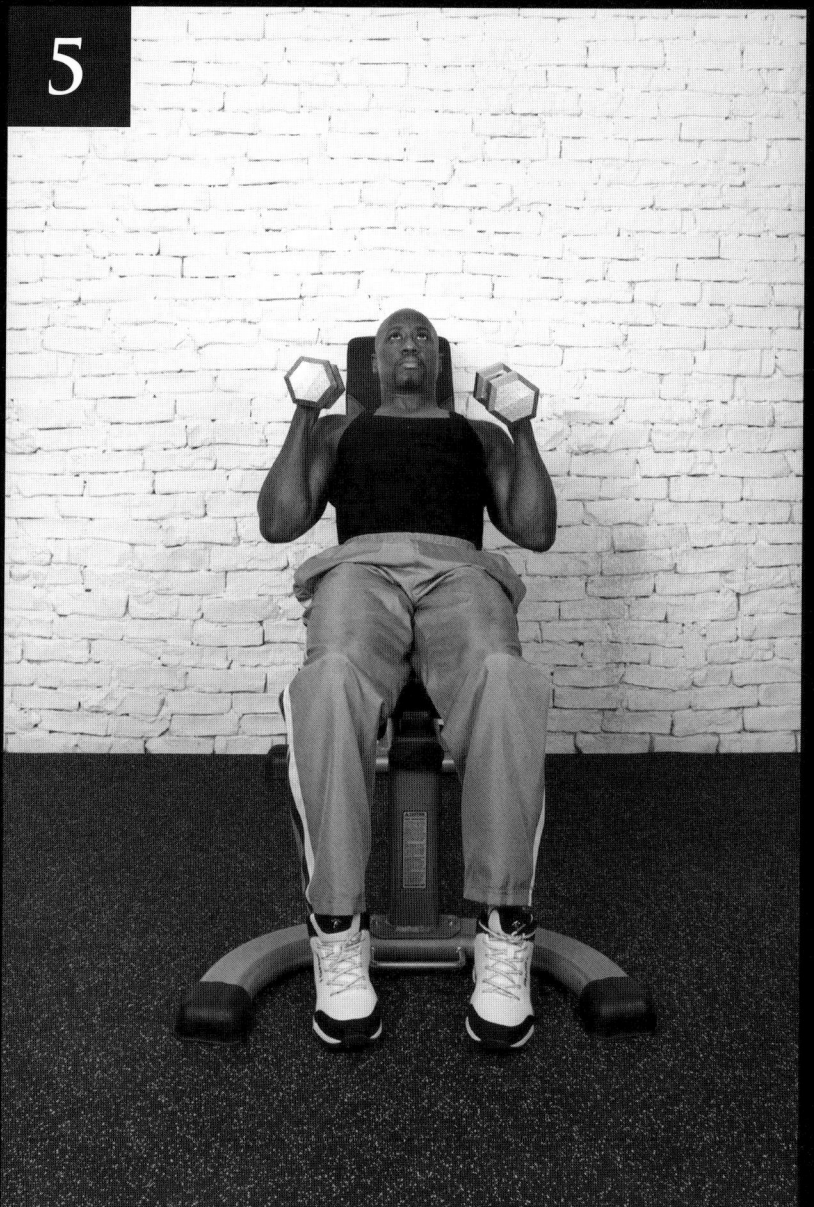

6

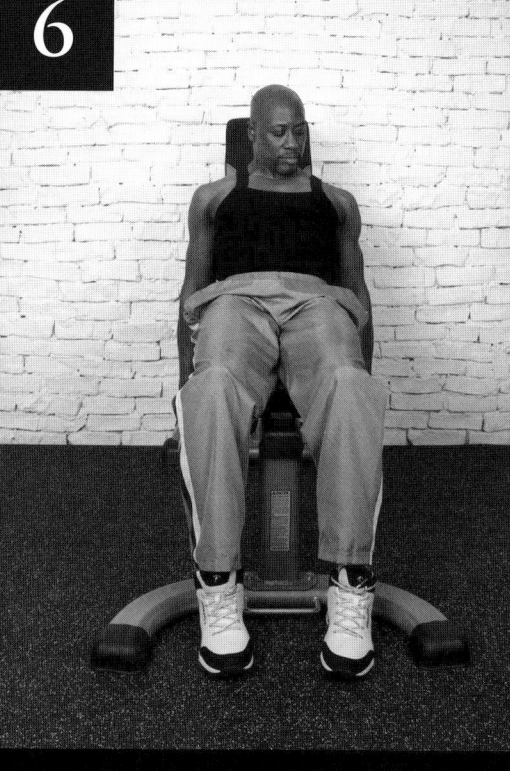

The weights should be brought back together again above the chest. Next slowly lower the weights back toward the chest and then to the sides in a safe manner.

Declined Bench Press Flys

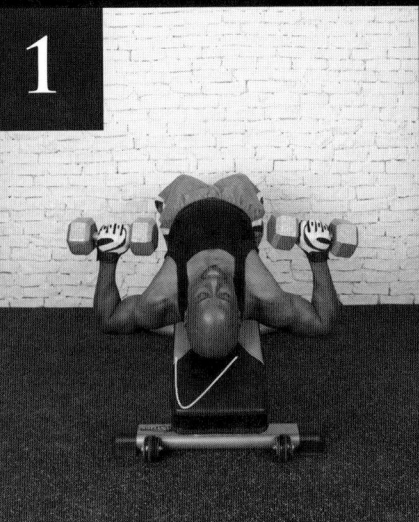

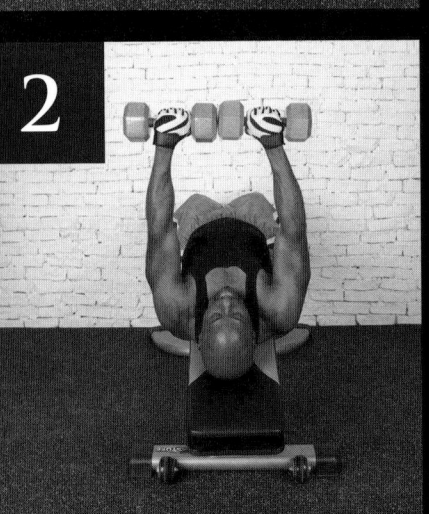

The standard declined bench press is started by lying flat on the bench with the weights in hand. The weights are lifted over the chest by extending both elbows synchronously with the weights balanced. The weights are then turned toward each other with the palms facing.

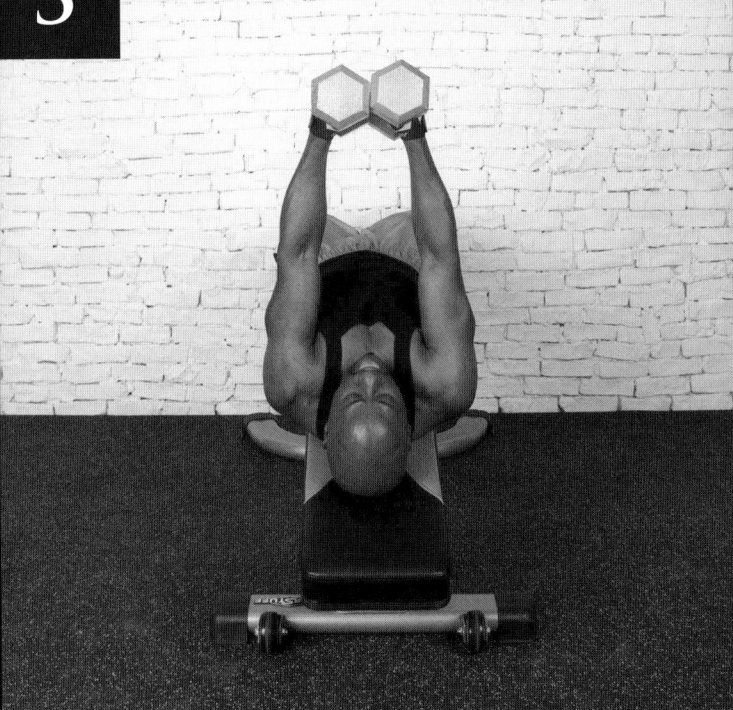

The arms stay with a minimal break at the elbows of less than 5-10 degrees. The arms are open as if hugging a barrel. The elbows are to go slightly past the shoulders and then the weights are to come together over the chest.

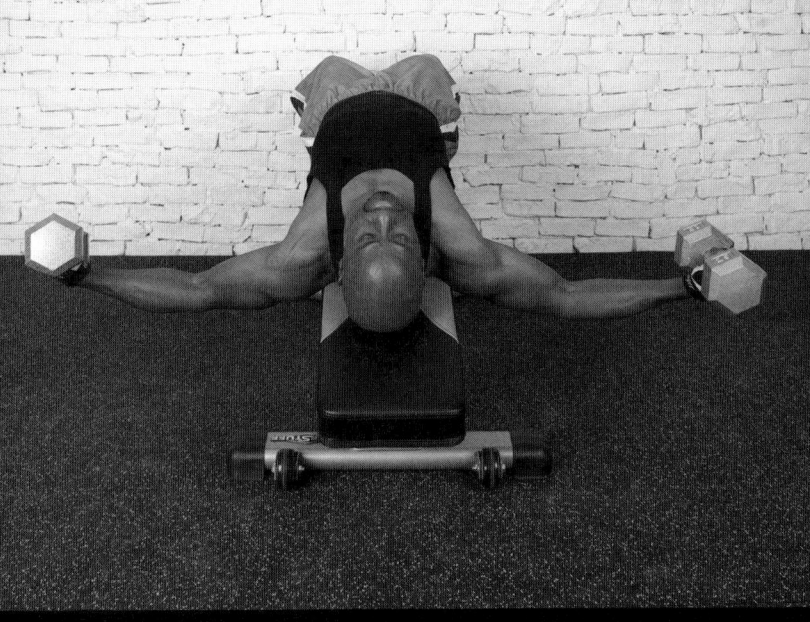

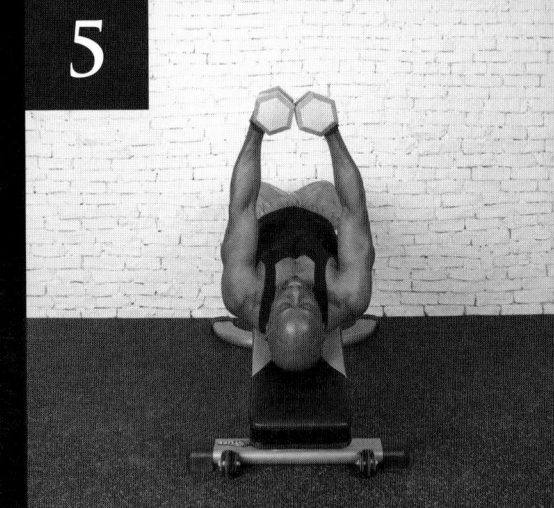

Side Views of the Declined Bench Press Flys

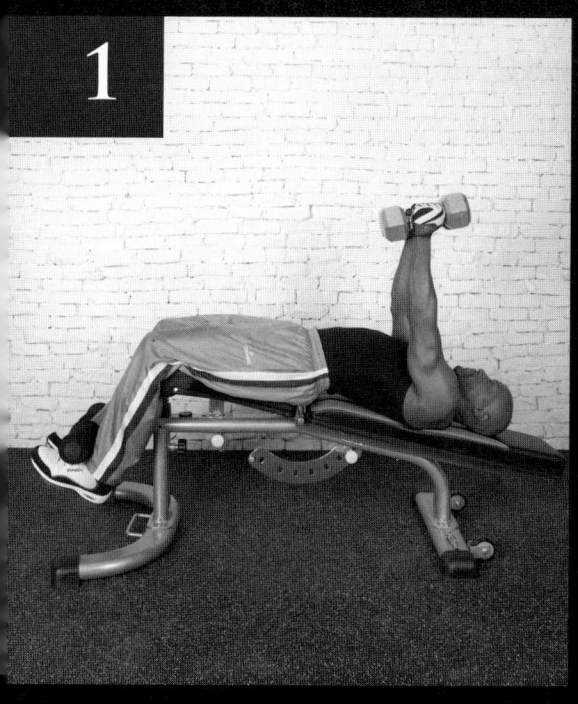

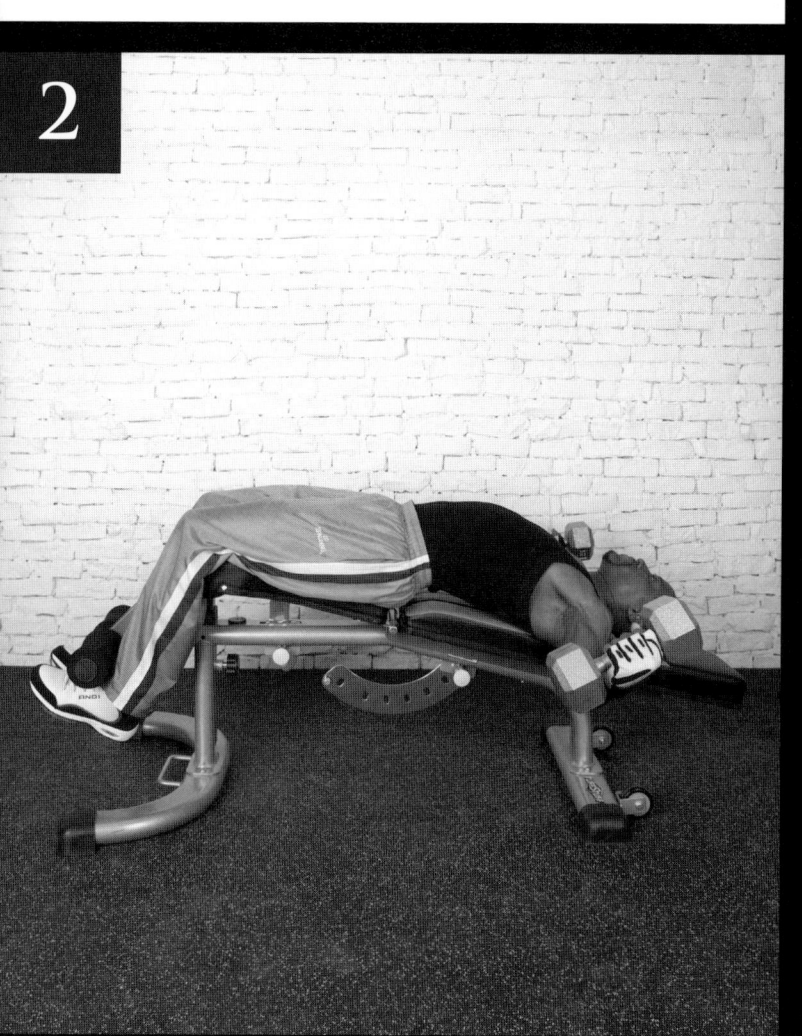

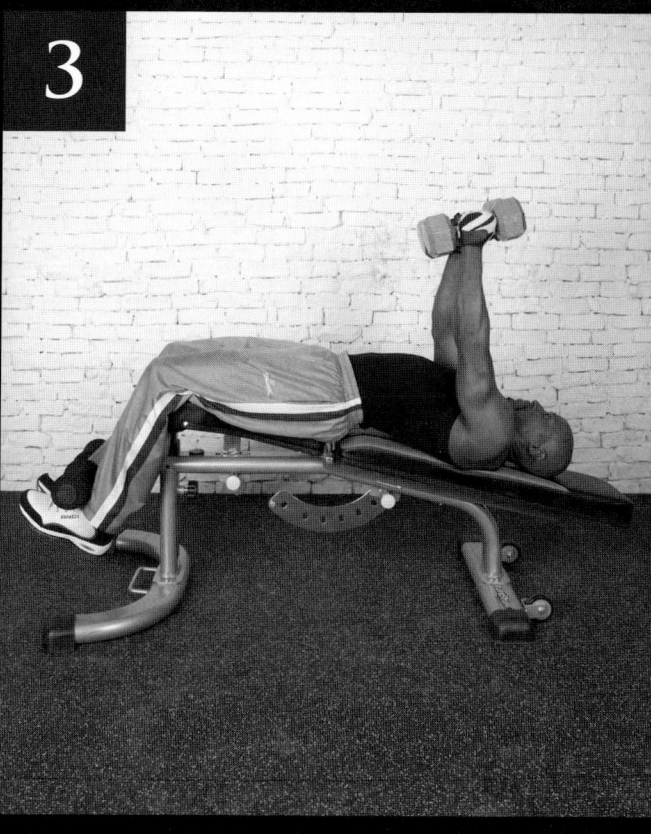

FIT TIP:

The bench should be at a 30 degree incline to the floor. This exercise is for the lower chest.

Seated Safe Shoulder Shrug

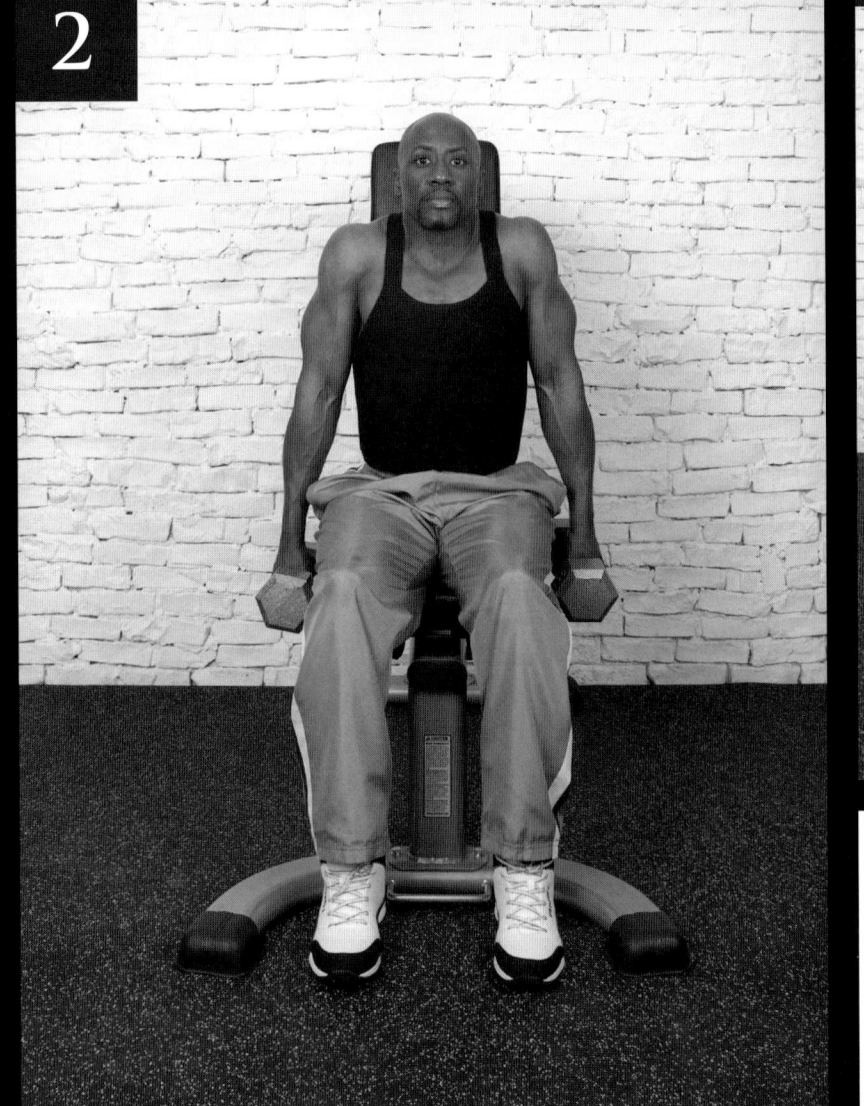

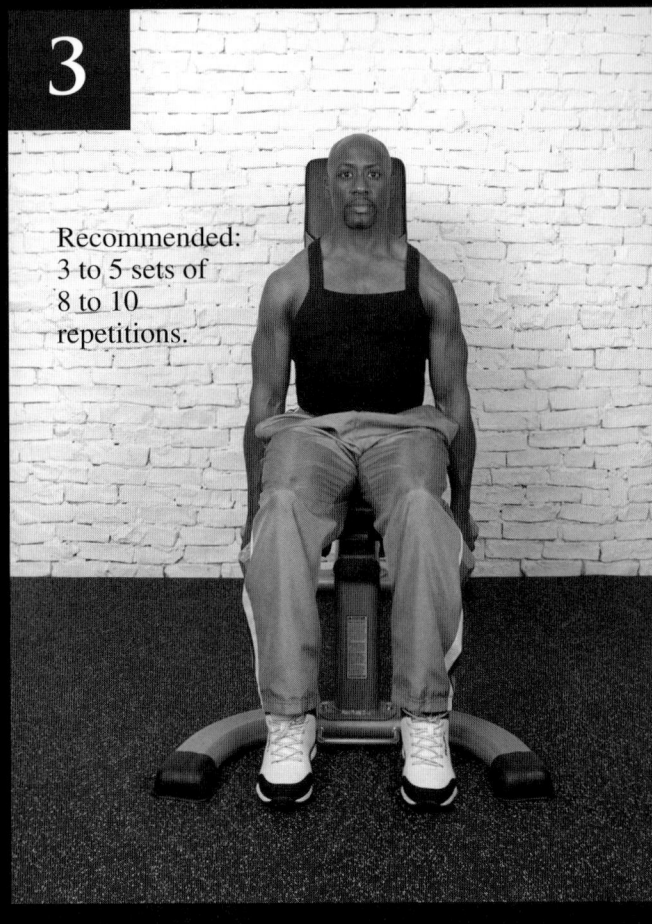

The seated safe shoulder shrugs are done in the seated position holding both weights at your side and palms of your hand toward your thighs. Elevate your shoulders upward with the weights in your hands and then relax your shoulders downward.

Recommended: 3 to 5 sets of 8 to 10 repetitions.

FIT TIP:

Inhale when bringing the weights upward and exhale when lowering the weights.

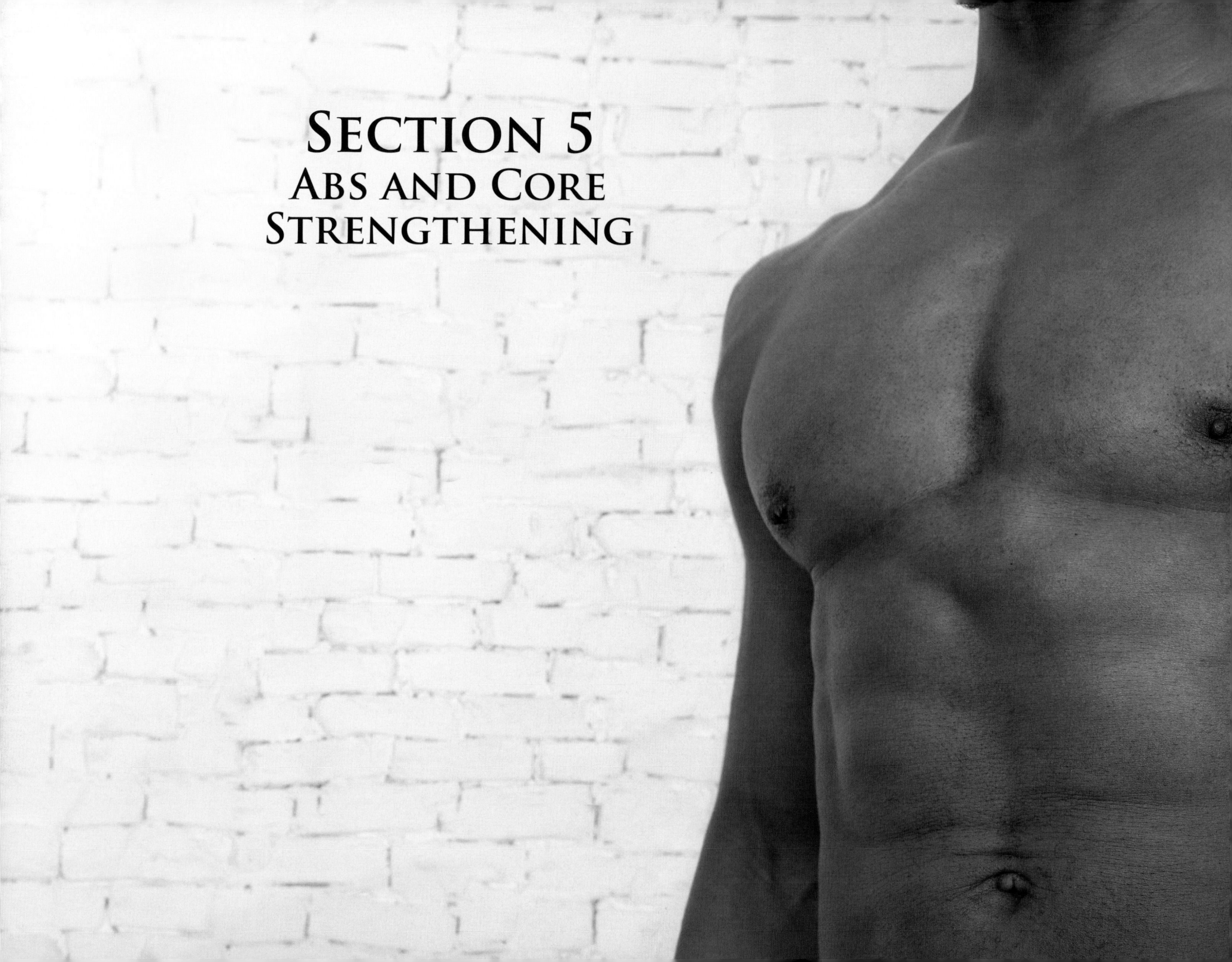

Section 5
Abs and Core Strengthening

Medicine Ball Side Twist

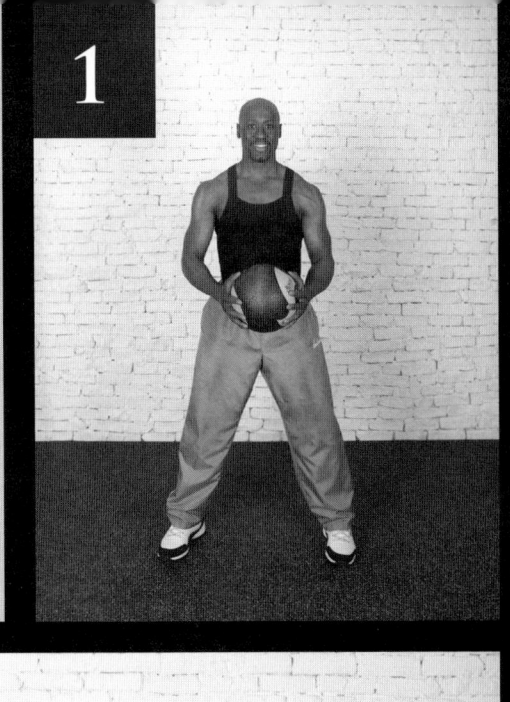

1

2

3 The abdominals should be contracted, and the neck should be upright and the shoulders upright.

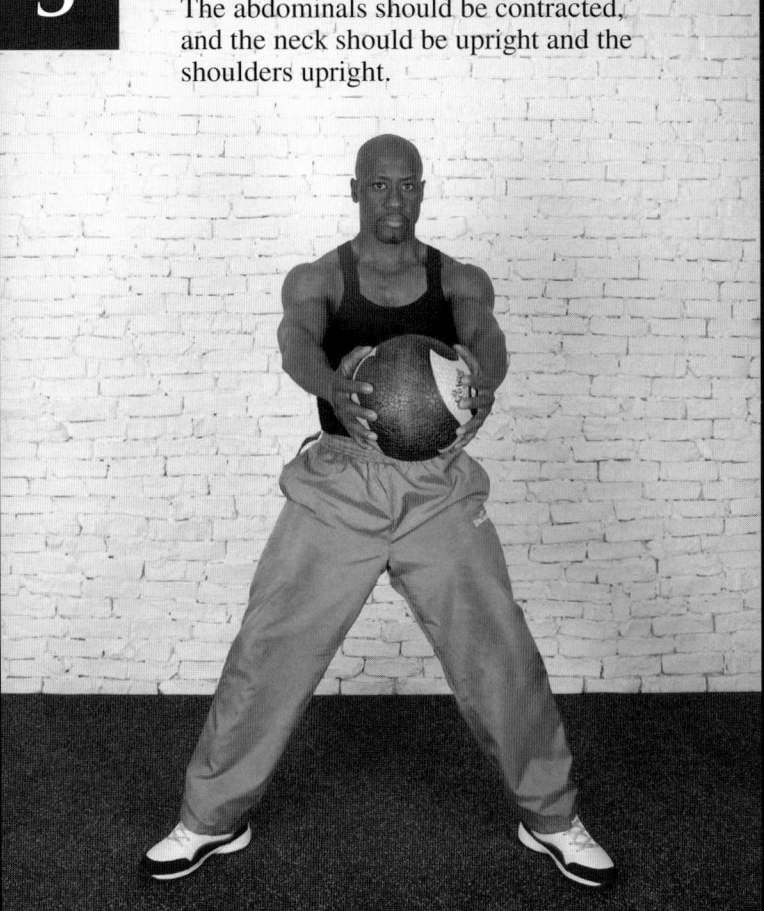

The exercise is done by having the feet wide apart. The medicine ball is held in front of the body. Both knees are bent as the twist occurs to the right. Then, you are to come back to center position. Hold the ball upright and high in front of your chest and then twist to the left.

4

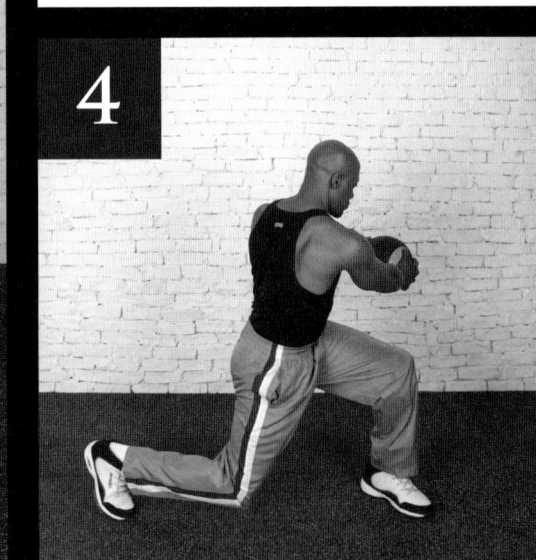

SHORT MEDICINE BALL TWIST

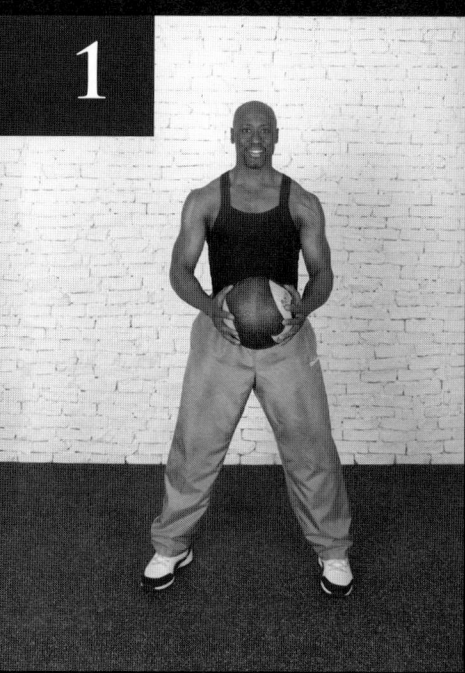

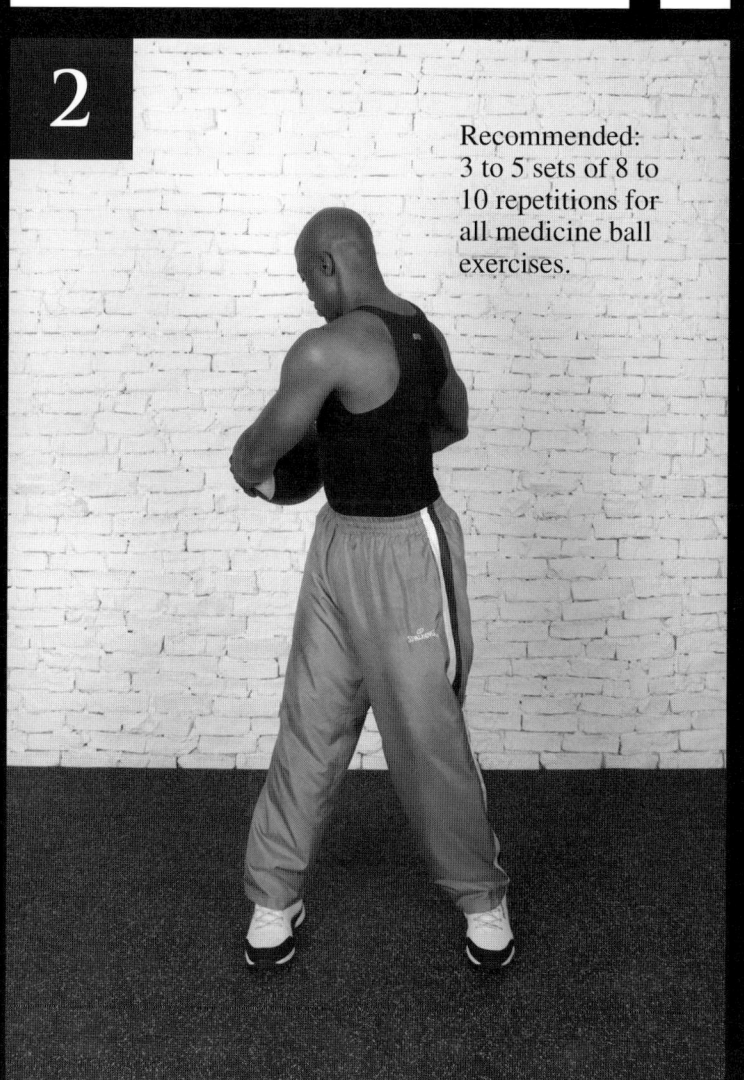

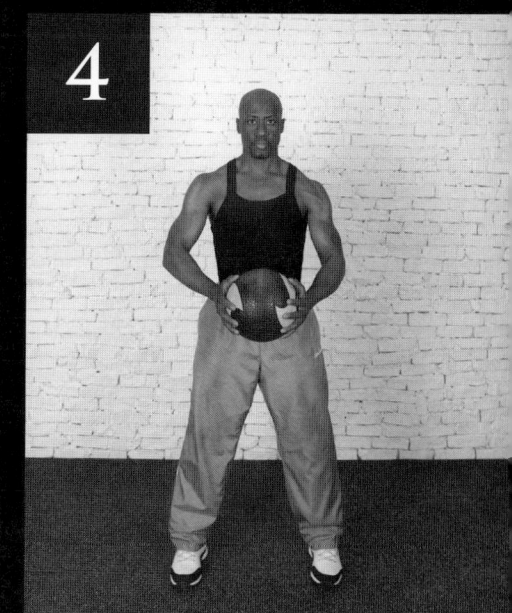

Recommended: 3 to 5 sets of 8 to 10 repetitions for all medicine ball exercises.

This can also be done without stopping at the center or neutral postion for a more focused, fluid twisting motion. I recommend 1 or 2 sets of 60 repetitions.

FIT TIP:
Do not torque your back (spine) quickly. Use slow, controlled movements.

The starting position is with the medicine ball held in front of the body with the elbows slightly bent. The feet are flat. The knees are slightly bent. Twist the torso to the right, then back to the center, then back to the left.

Standard Bosu Ball Plank and Push-up

Mount the BOSU ball in a standard push-up position and hold for 2 to 3 minutes, keeping the back flat without any sagging of the hips or without letting the back curve downward. The second part of this is a regular push-up done directly on the BOSU ball.

Recommended: 3 to 5 sets of 8 to 10 repetitions.

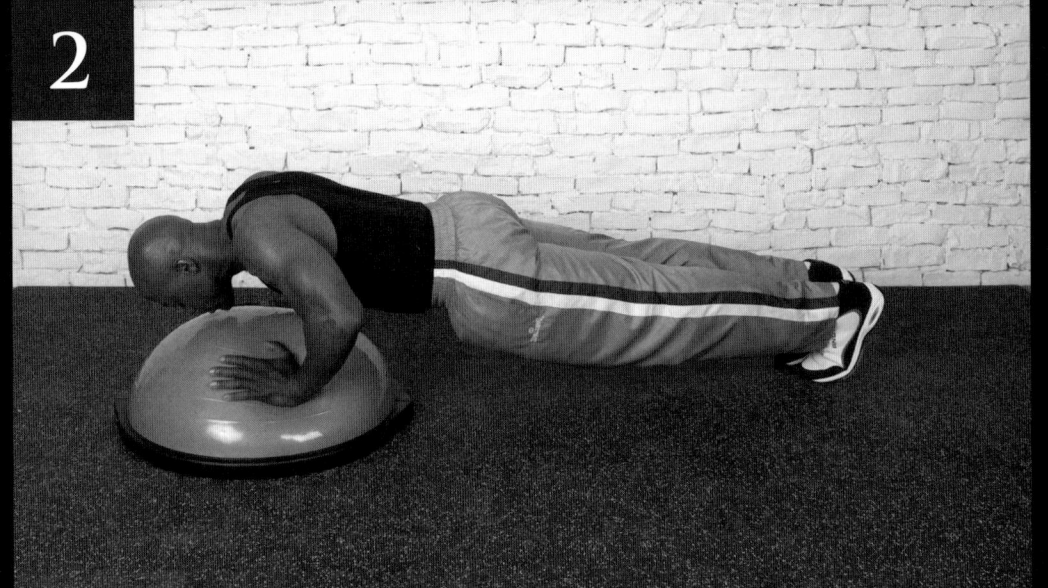

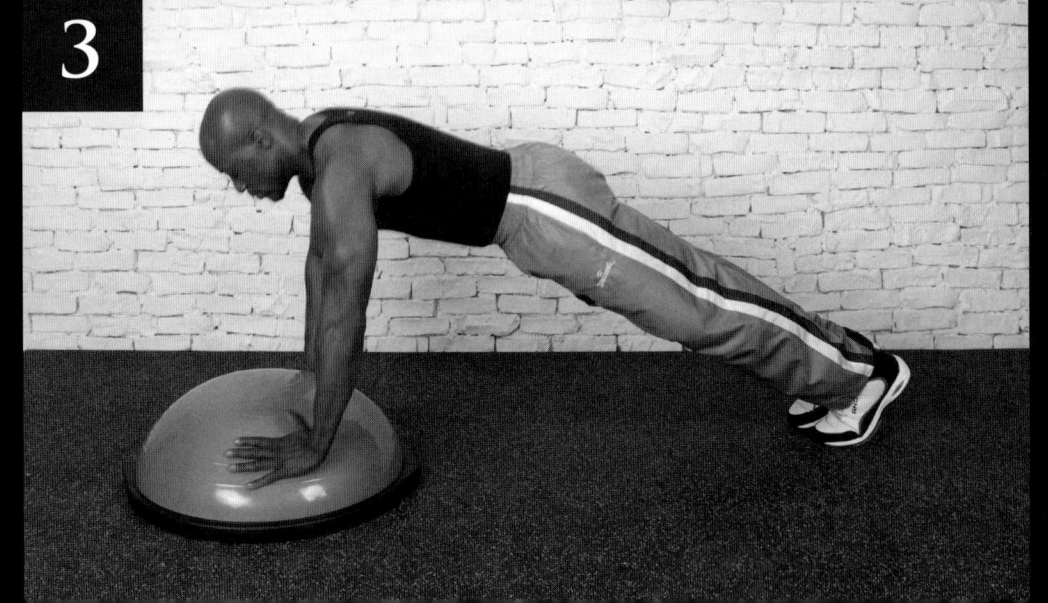

BOSU BALL FLYING PUSH-UP

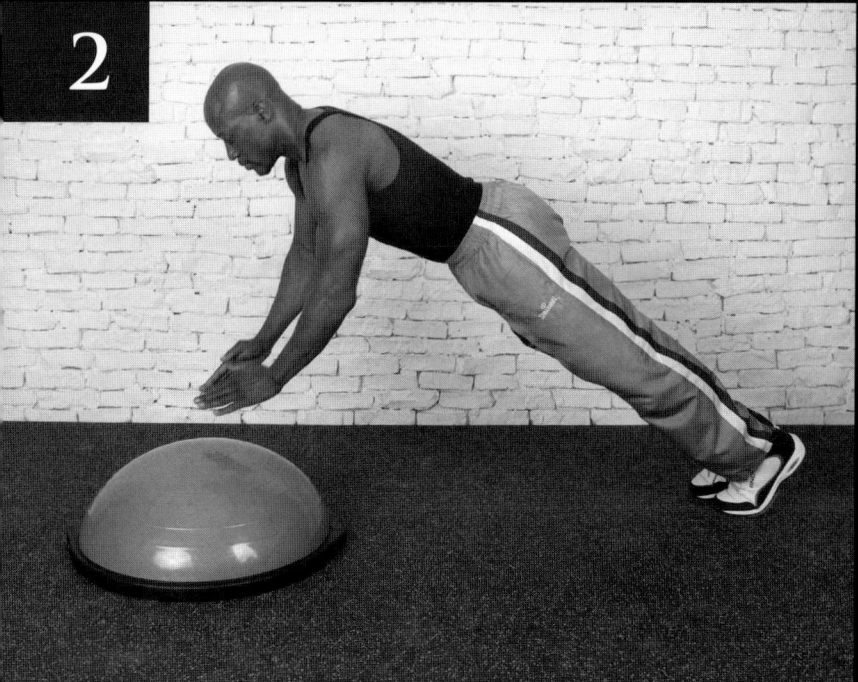

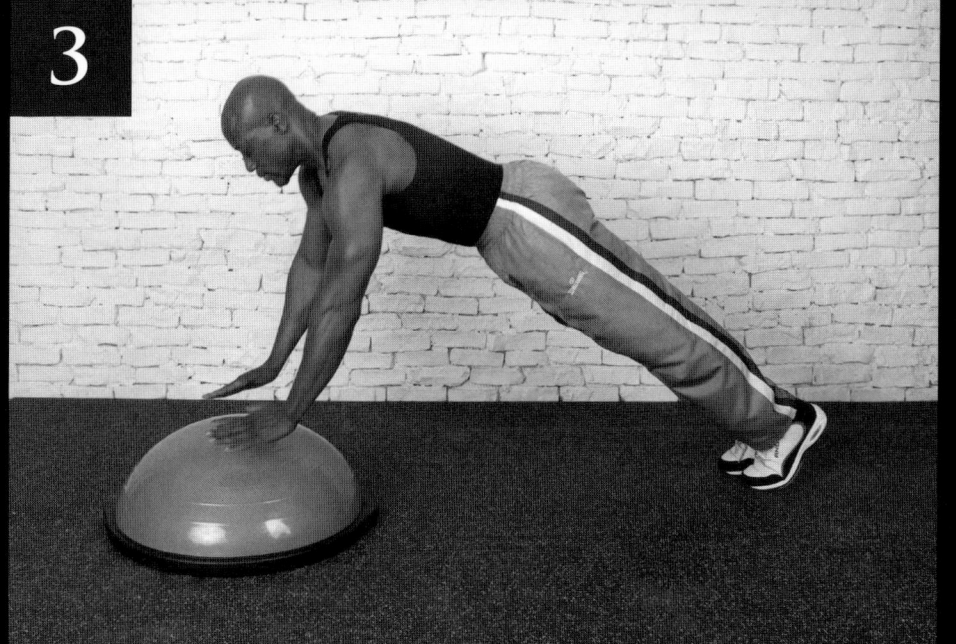

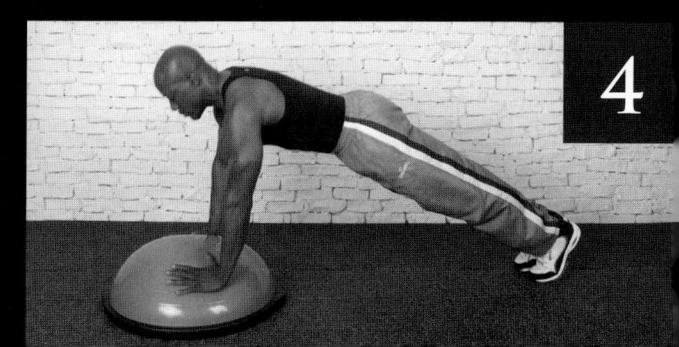

Start from the standard push-up position on the BOSU ball. Complete a standard push-up. While down on the BOSU ball, push up off the BOSU ball and clap your hands.

FIT TIP:
Keep your back straight during this exercise.

Advanced "Superman" Bosu Ball Push-Up

Starting in the regular push-up position, as the push-up is being executed by letting the body drop downward, the BOSU ball is pushed off very methodically and very evenly, and the hands are clapped very high above the BOSU ball.

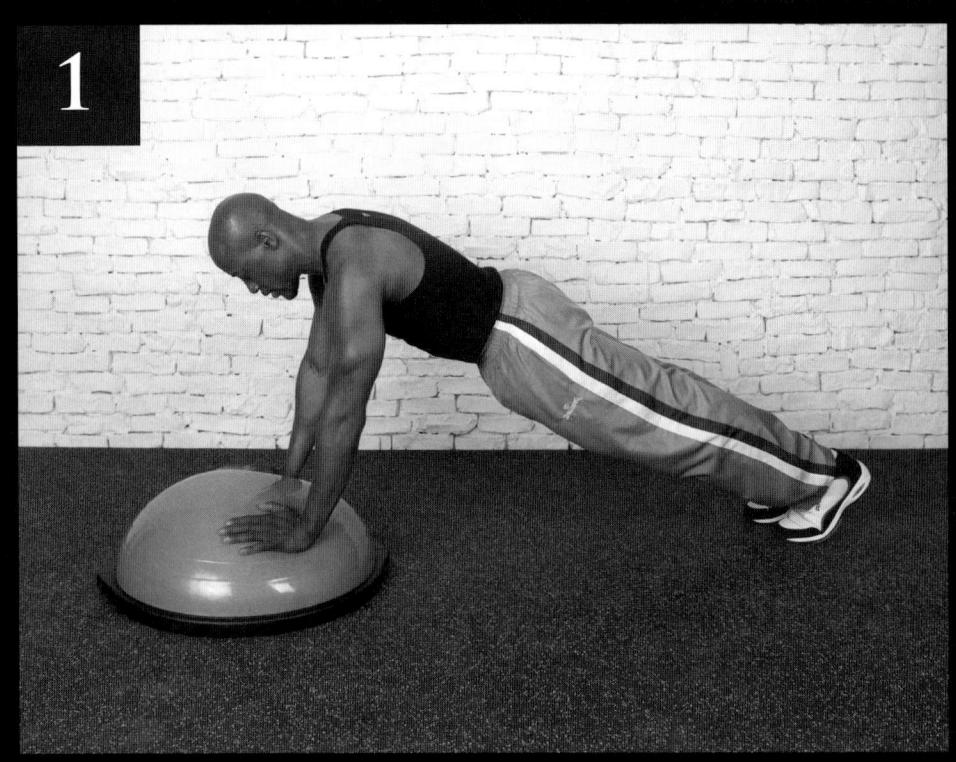

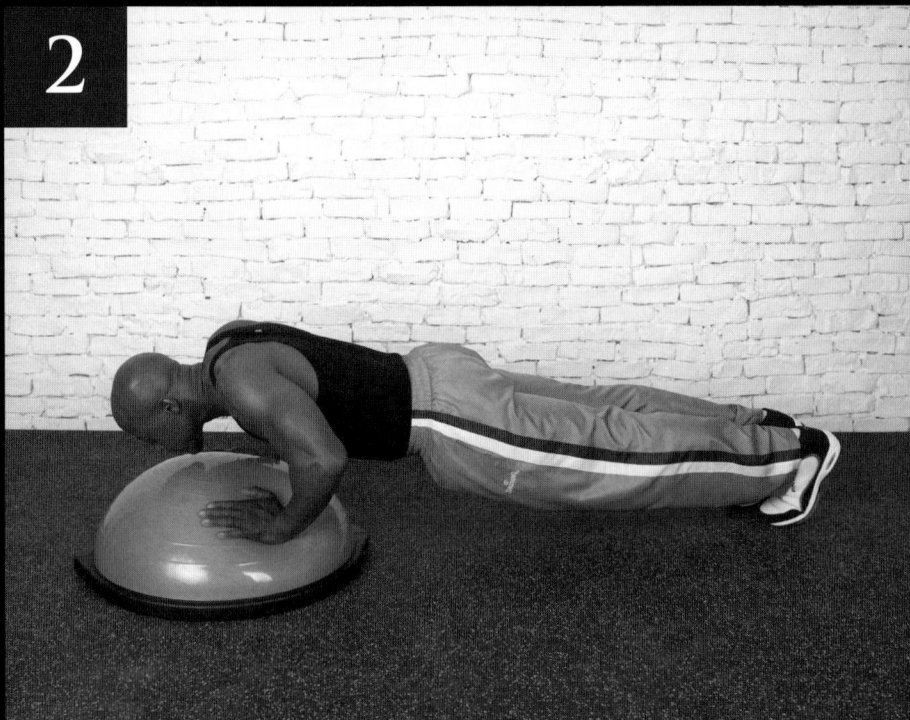

4

The key is to keep the back straight throughout the execution of this exercise.

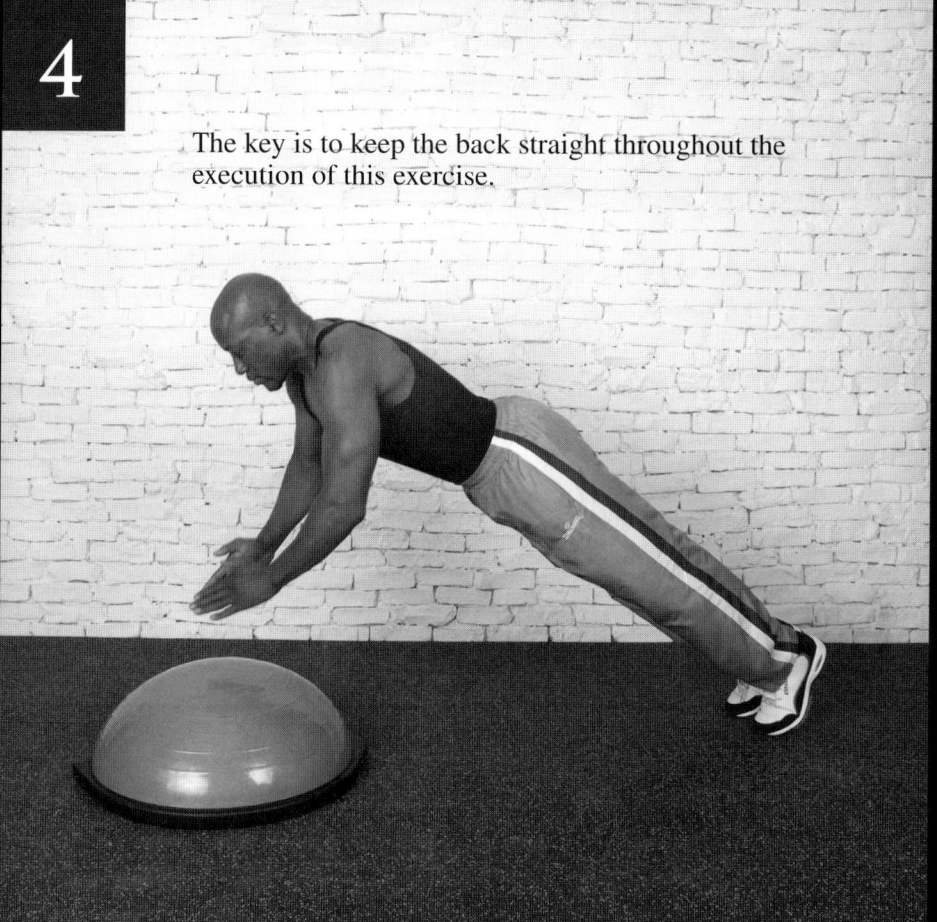

3

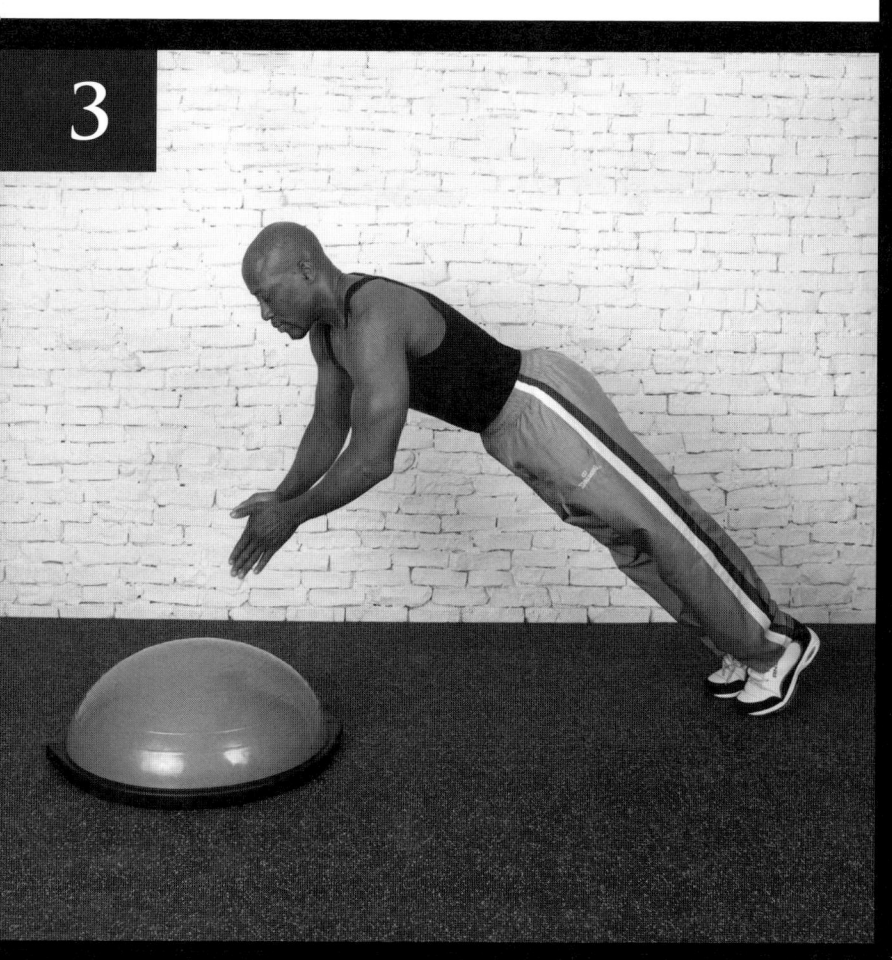

The key is to push off very aggressively from the BOSU ball to get elevated and to clap the hands once or twice while in the air and to safely land with the hands on the BOSU ball.

Recommended:
3 to 5 sets of
8 to 10 repetitions.

5

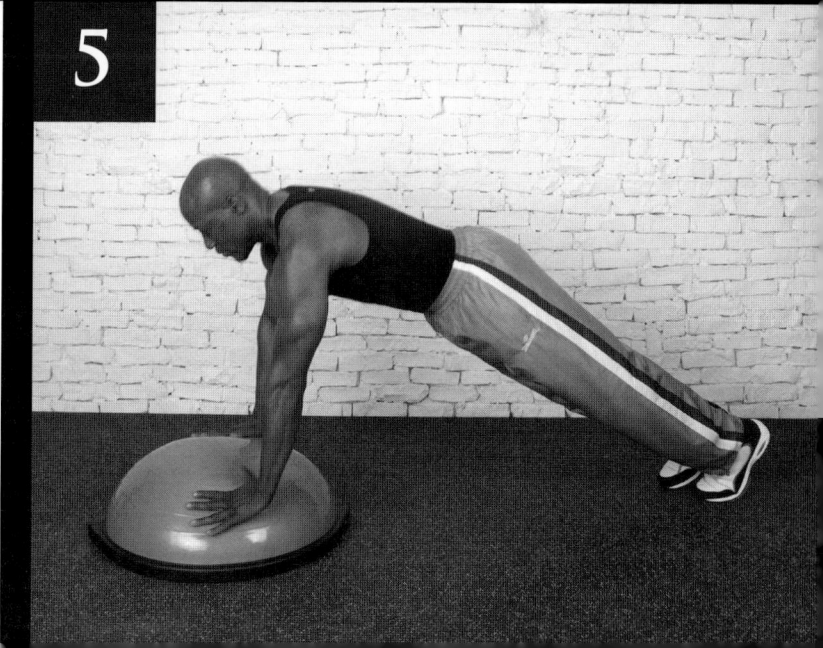

BOSU BALL TRIANGLE PUSH-UP

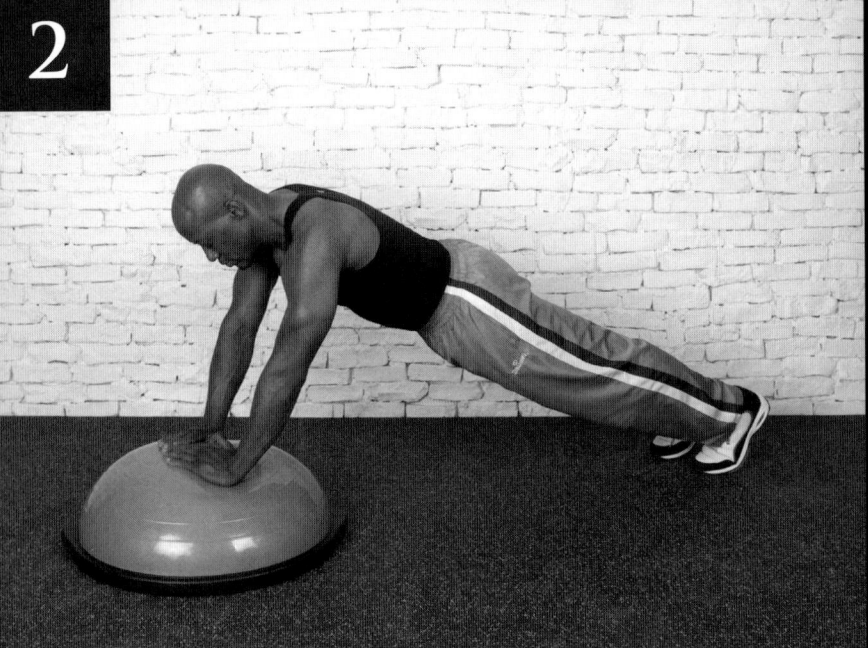

With the hands remaining in the triangle position on the BOSU ball, the goal is getting the chin to touch the BOSU ball inside the diamond or to have the chin touch the fingers.

The hands are placed in a triangle-type position onto the BOSU ball in the basic push-up position. The push-up is executed by bending the elbows and letting the body come down towards the BOSU ball and then extending your elbows and straightening your arms for the completion of the push-up.

Recommended:
3 to 5 sets of
8 to 10 repetitions.

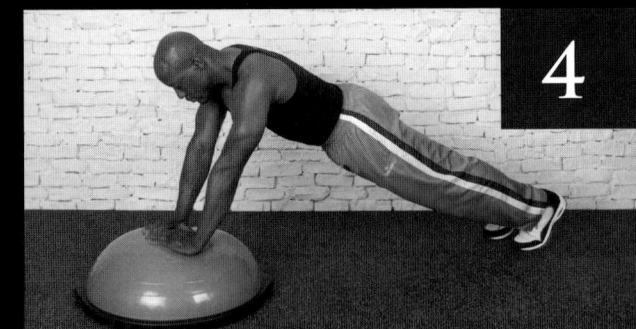

BOSU BALL MODIFIED TRIANGLE PUSH-UP

FIT TIP:
The regular standard push-up without the BOSU ball can also be done in the modified kneeling position.

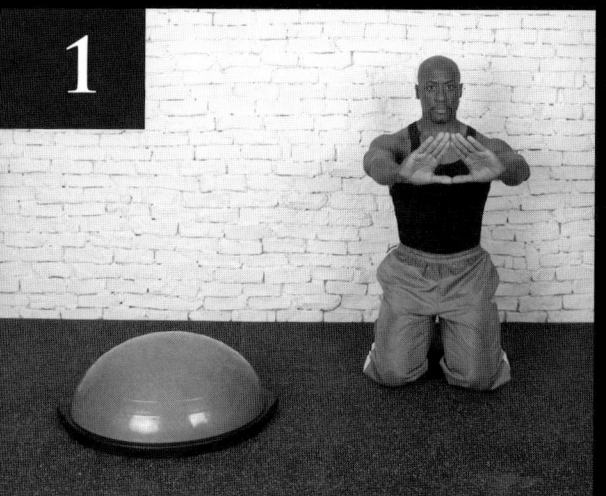

The fingers are placed in a triangle position on the BOSU ball. This is done from a kneeling position. The body is lowered as the elbows are flexed. Touch the chin to the fingers if possible and then straighten the arms by extending the elbows returning to the kneeling position.

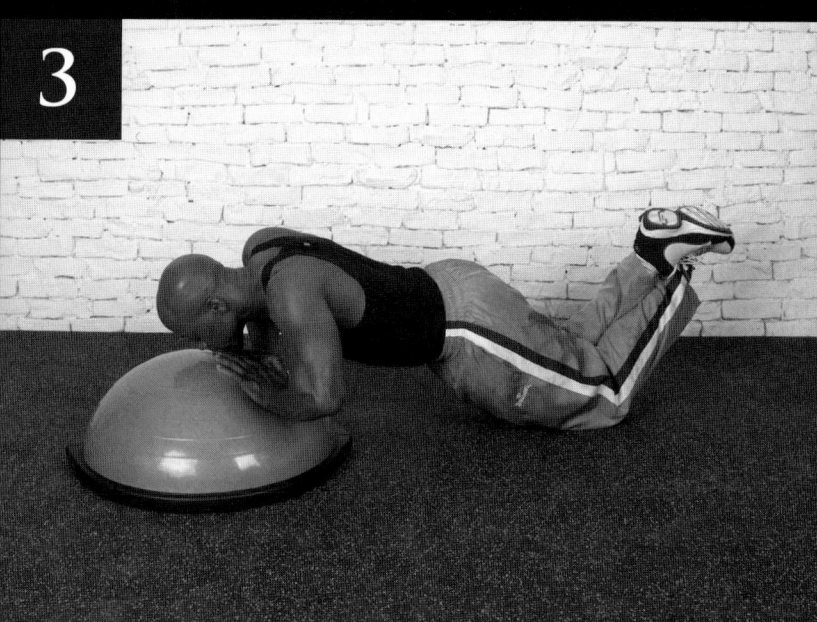

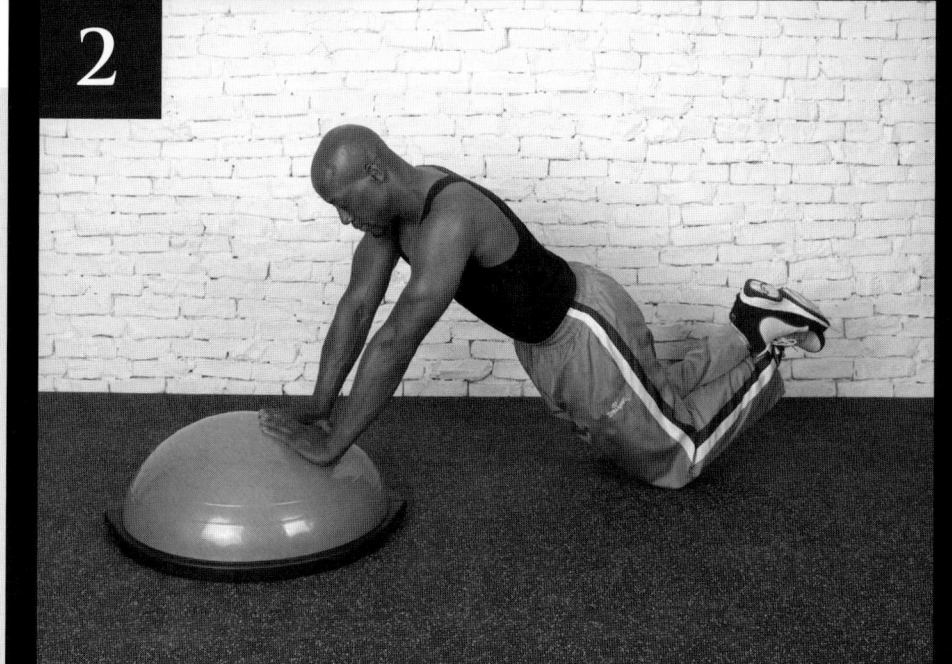

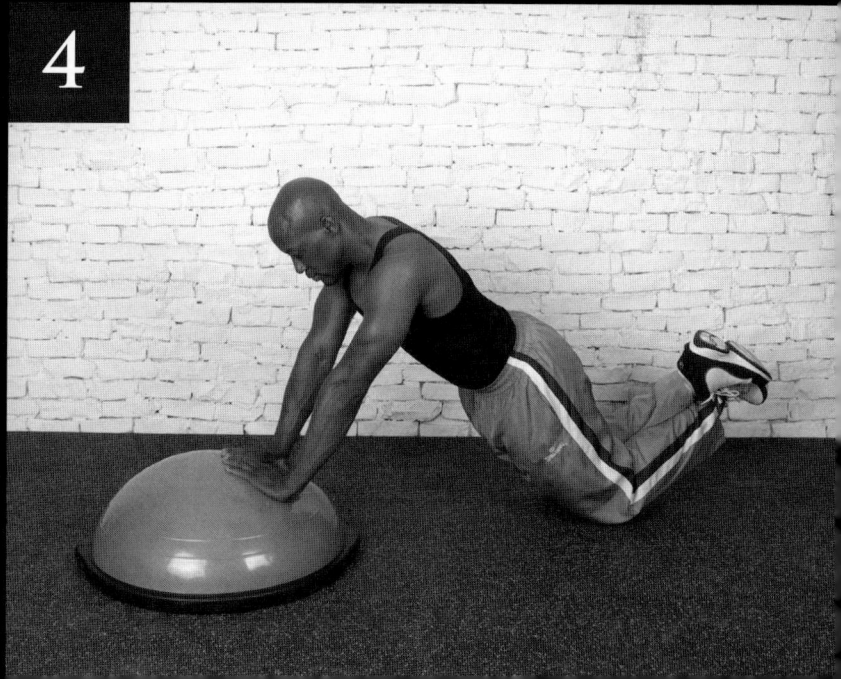

Oblique Mountain Climbers

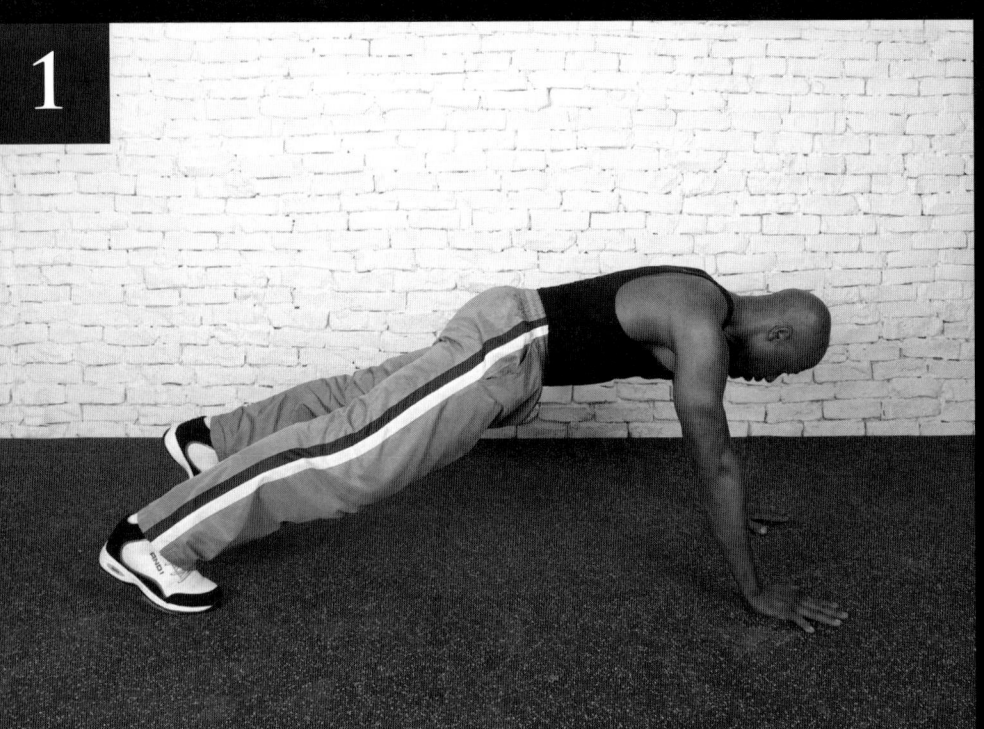

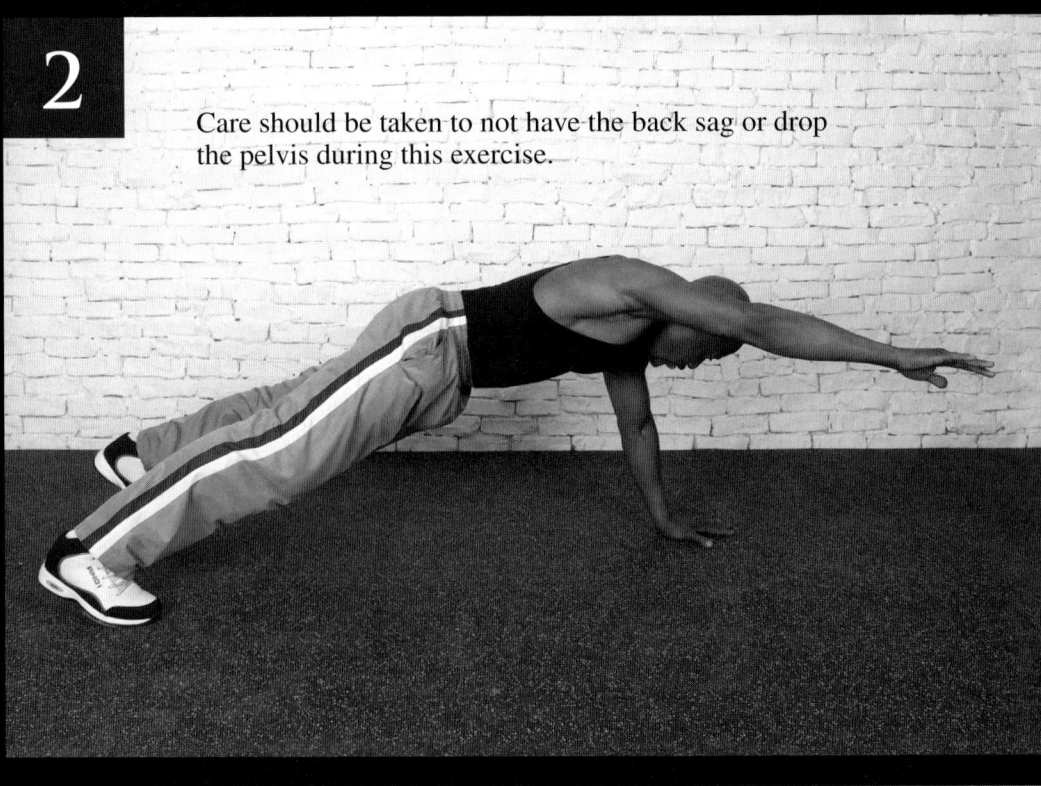

Care should be taken to not have the back sag or drop the pelvis during this exercise.

The initial position is a wide-based push-up position. Care is then taken to extend one arm forward, and the knee is brought to the opposite leg and arm. The knee of the opposite leg should be brought to the elbow of the other side of the body, crossing the midline of the body with the knee and the elbow.

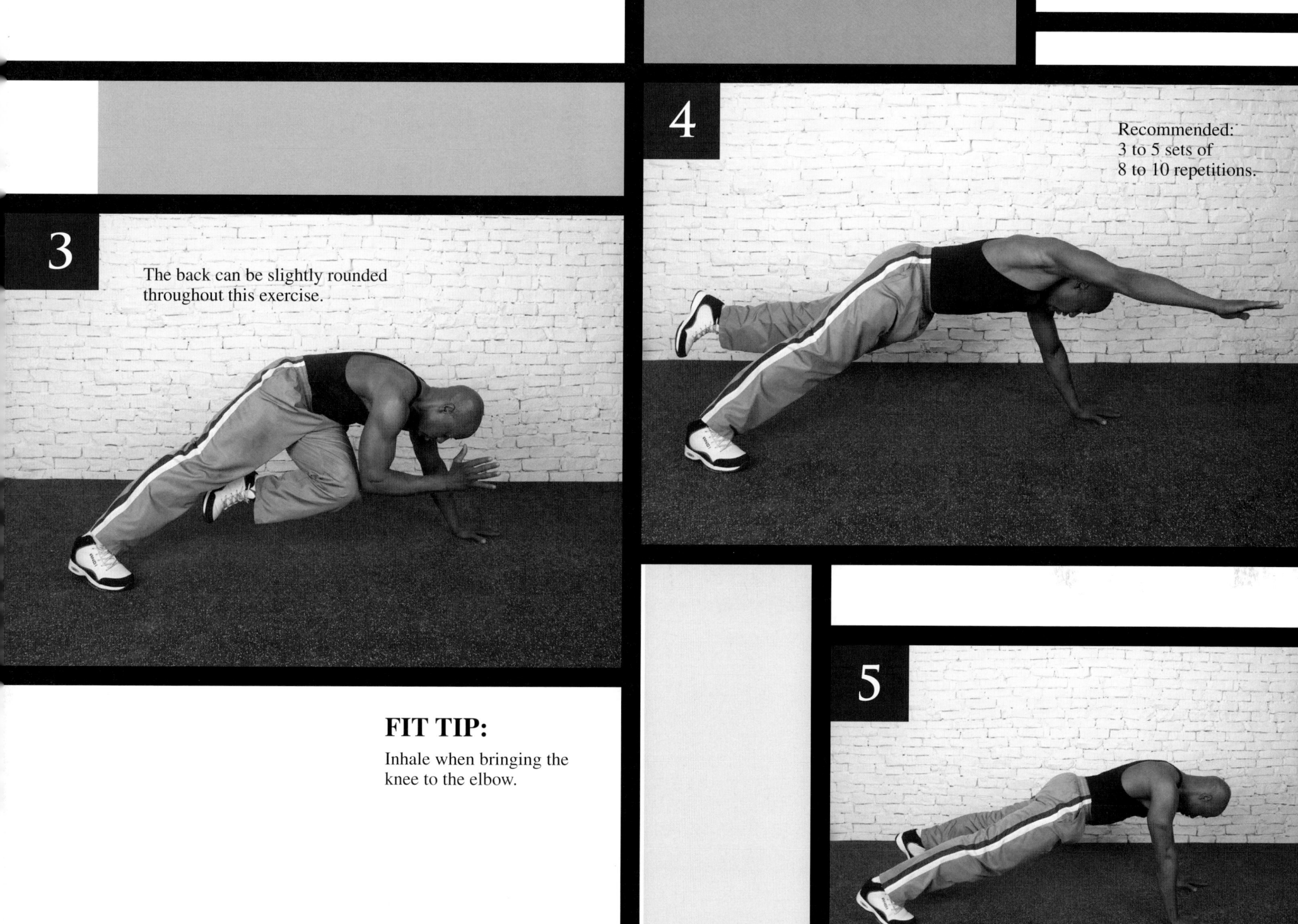

3 The back can be slightly rounded throughout this exercise.

4 Recommended: 3 to 5 sets of 8 to 10 repetitions.

FIT TIP:

Inhale when bringing the knee to the elbow.

Wide Based Spider Push-Up

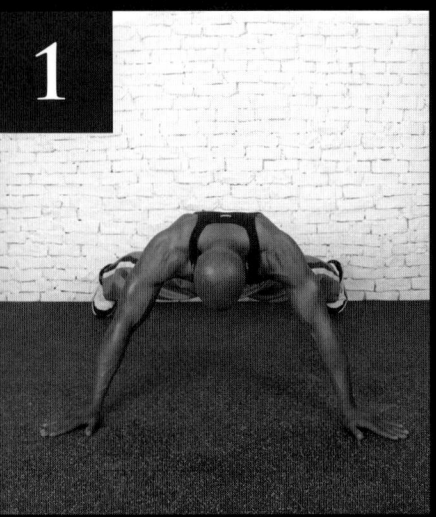

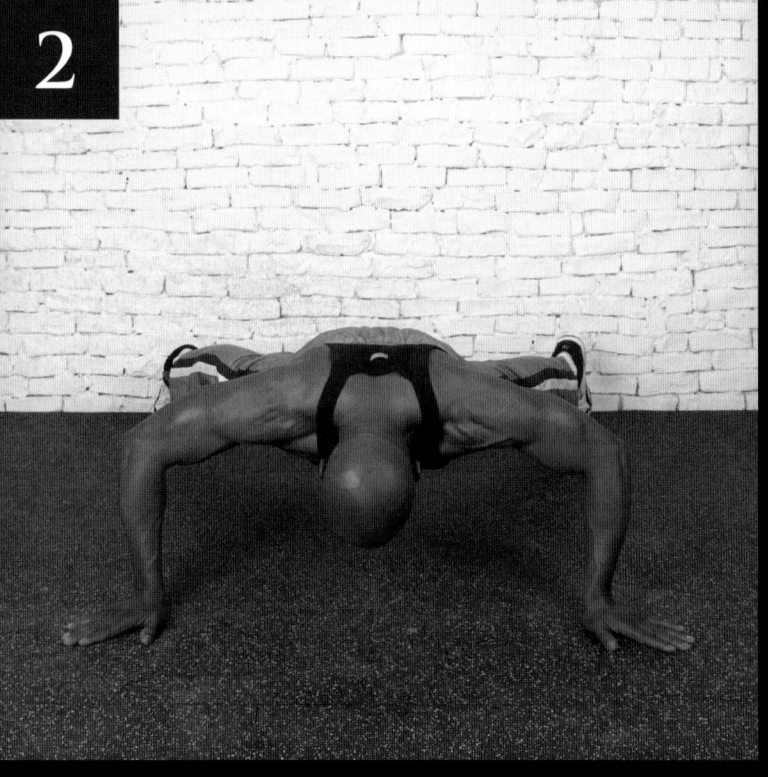

In a standard push-up position with the hands, feet and legs wide apart, perform a push-up.

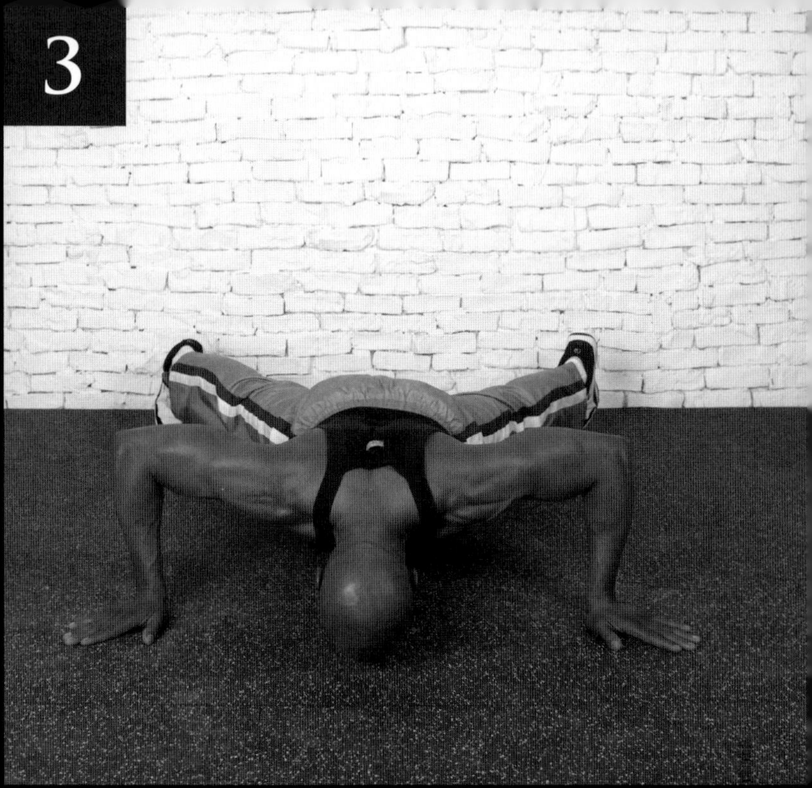

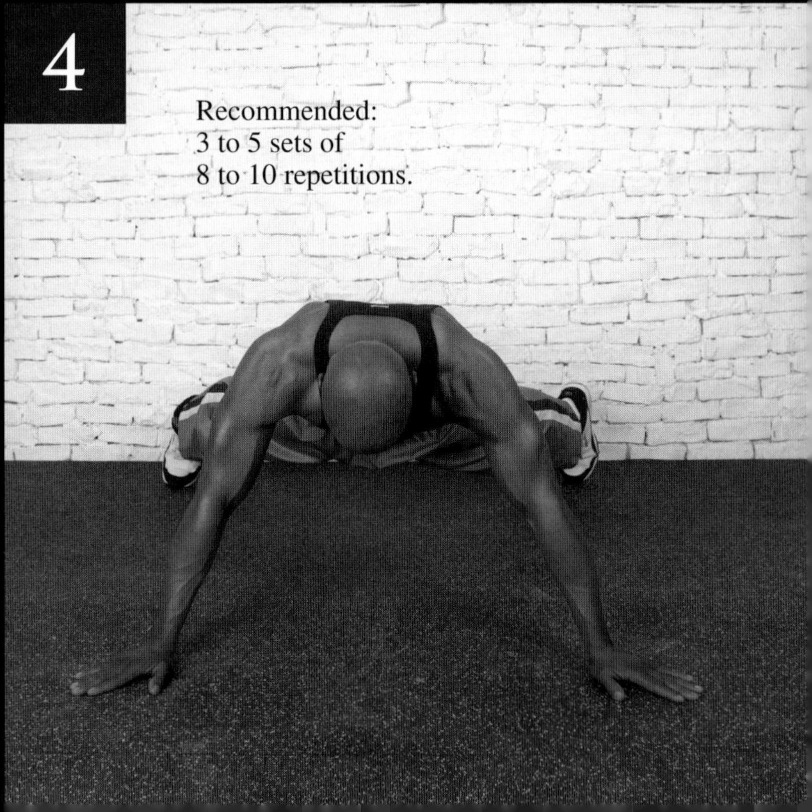

Recommended:
3 to 5 sets of
8 to 10 repetitions.

Mountain Climbers

In a runner's type position, alternate the legs in climbing-type style.

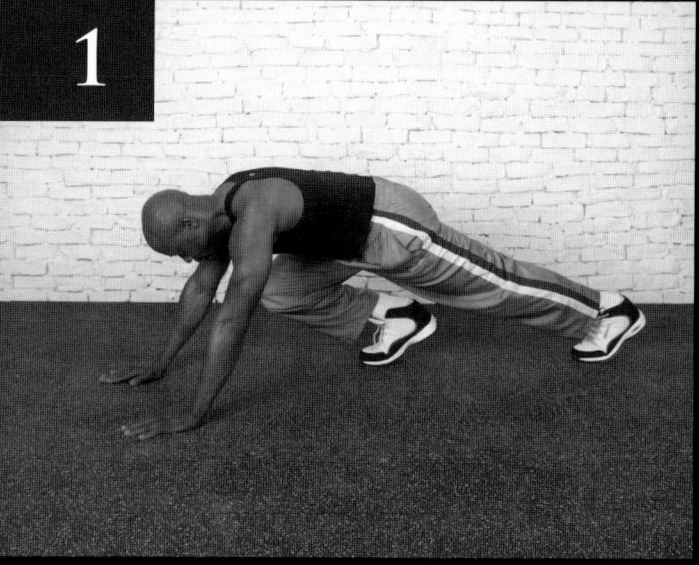

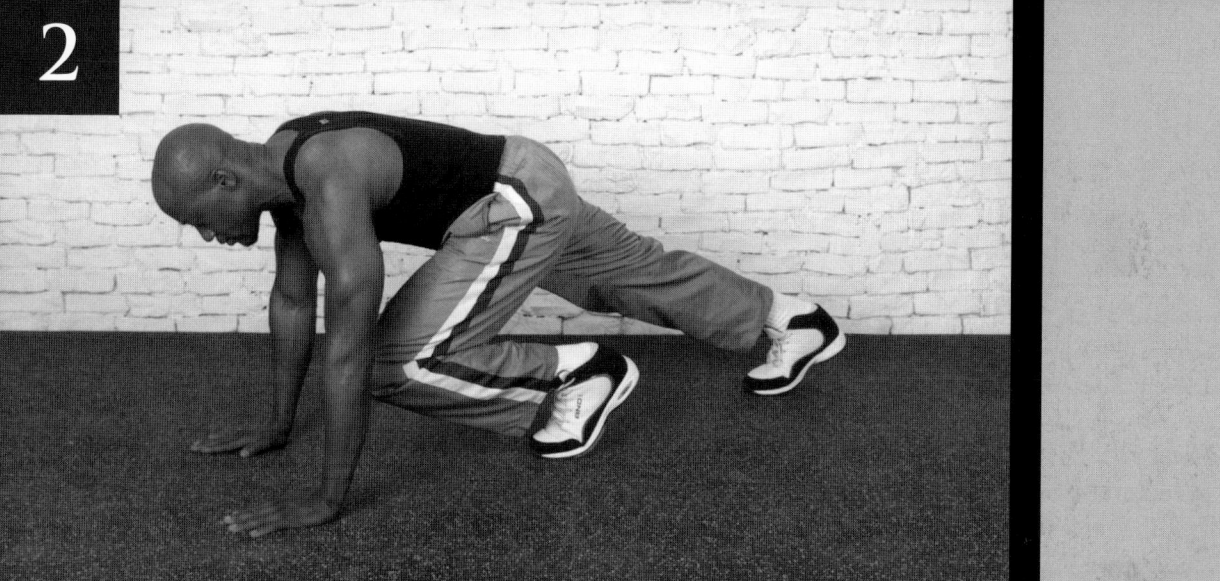

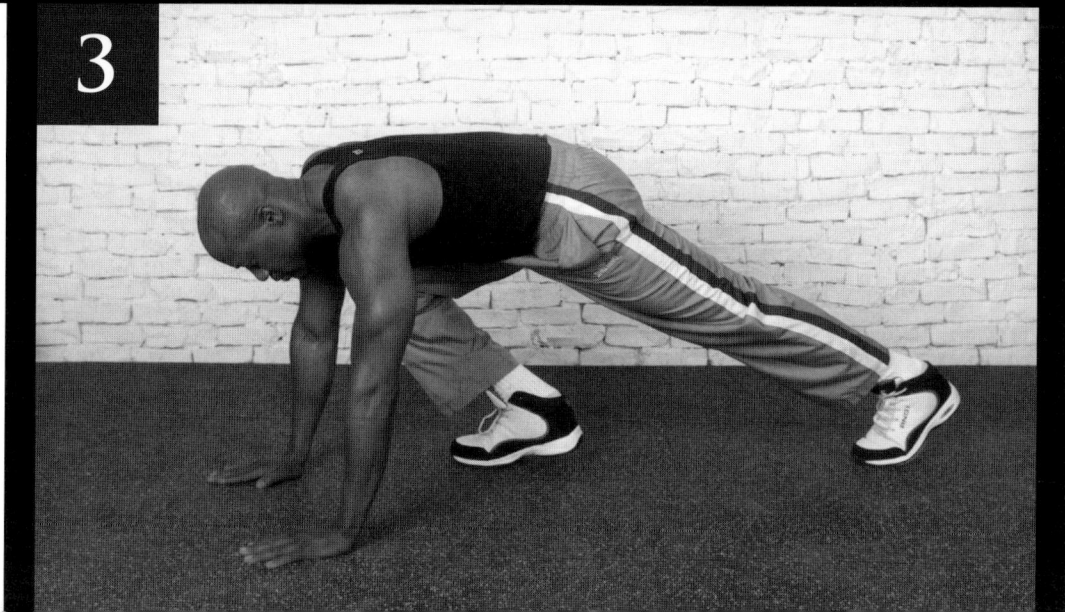

FIT TIP:
Keep the palms of the hands flat on the floor during this exercise.

Medicine Ball Exchanged Push-Ups

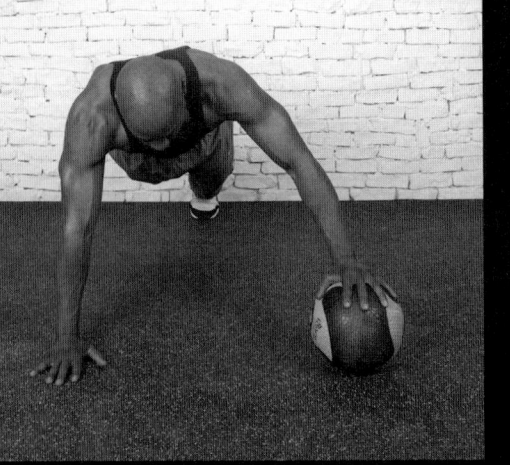
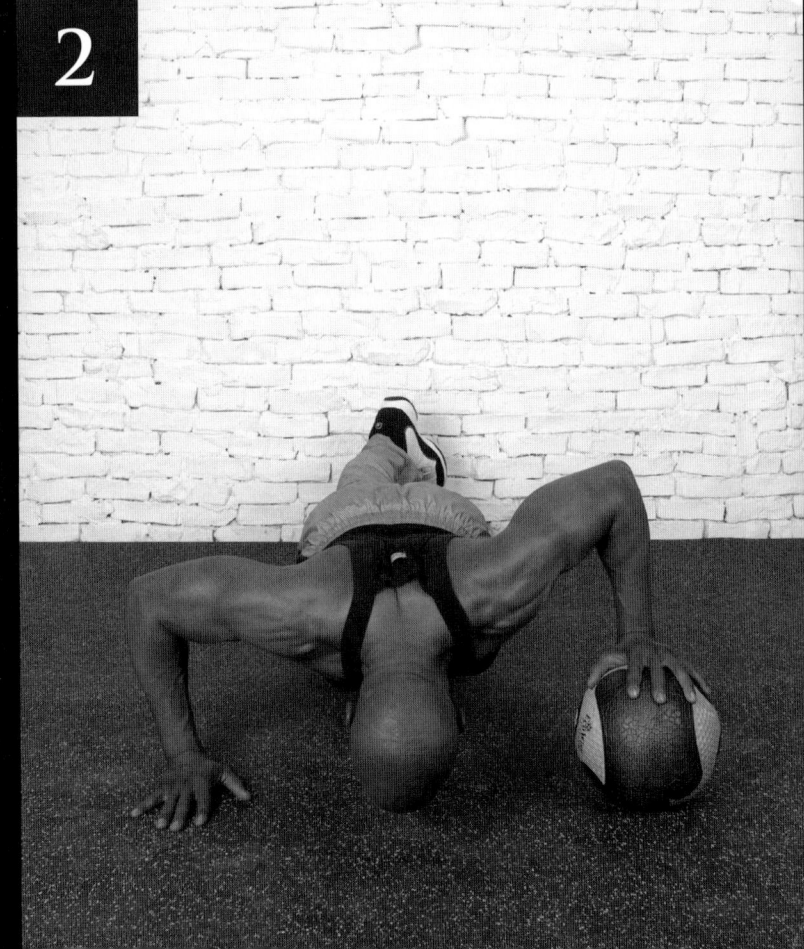
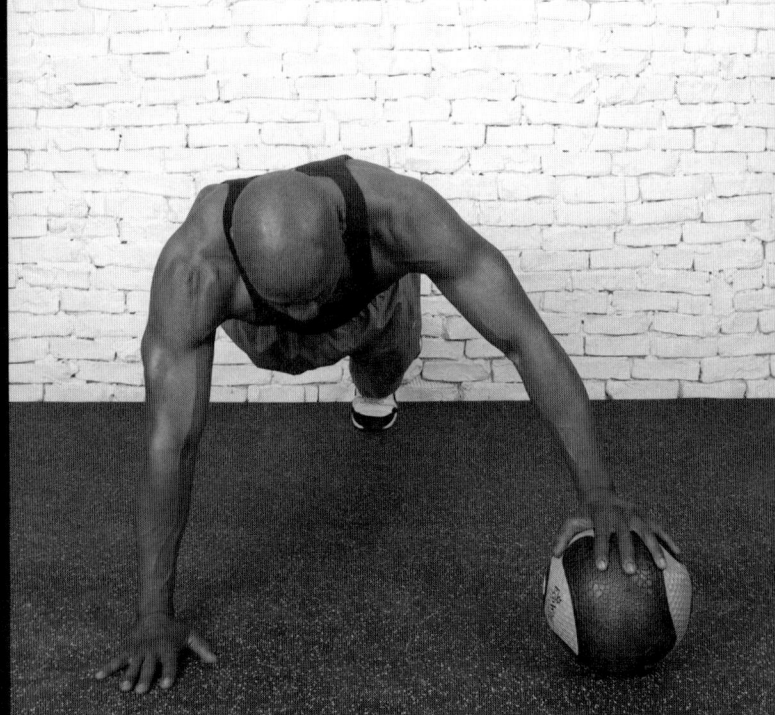

Starting off in a standard push-up position with the medicine ball under one hand as balance, care is taken to execute a regular push-up. After that push-up is done, release the medicine ball and push it over to the opposite side, exchanging hands. Catch it with the opposite hand and then another push-up is executed. Then roll the ball back to the other side.

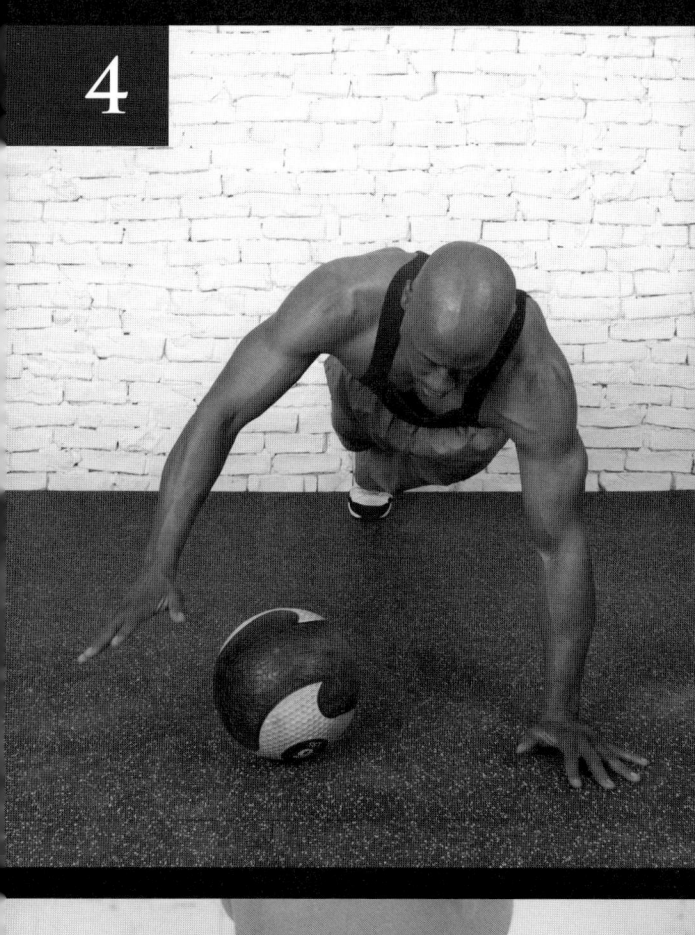

This should be a very fluid, continuous motion with no stop and go action. This can also be done from the modified position.

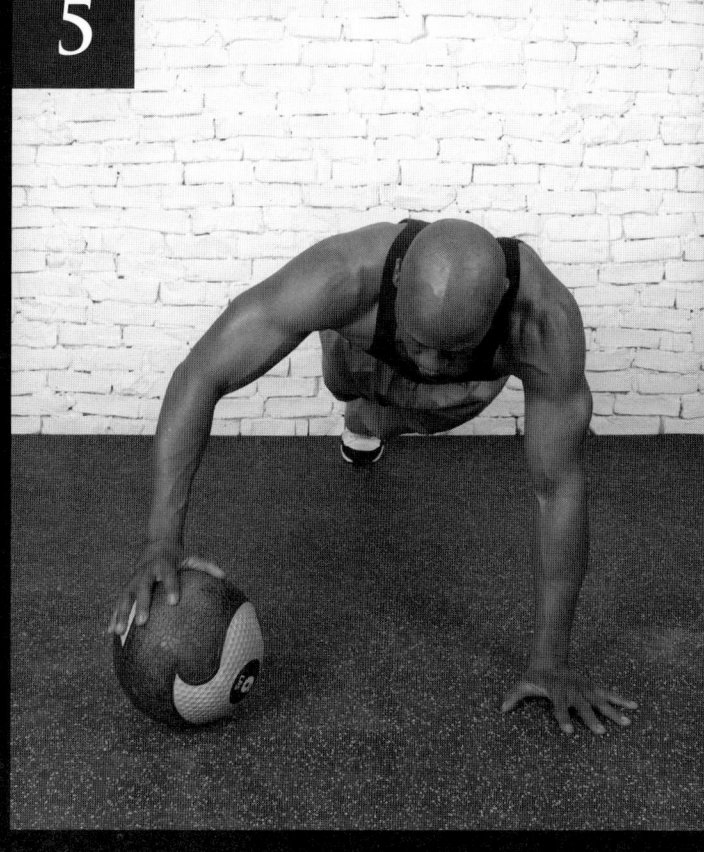

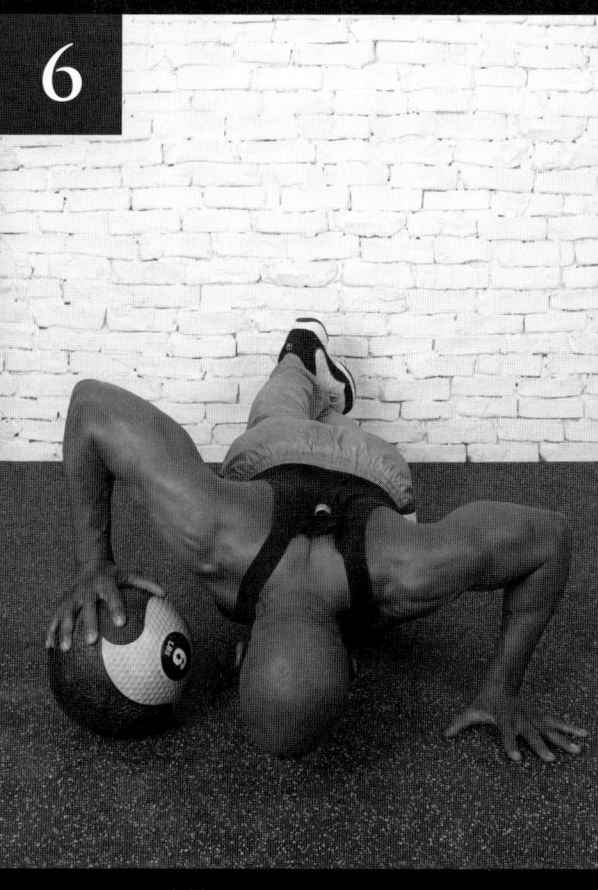

Medicine Ball Modified Push-Up with Extension

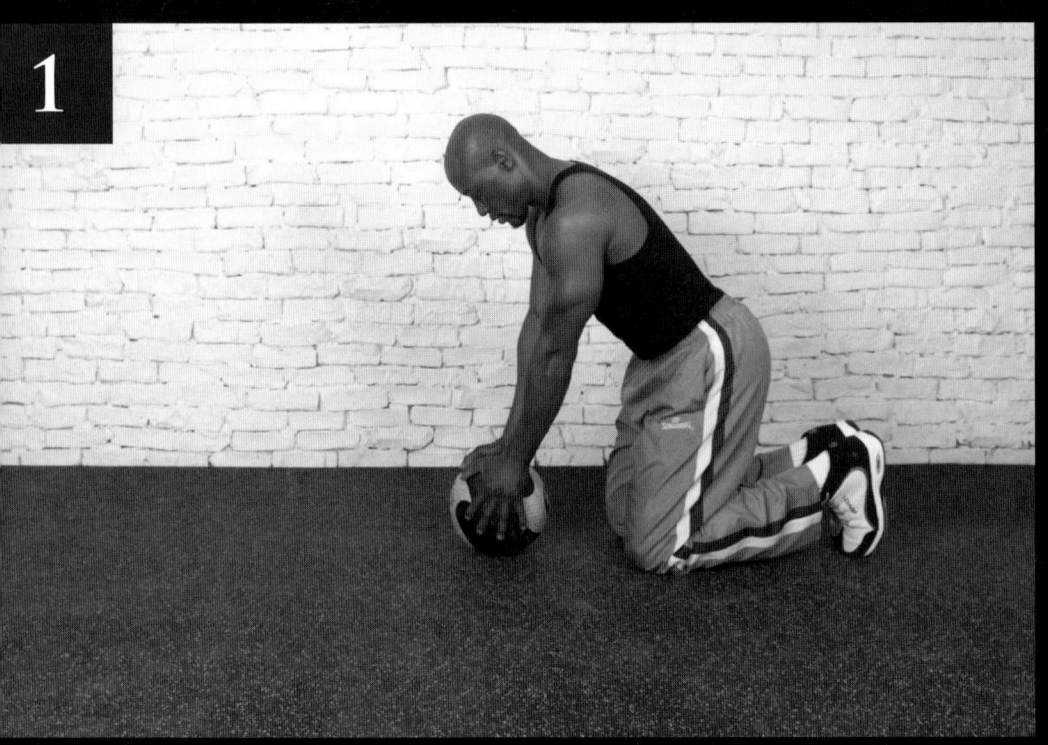

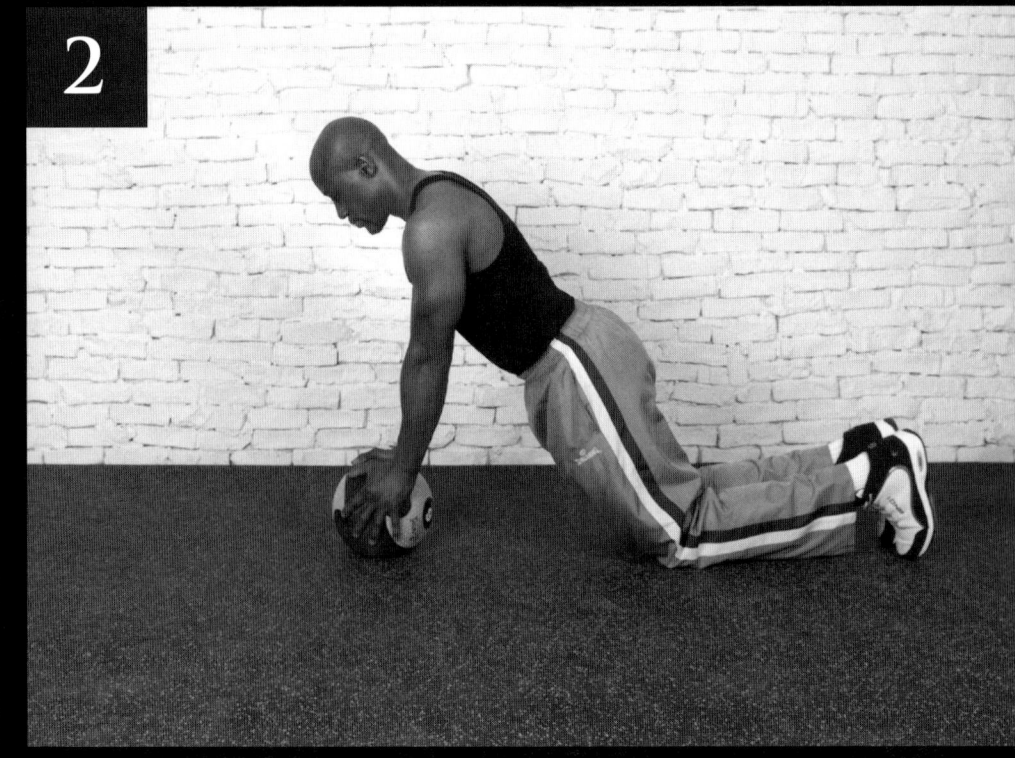

The exercise is done using the medicine ball in front of the body with the arms extended in front of the torso. A push-up is done from the modified position from the knees. After the push-up is done, the medicine ball is rolled forward and the body must be extended as the medicine ball rolls forward.

The medicine ball is then brought back to the starting position after the body has been extended. Care must be taken not to sag the back or to have your lower back arch during this modified medicine ball push-up with extension.

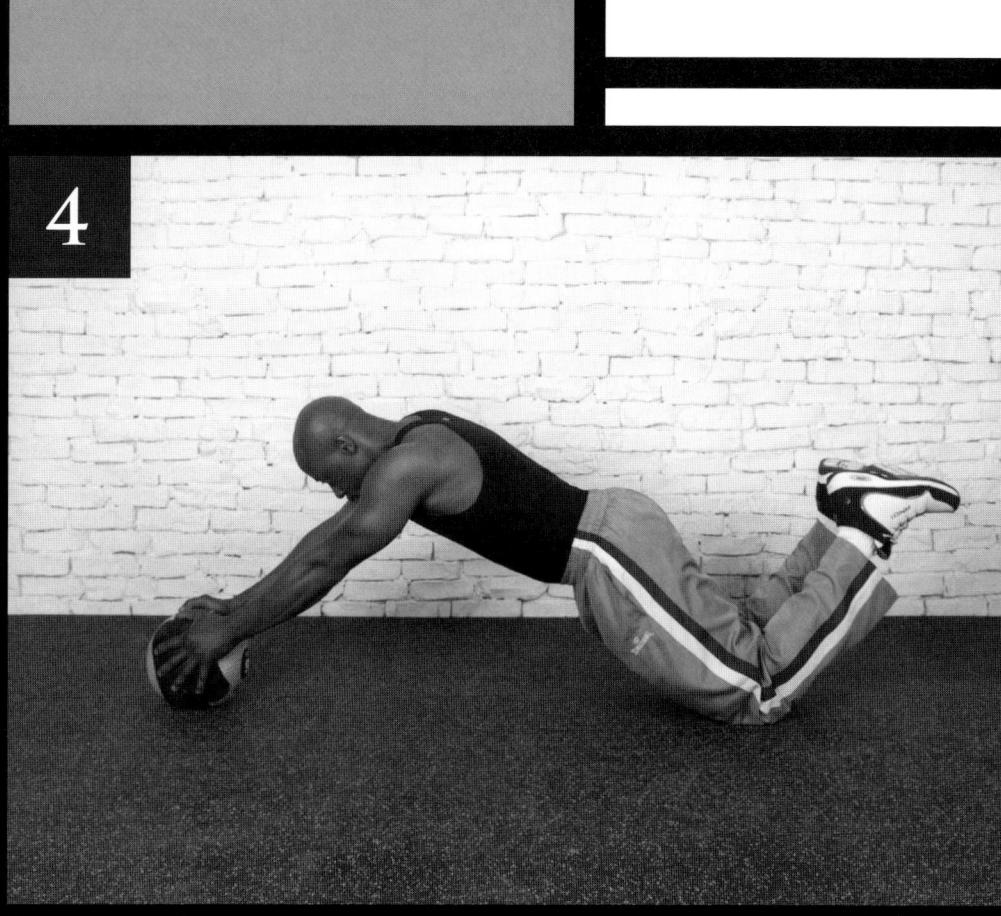

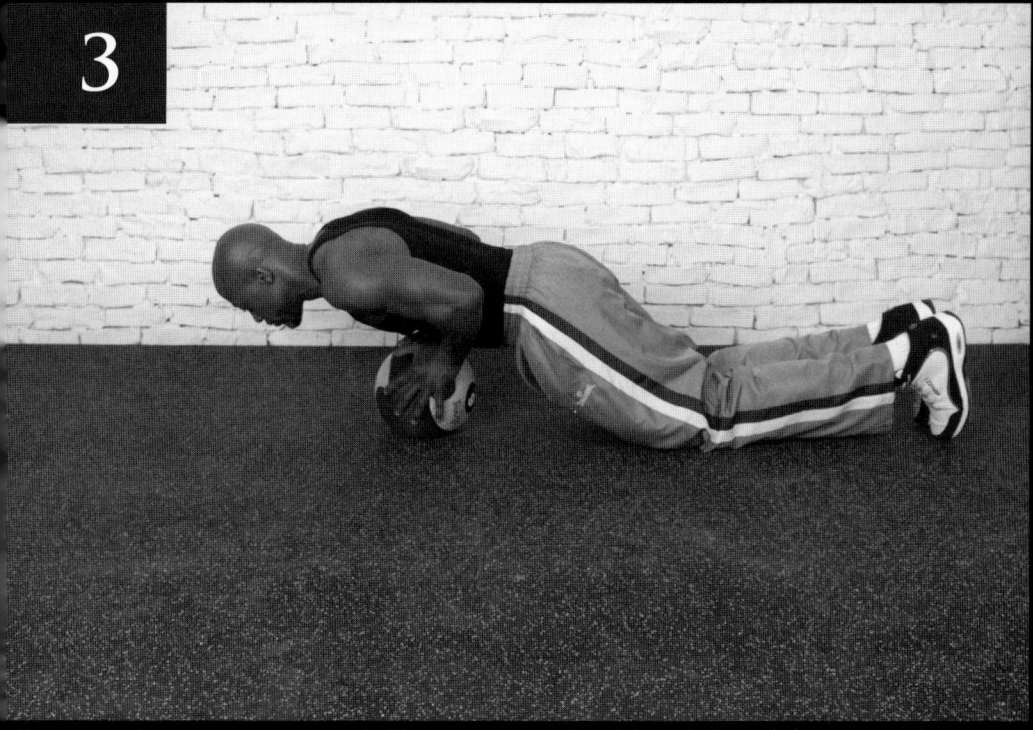

FIT TIP:

Contract the abdominal and gluteal muscles when rolling the ball forward.

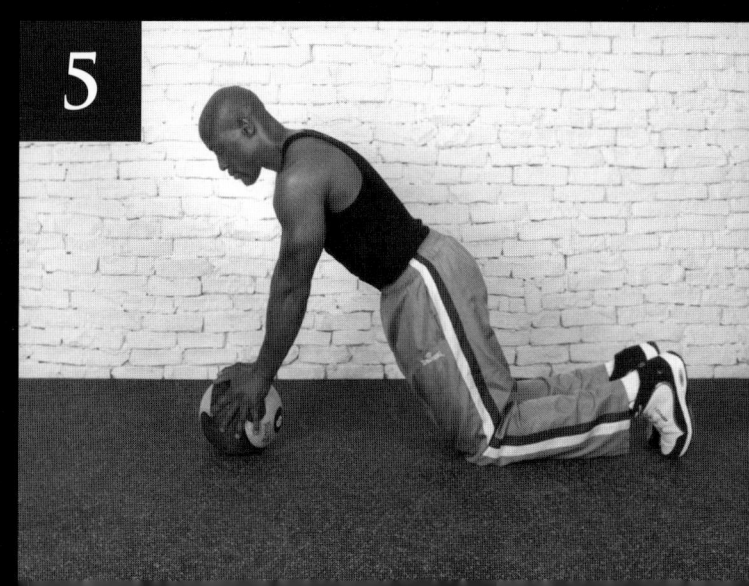

Side Perspective Triangle Push-Up

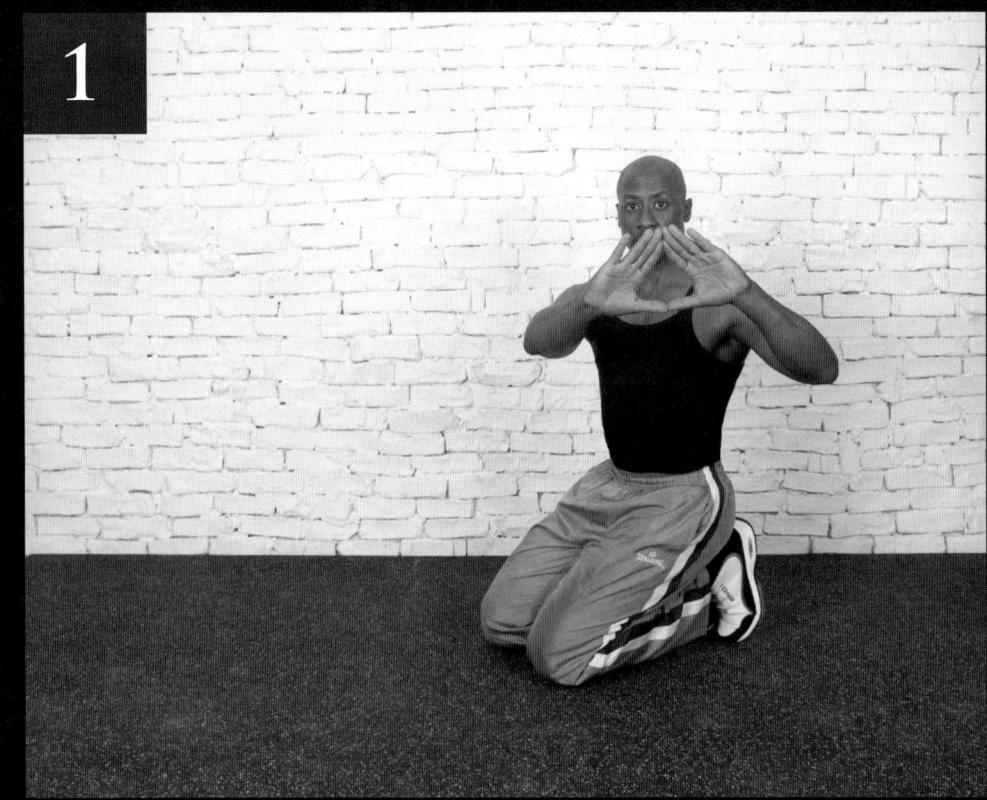

The exercise is done by first, putting the fingers together, thumbs together, and index fingers together in a triangle pattern. The hands are then placed on the floor while on your knees. The body is then elevated. The legs can be crossed behind you with the back flat, and the stomach tight.

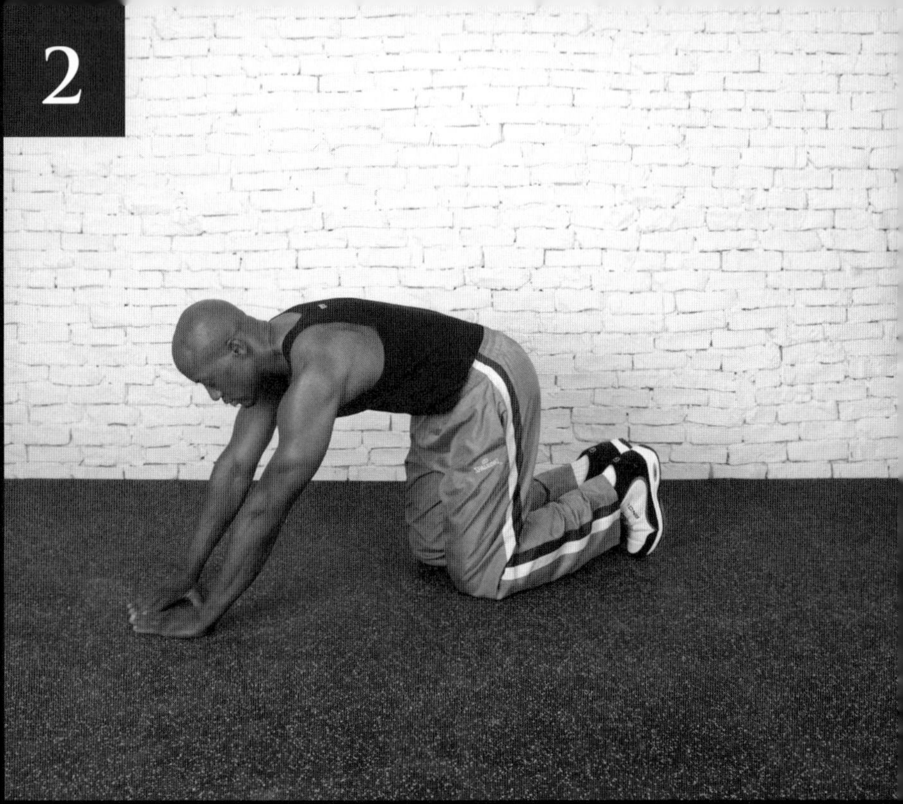

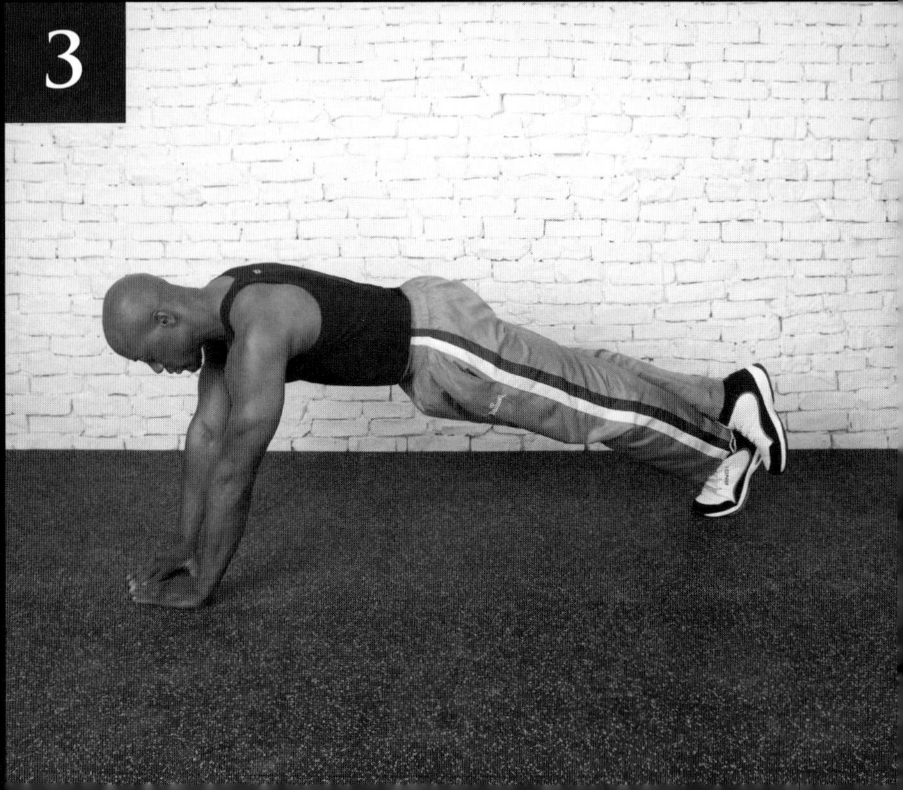

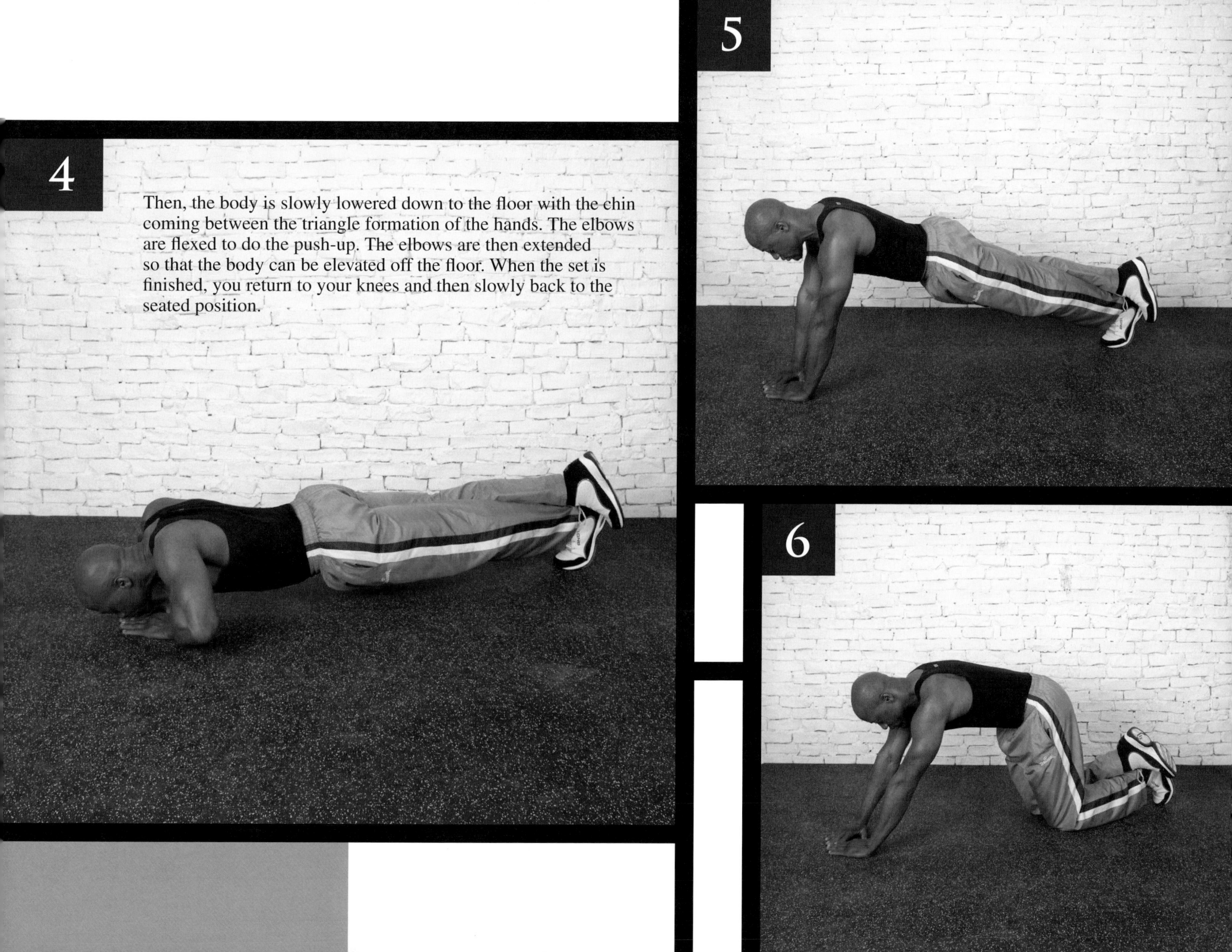

4 Then, the body is slowly lowered down to the floor with the chin coming between the triangle formation of the hands. The elbows are flexed to do the push-up. The elbows are then extended so that the body can be elevated off the floor. When the set is finished, you return to your knees and then slowly back to the seated position.

Modified Triangle Push-Up

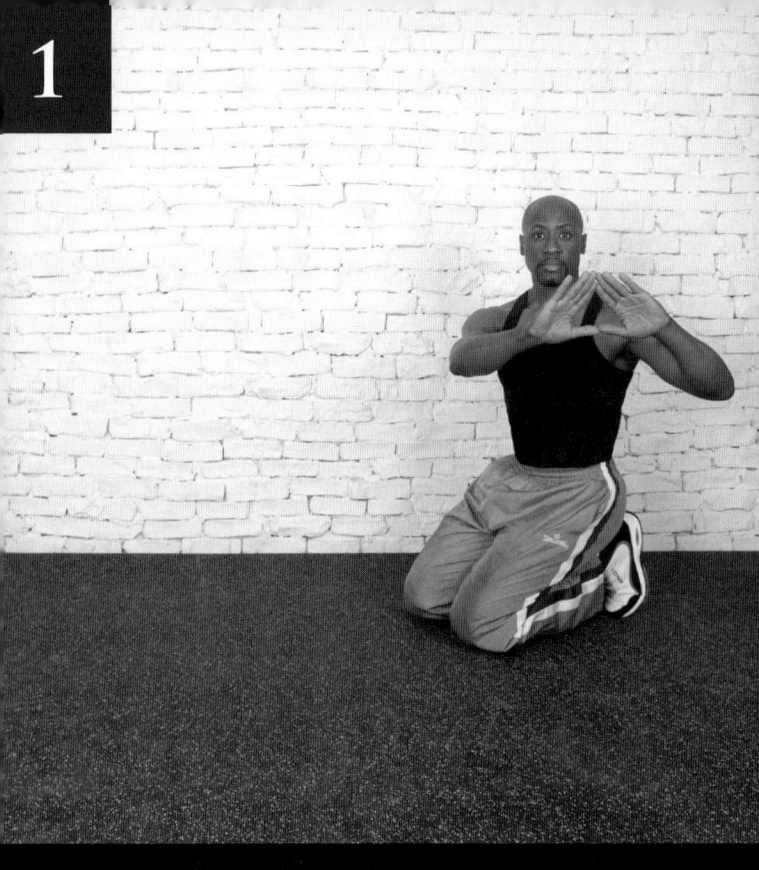

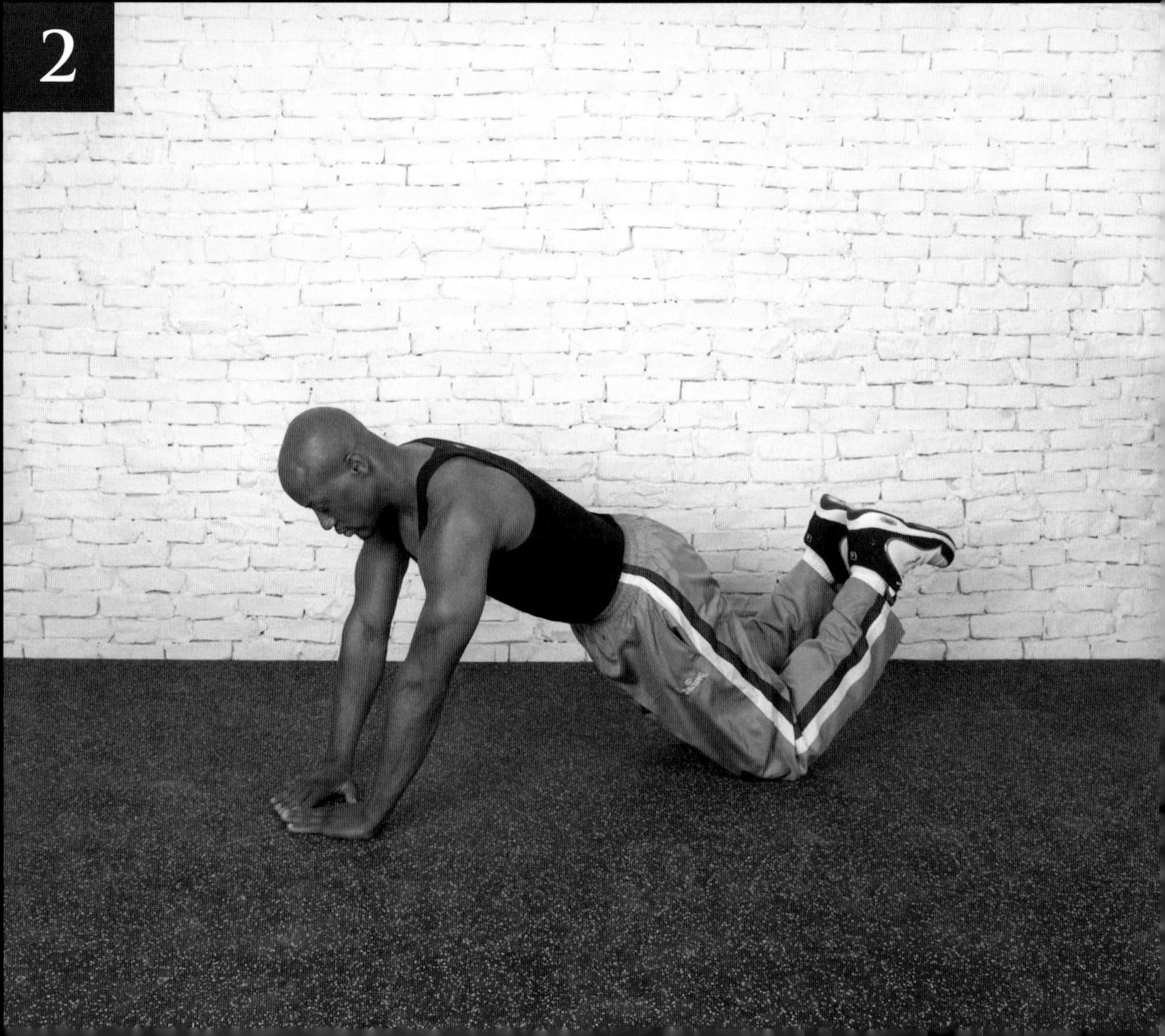

Start with the knees together. Put the fingers together in a triangle formation. The hands are placed on the floor with the hips extended behind your torso.

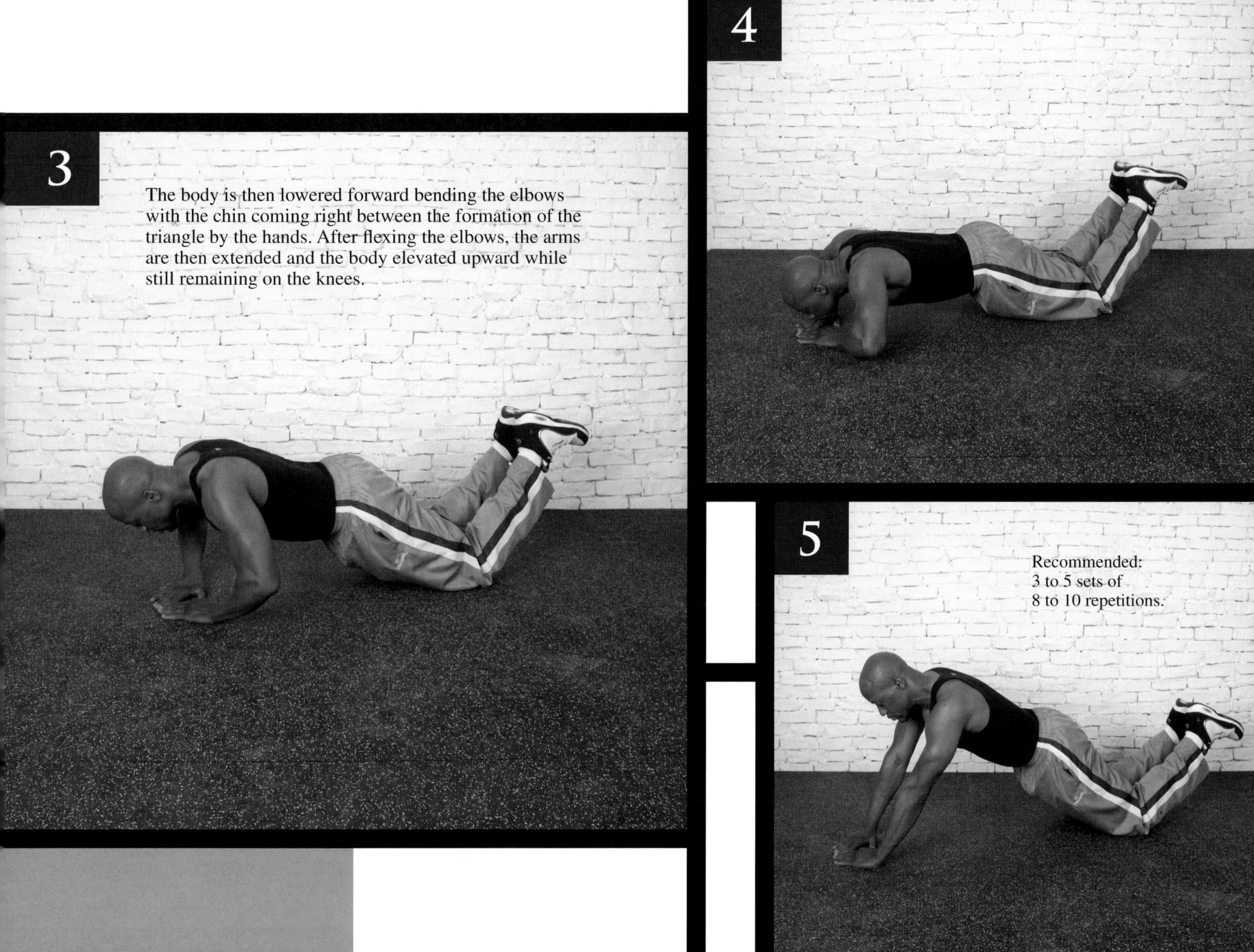

3 The body is then lowered forward bending the elbows with the chin coming right between the formation of the triangle by the hands. After flexing the elbows, the arms are then extended and the body elevated upward while still remaining on the knees.

4

5 Recommended: 3 to 5 sets of 8 to 10 repetitions.

Front Perspective Standard Triceps Push-Up

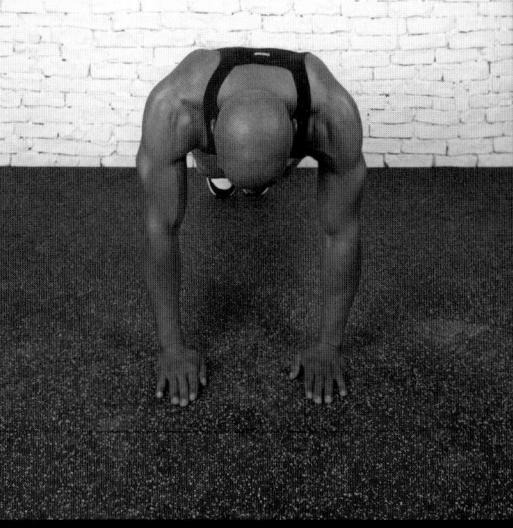

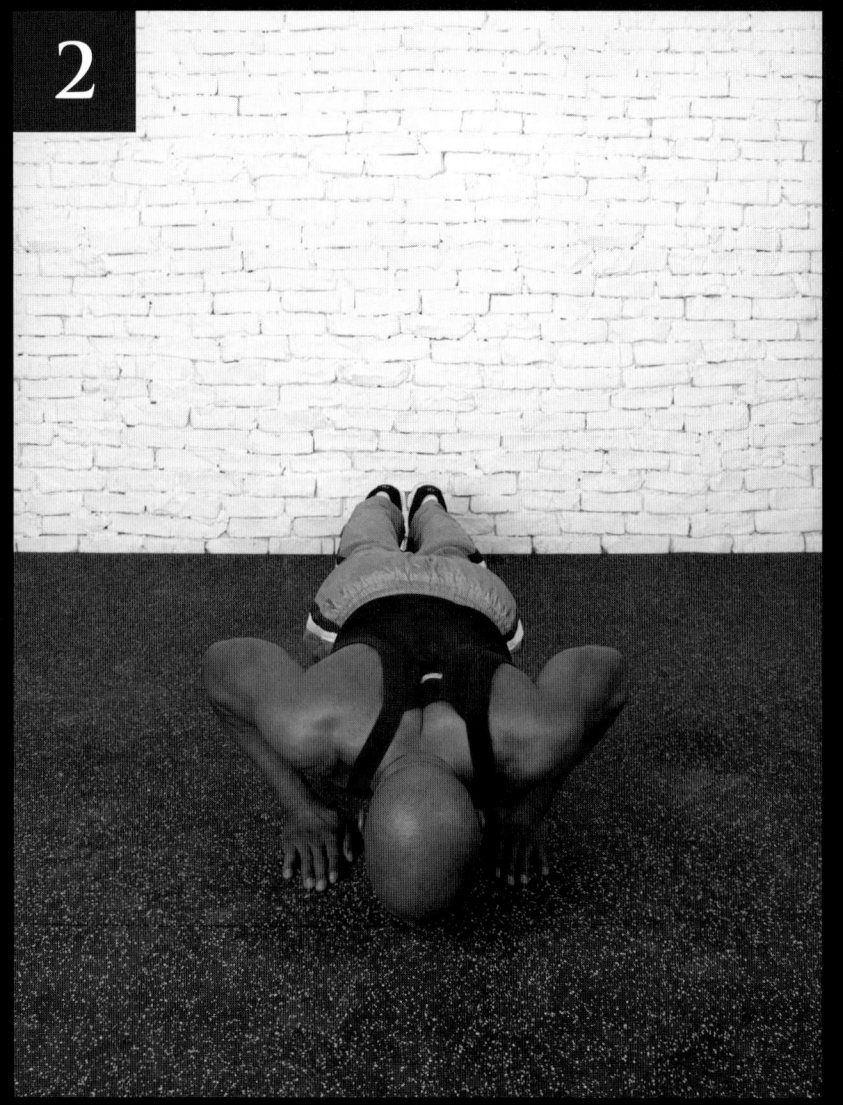

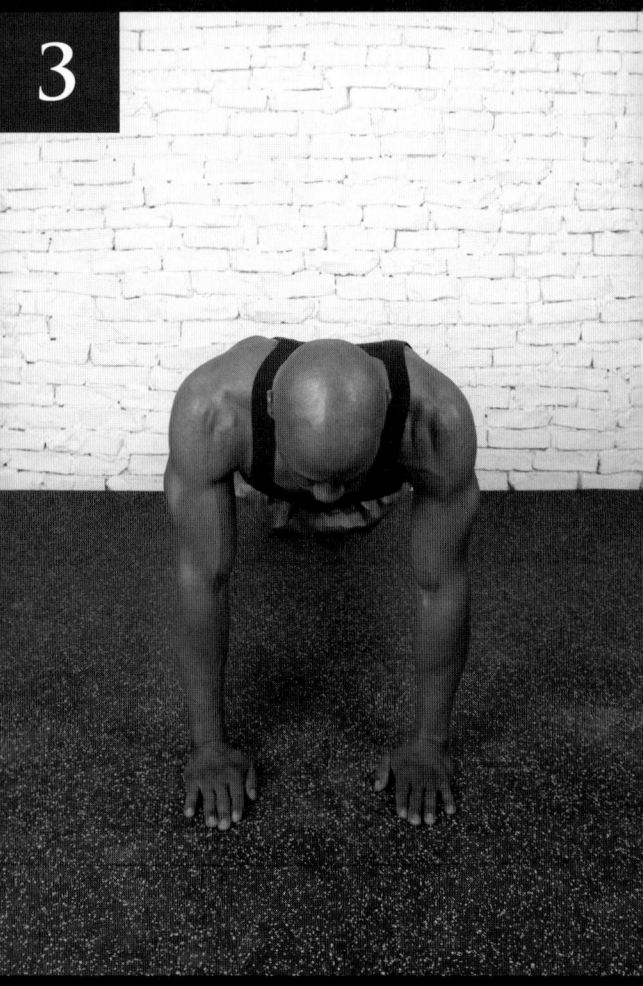

Starting position is prone with the body elevated and in a suspended position. The body is then slowly lowered, flexing the elbows with the face toward the floor. The body is elevated by pushing downward on the floor and lifting the body.

FIT TIP:

Keep the back flat.

Same Side Plank and Knee Lift

1

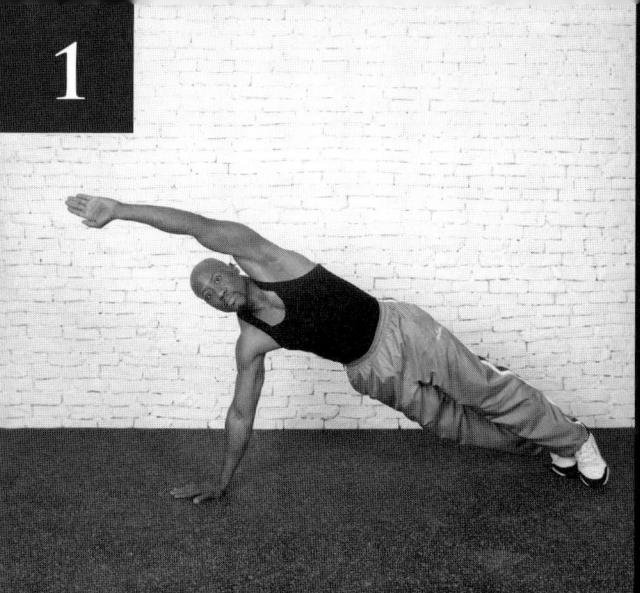

2

FIT TIP:

This is a strong core and abdominal building exercise.

Recommended: 2 to 5 sets with a minimum of 15 repetitions.

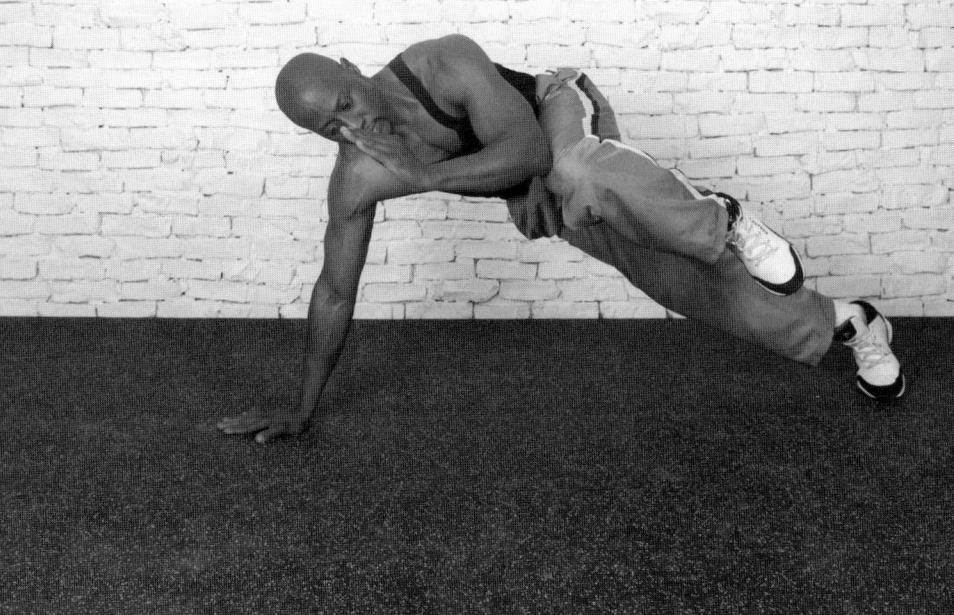

3

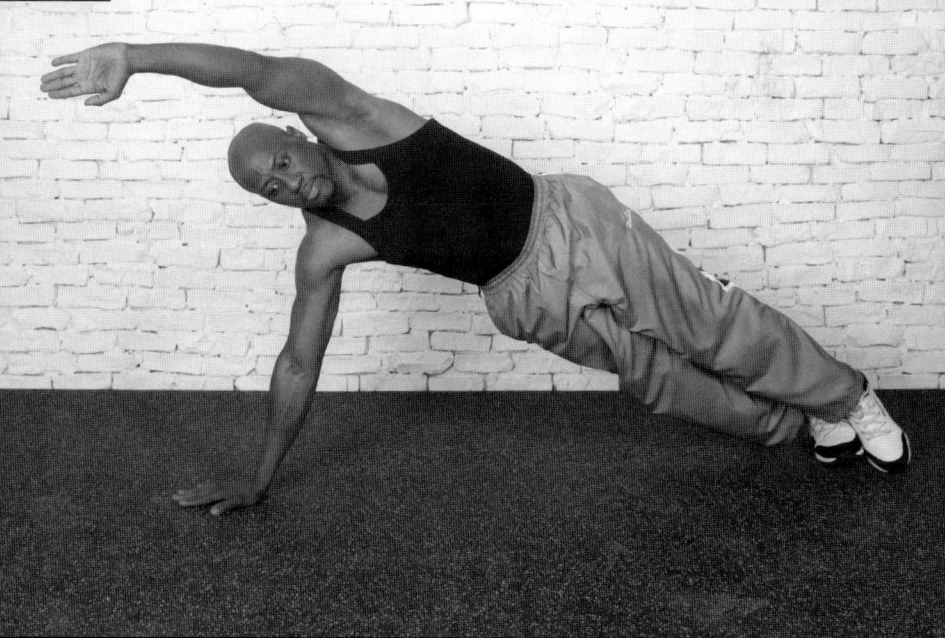

The exercise is done by starting in a side plank position as shown with one hand above the head and extended. If the right hand is downward then the left hand is above the head and the left elbow is brought to the left knee in a balanced manner. Again, the left elbow is brought to the left knee while remaining in the side plank position.

Half-Ups

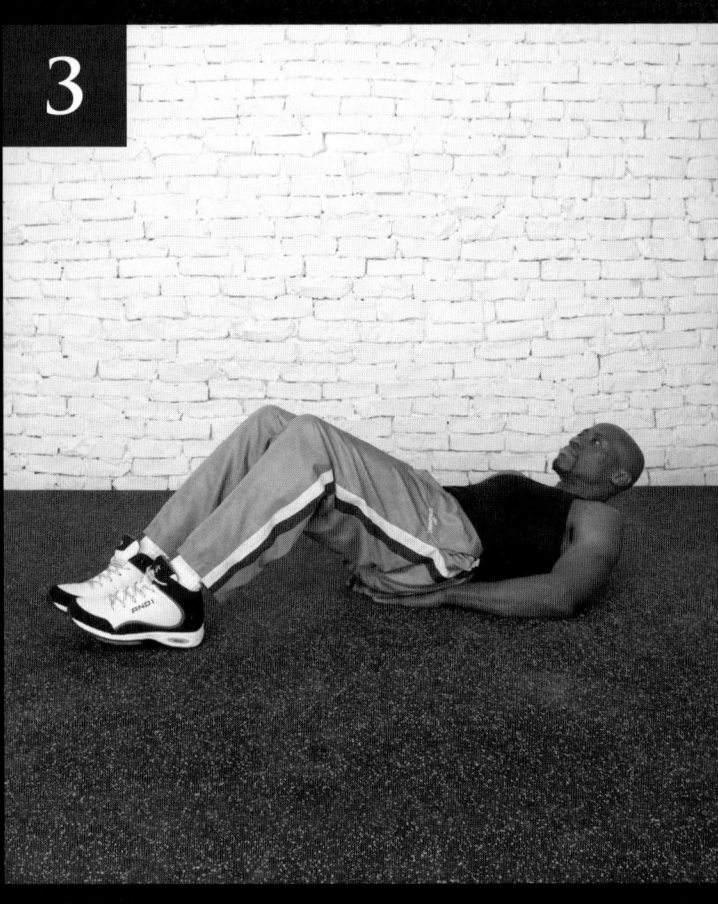

The exercise is started by lying on your back flat with your knees flexed and your hands under your buttocks. The knees are then lifted up approximately 6 inches off the ground and held. The feet are slowly lowered back down to the ground after the count of 15.

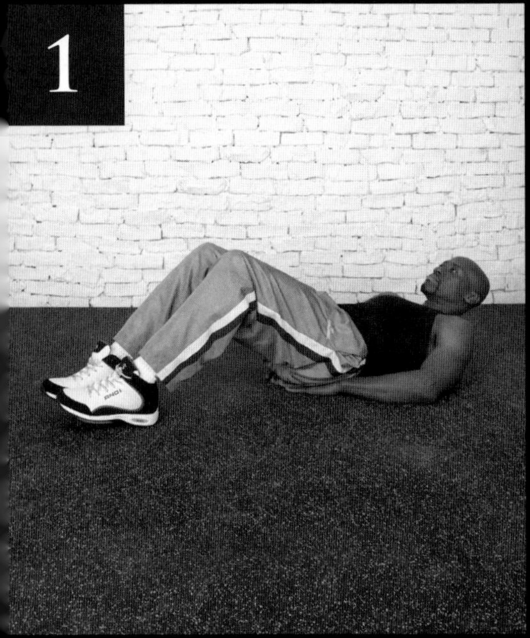

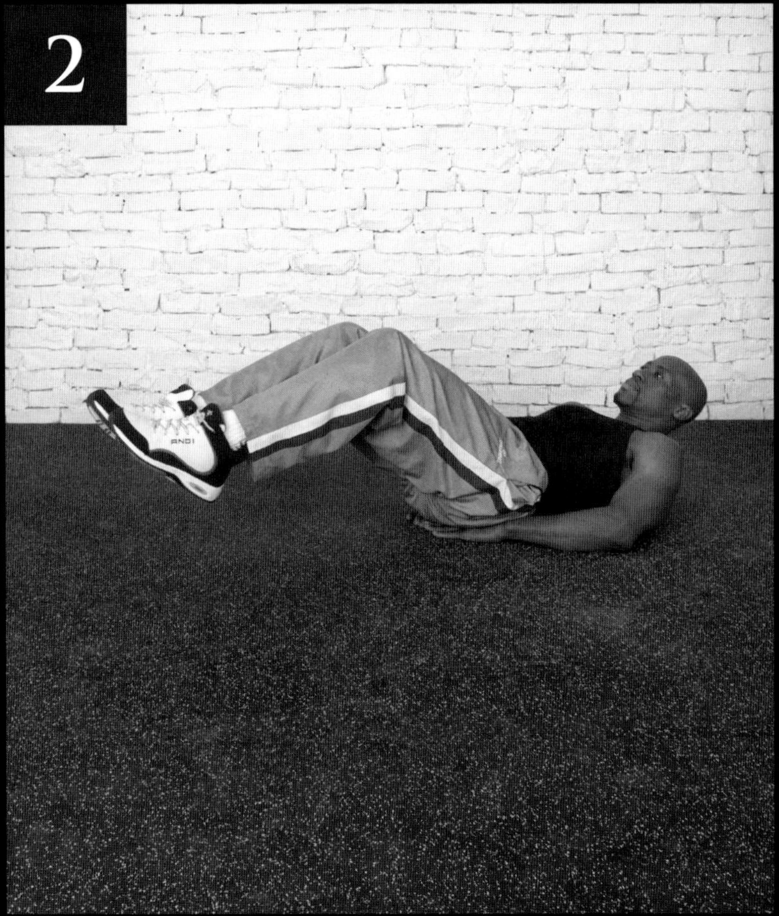

KNEE RAISES FROM THE 6-INCH POSITION

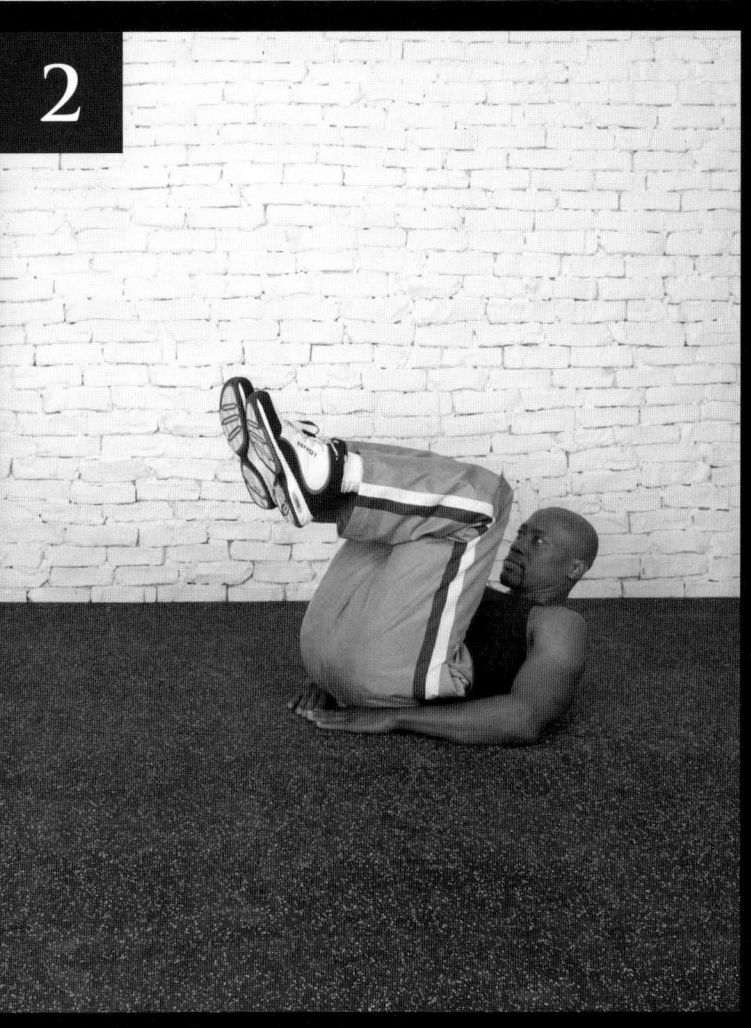

This exercise is done by starting with the hands under the buttocks, and the legs extended in front, 6 inches off the floor. This position is held. Next, the knees are brought toward the face and the shoulders are rolled forward toward the knees. Keep the neck relaxed and the hands under the buttocks. The knees are then extended. The feet are then placed back onto the floor.

FIT TIP:
Protect your lower back with your hands under your hips and buttocks.

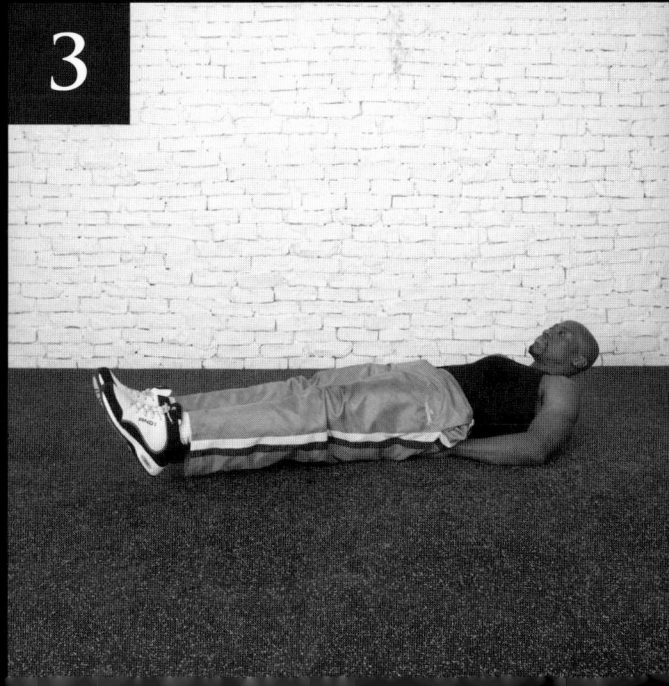

BALANCE PLANK

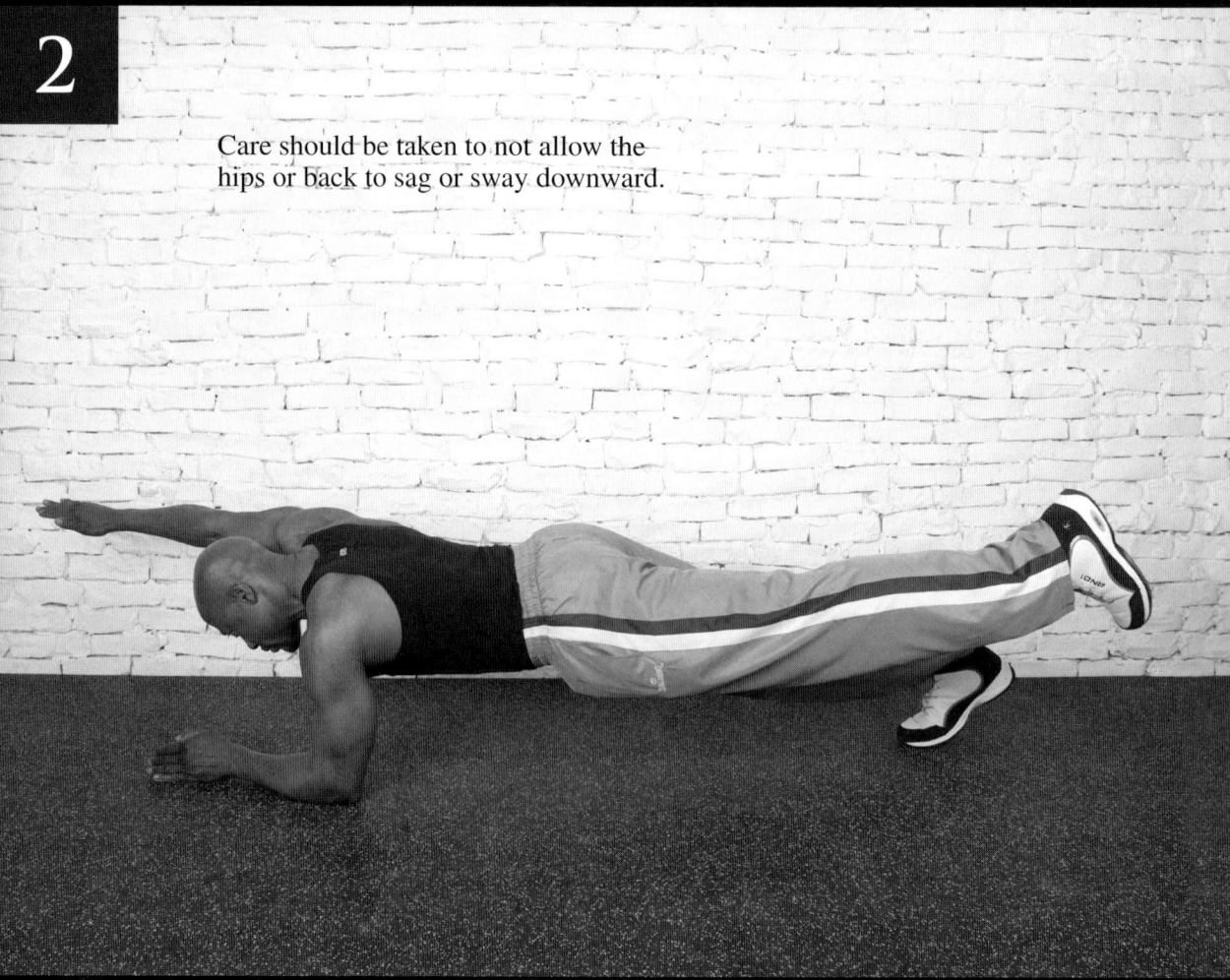

Start out in the regular plank position. The right arm should be elevated off the floor. The left leg should be elevated off the floor and the back should be kept straight, balancing on the floor with the left elbow and the right foot.

Care should be taken to not allow the hips or back to sag or sway downward.

BOSU Ball Plank

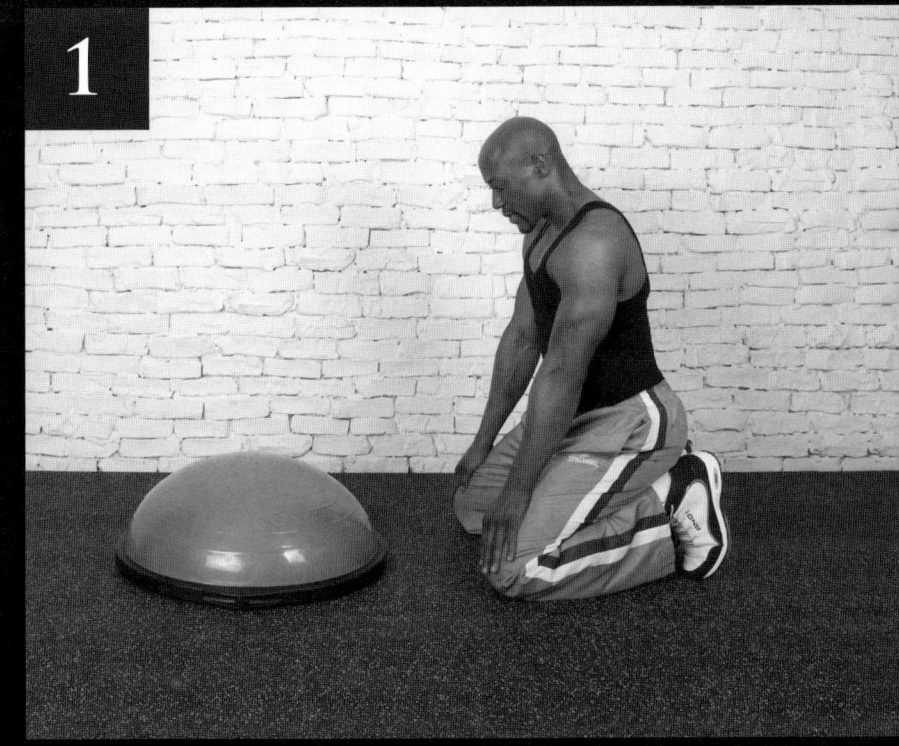

Recommended:
3 to 5 sets of
8 to 10 repetitions.

This exercise is executed by first beginning with the knees bent, hands and arms extended on top of the BOSU ball. The legs are straightened and this position is held for 30 seconds to 1 minute.

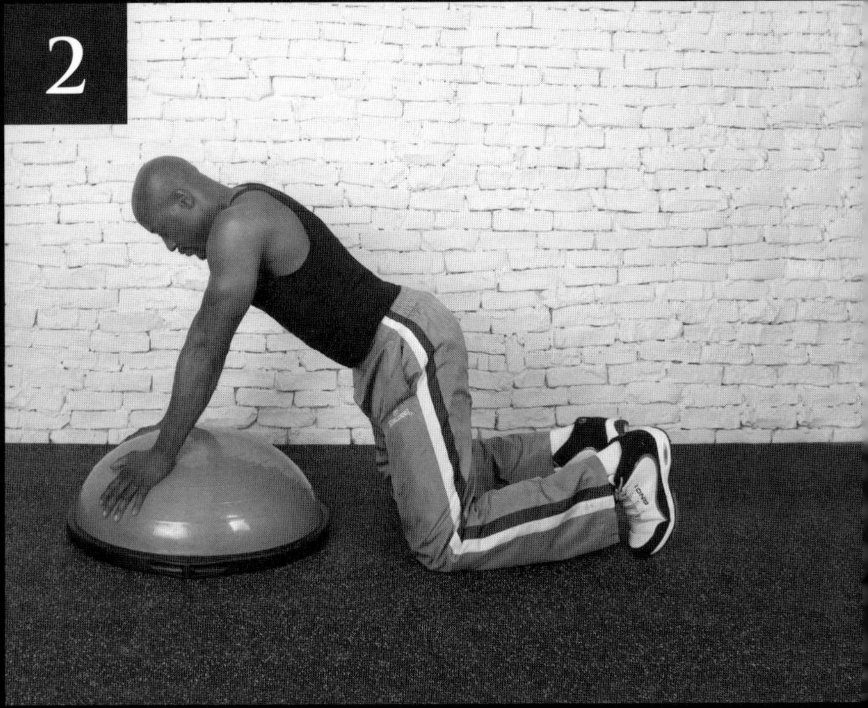

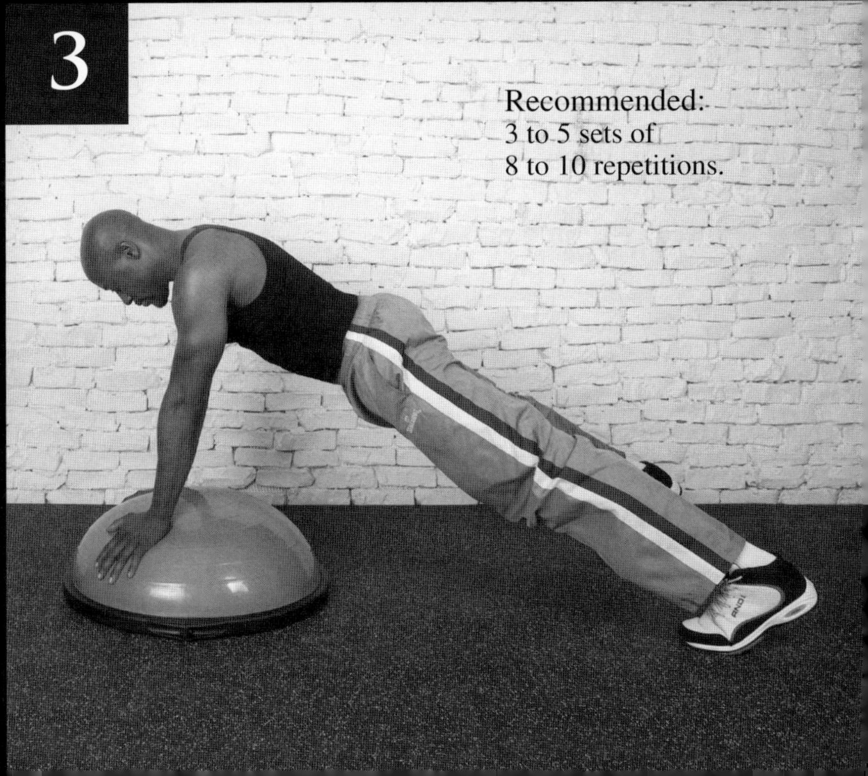

BOSU BALL HYPEREXTENSION BALANCE PLANK

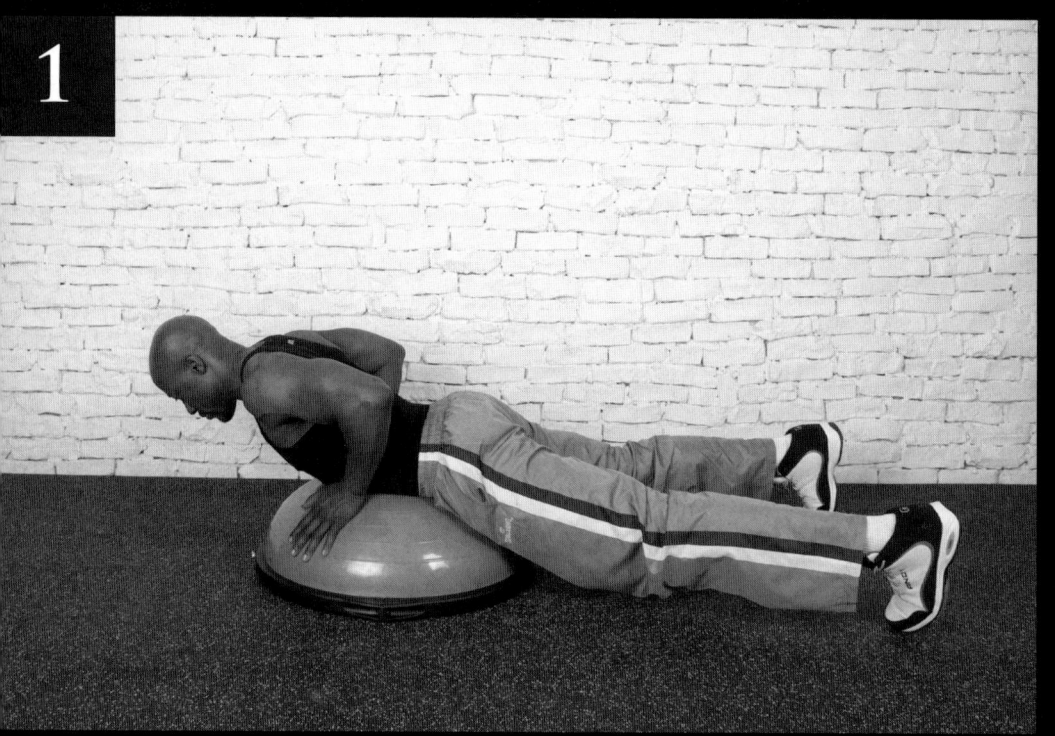

FIT TIP:
Hold this position for 15-30 seconds for 2 to 3 sets of 3 repetitions.

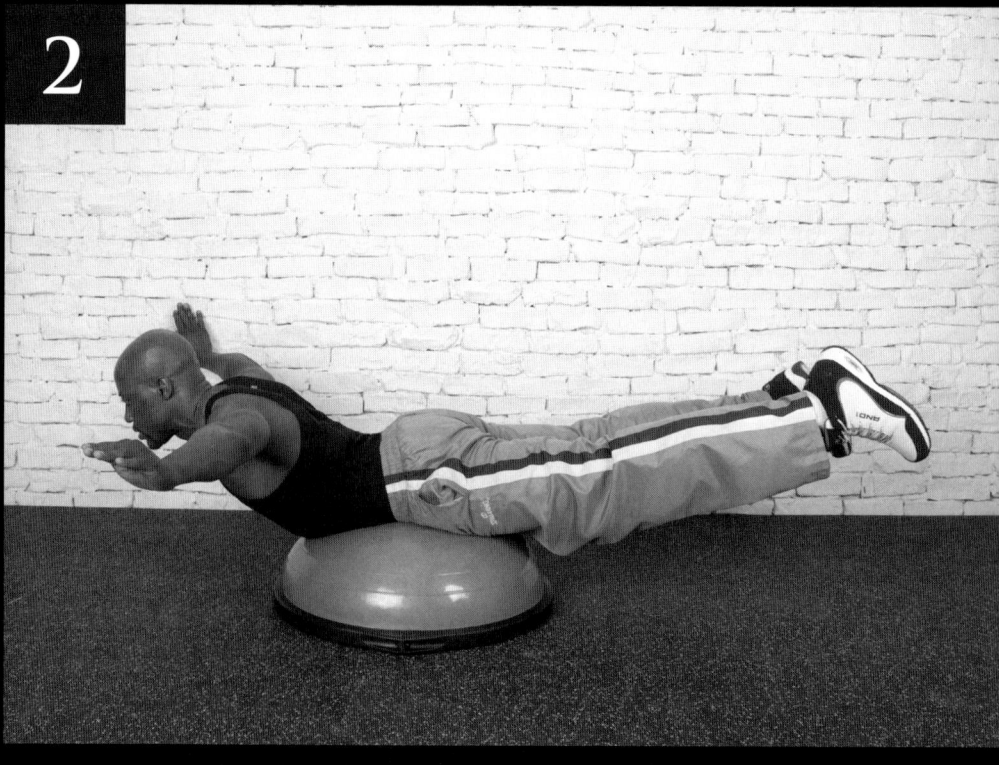

The exercise is done by initially placing the hips directly over the center of the BOSU ball, the arms are extended in front, and the legs are then lifted behind, and this position is held with mild hyperextension of the back and contracture of the abdominal core muscles.

One-Arm Side Plank

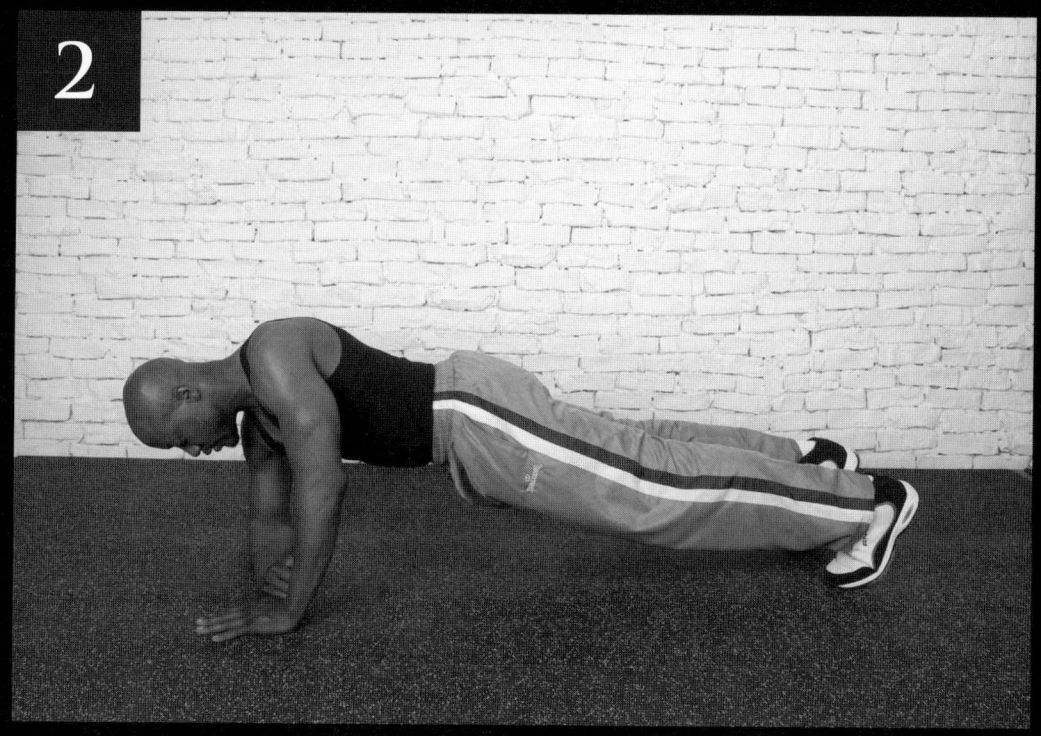

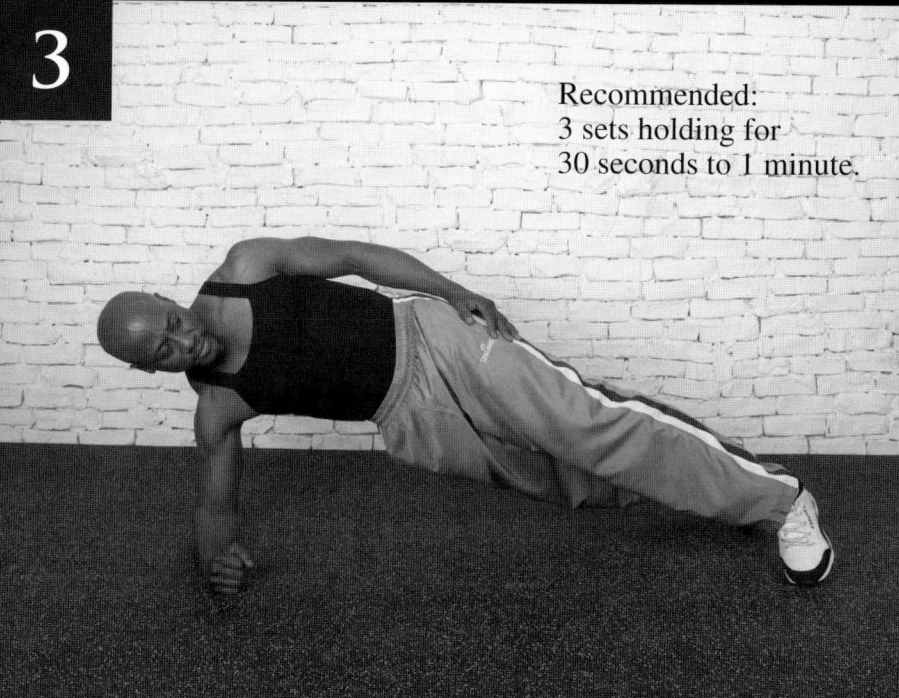

Recommended: 3 sets holding for 30 seconds to 1 minute.

This exercise starts by lying on your side or hip. Then, lift your body upright onto your elbow. The feet can be slightly separated or you can have your feet together. Hold position for 30 seconds to 1 minute. This exercise can be done by starting out in the regular push-up position, then place one elbow down on the ground and then lift the other arm to the side. The feet can be together or slightly apart.

Double Balance Elbow Plank

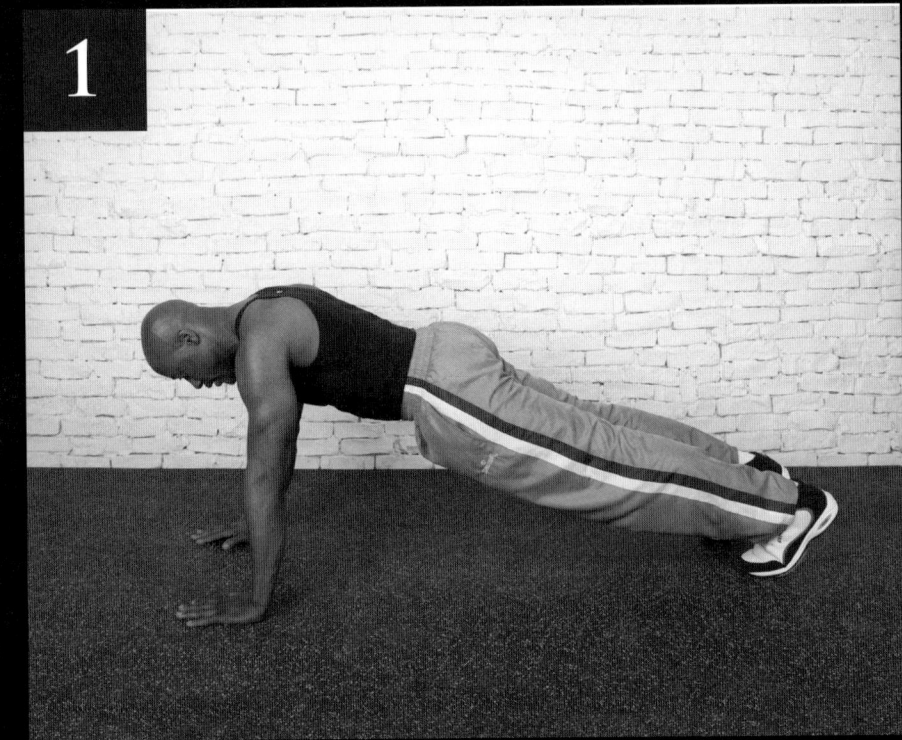

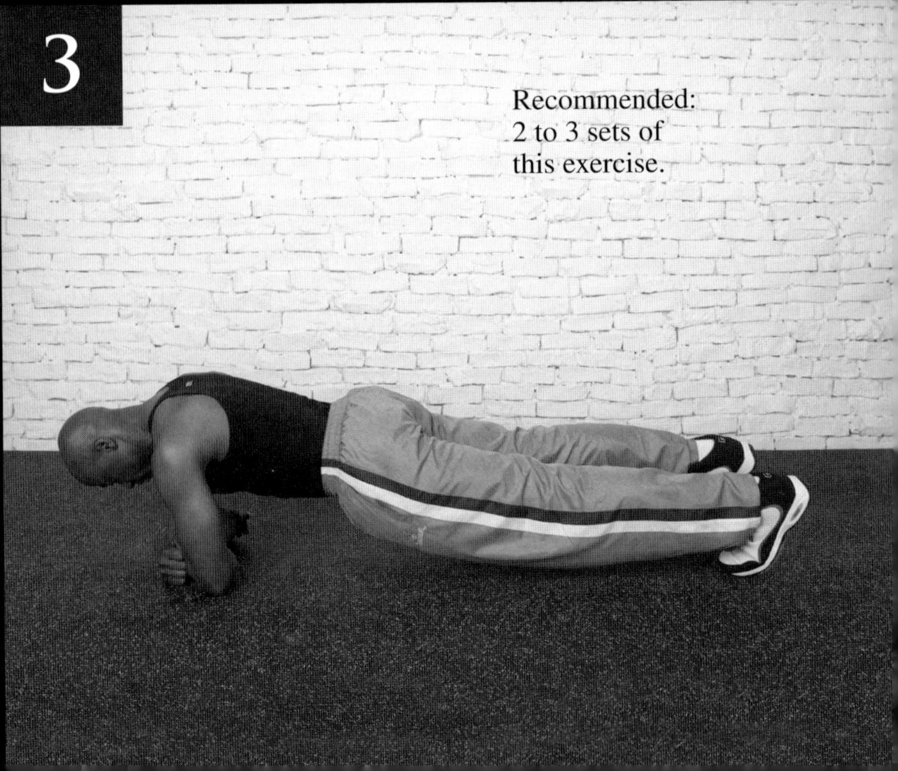

Recommended: 2 to 3 sets of this exercise.

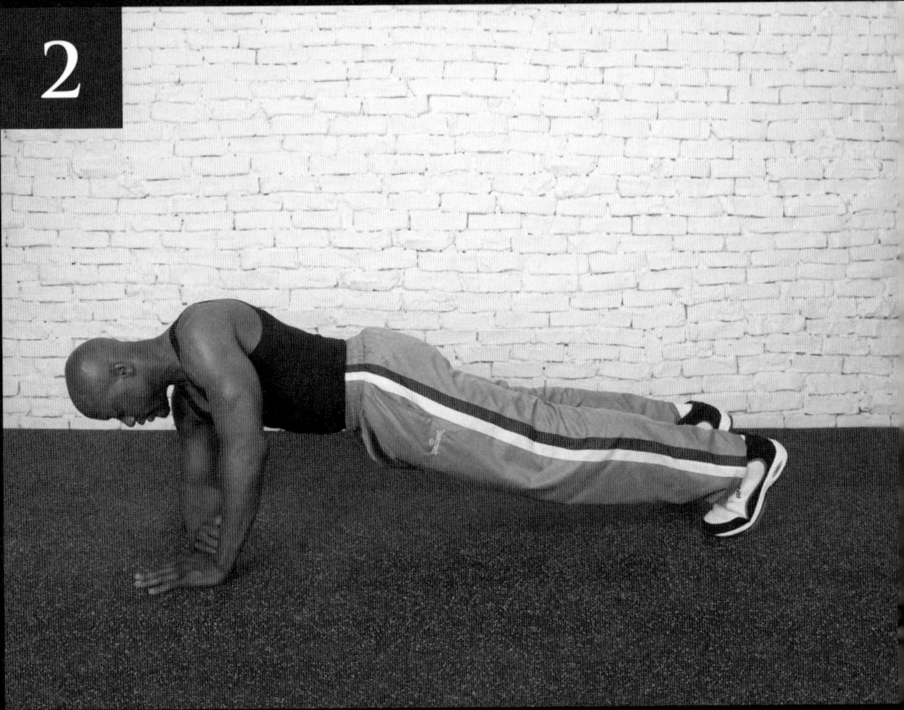

Start in the regular push-up position. One elbow is placed on the floor followed by the other elbow on the floor and both forearms are under the chest. This position should be held for 30 seconds to 1 minute.

REGULAR ABDOMINAL CRUNCH

1

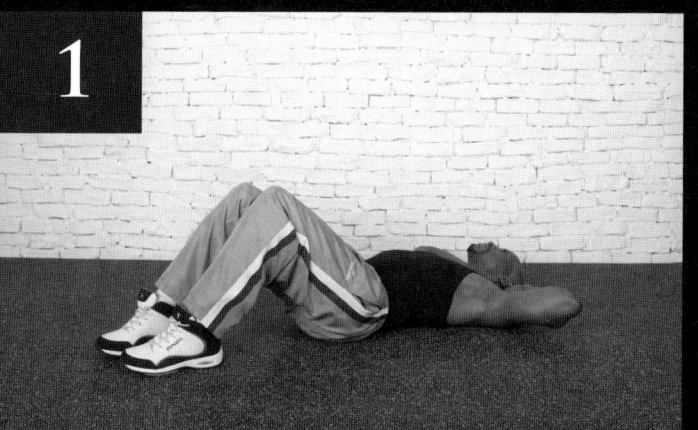

Lie on the floor with the knees together and flexed with the hands slightly below your ears. Do not place the hands on the neck.

2

The shoulders are curled forward toward the thighs, lifting the head with the chin off the chest. Avoid tucking the chin toward the chest. Lift the head up gently and then down. The shoulders should be curled forward toward the chest.

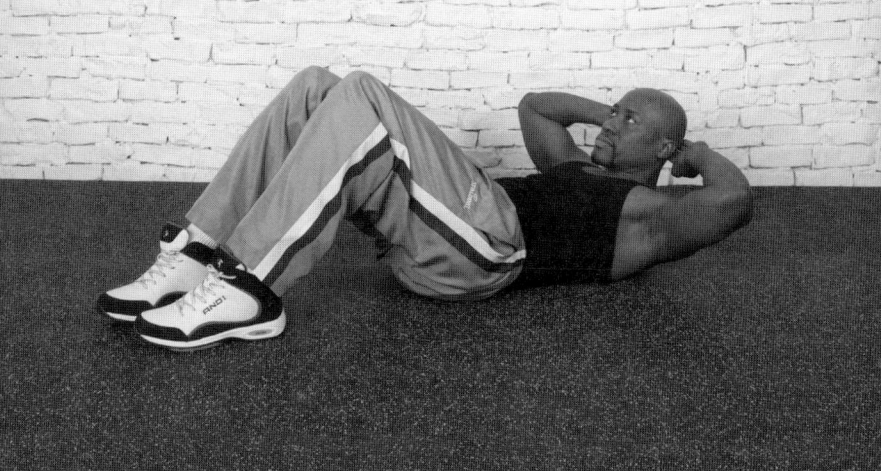

3

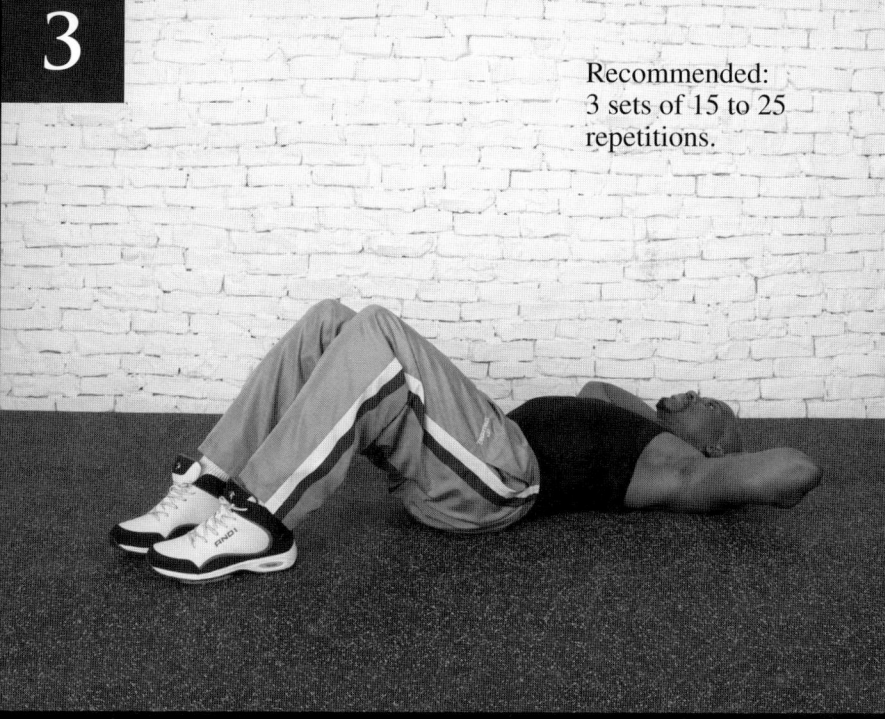

Recommended: 3 sets of 15 to 25 repetitions.

The key is curling the shoulders toward the pelvis and keeping the hands behind the ears. I recommend focusing on a mark on the wall or ceiling when you lift and curl upward and forward. Your hands can be placed to support the weight of the head; however, no force should be exerted on the neck during this exercise. As you come forward, you contract your abdominals. I recommend curling up 35 to 50 degrees forward.

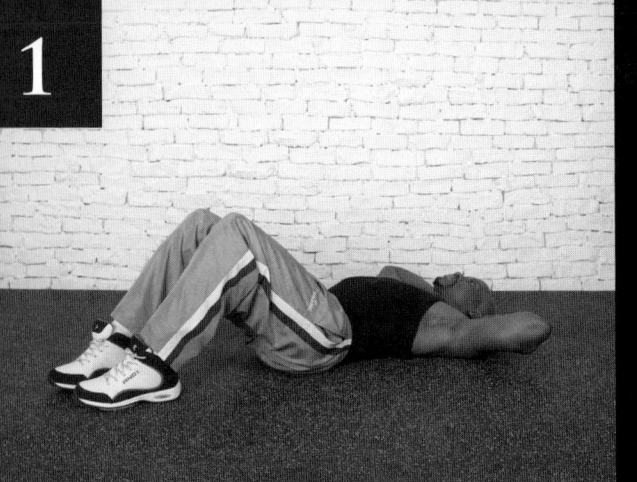

ELEVATED LEG CRUNCH

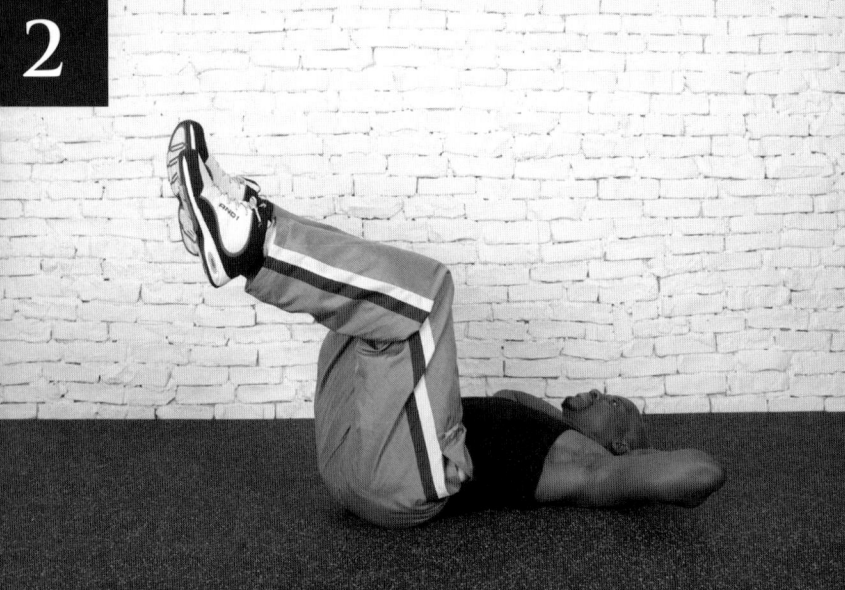

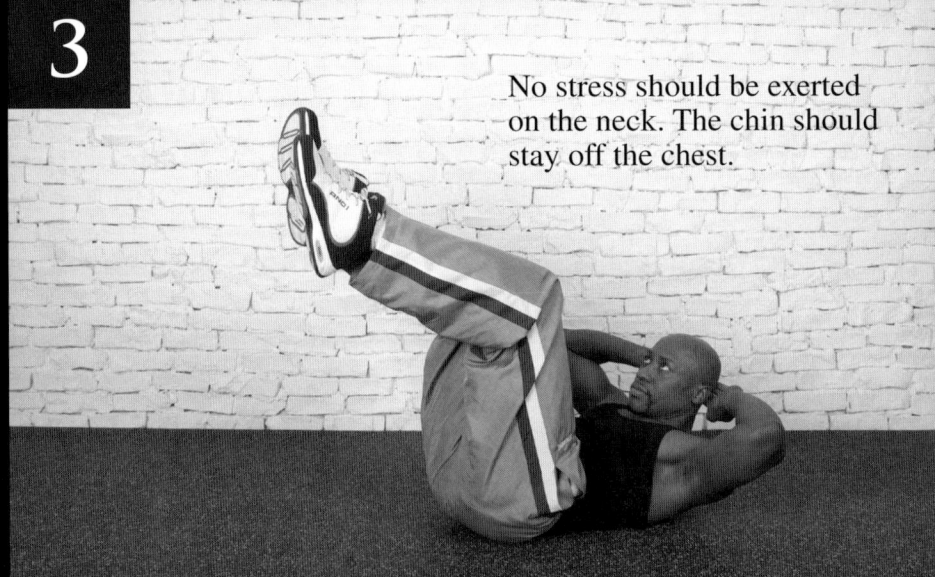

No stress should be exerted on the neck. The chin should stay off the chest.

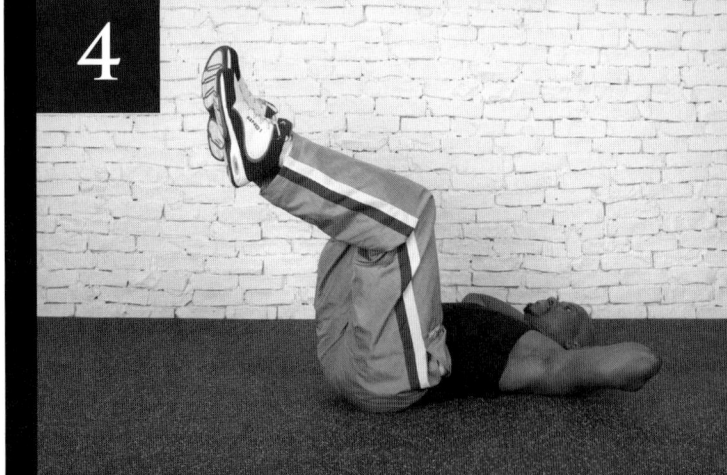

Start out in the regular sit-up position with the feet forward and knees bent or flexed. The hands should be behind the head at the level above or slightly below the ears. The knees are flexed to 90 degrees or 115 degrees, and the shoulders are curled forward toward the thighs.

Extended Leg Crunch

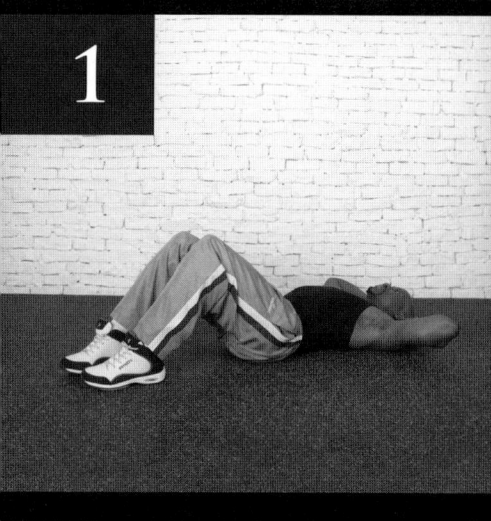

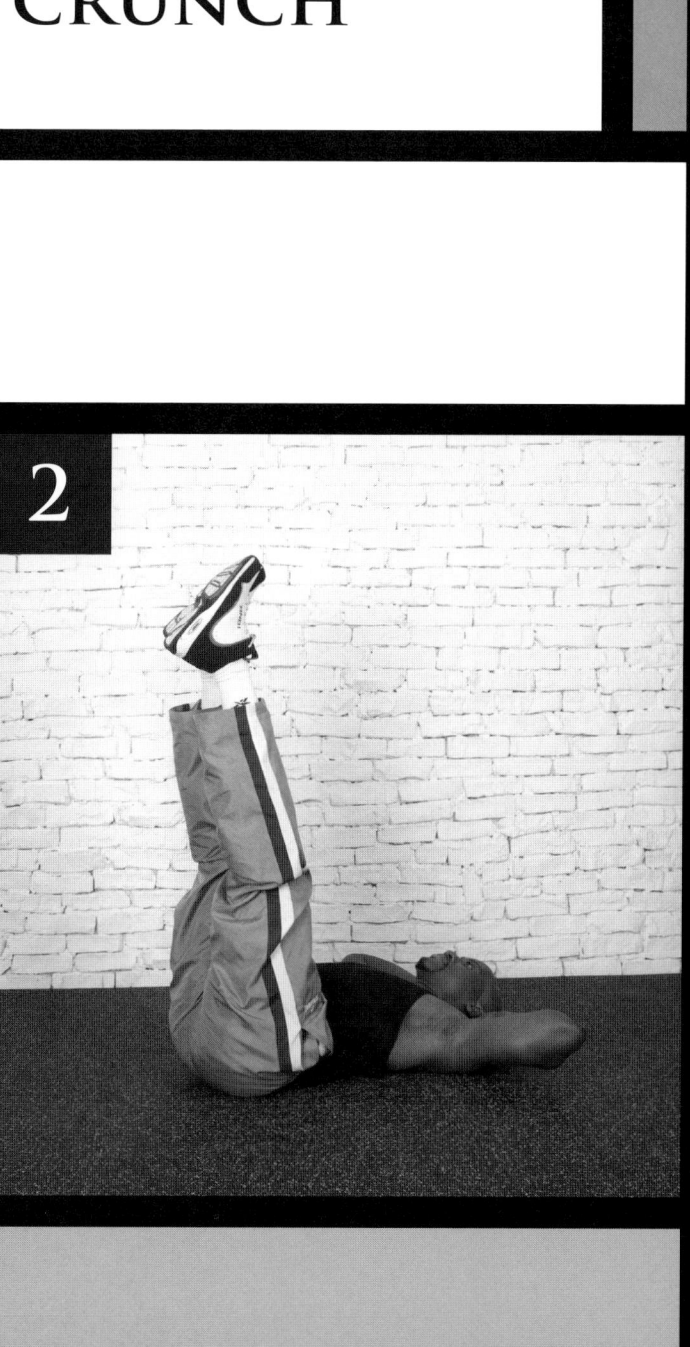

Starting out in a regular sit-up position, the legs are extended upward focusing on the toes. The shoulders should curl toward the thighs and knees, keeping the elbows bent without exerting pressure on the nape of the neck. The torso should be brought forward and then relaxed back downward. The legs should be brought back down to the floor.

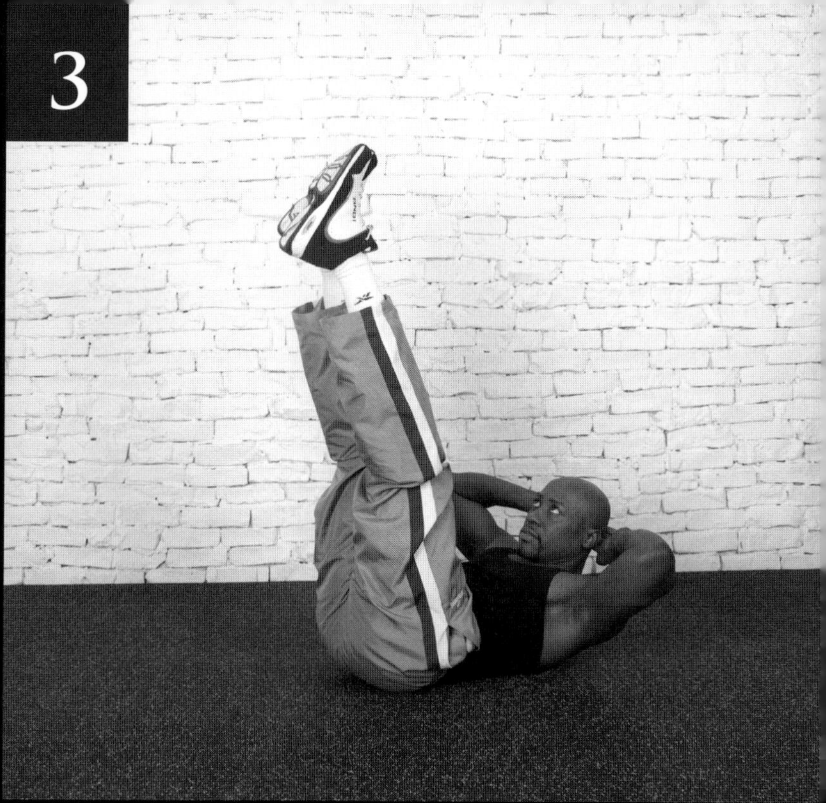

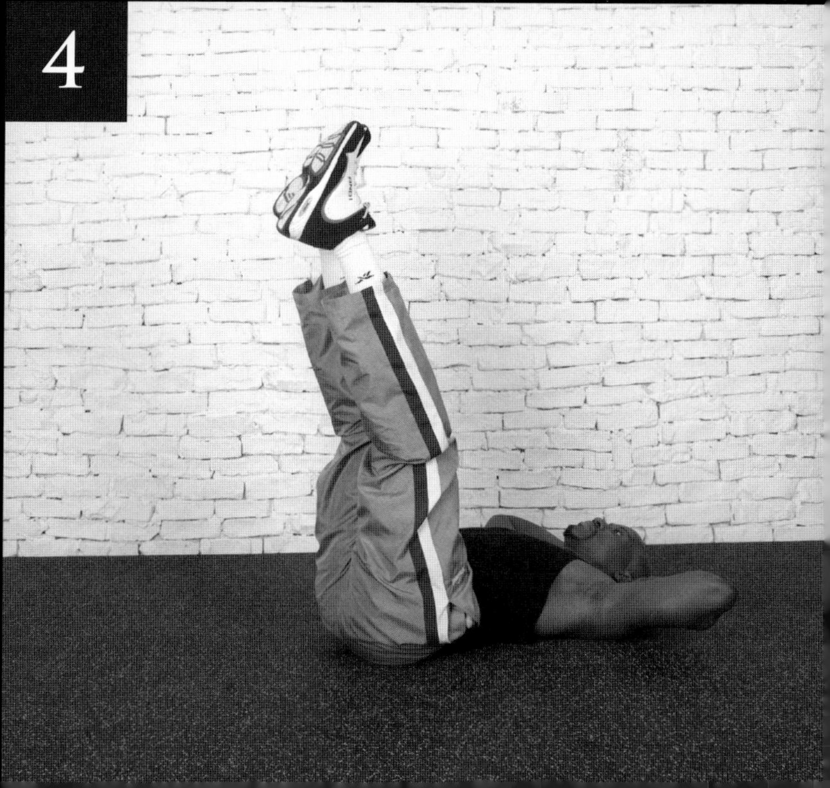

Seated Leg Lifts

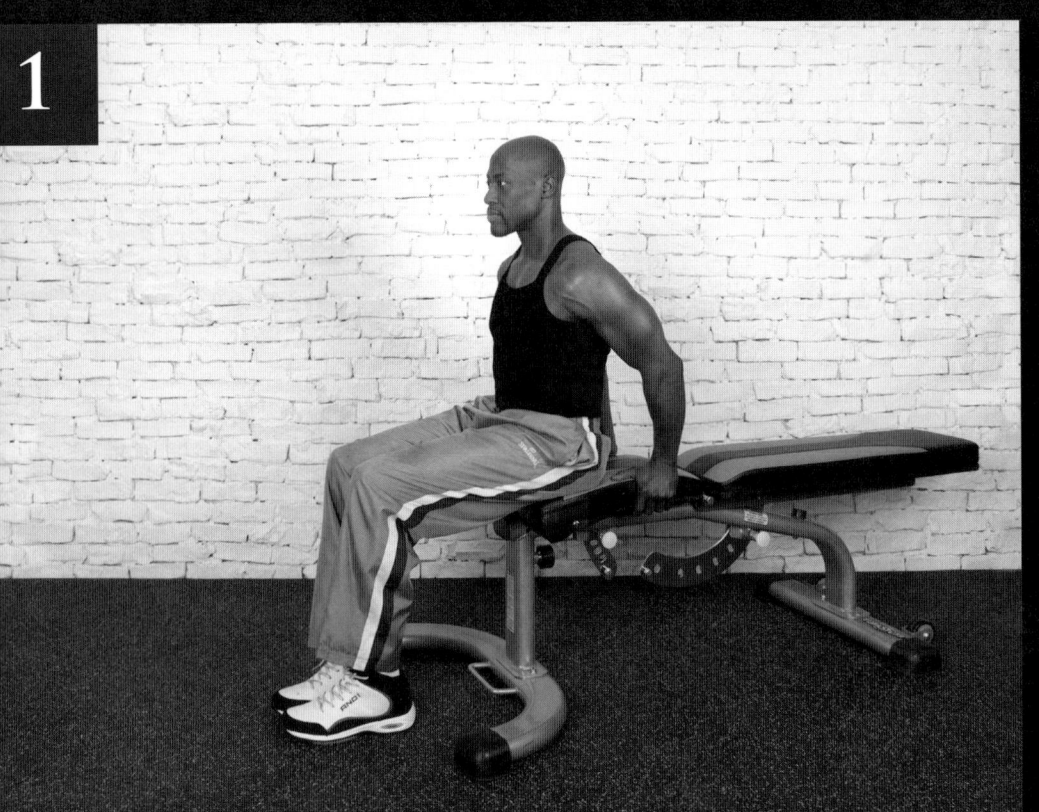

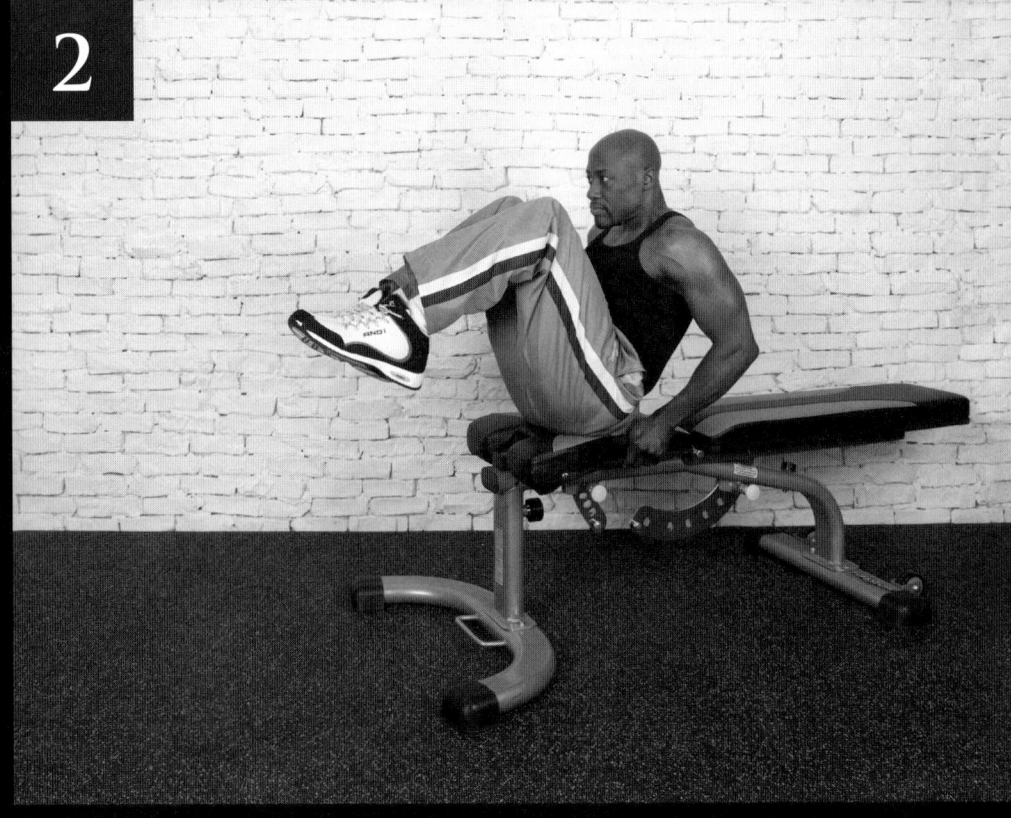

Sit at the edge of a bench or chair. The knees are brought to the chest. Then the legs are extended in front. The knees are then brought back up to the chest. The knees and the feet are then lowered to the floor.

Recommended:
3 sets of 15 to 25 repetitions.

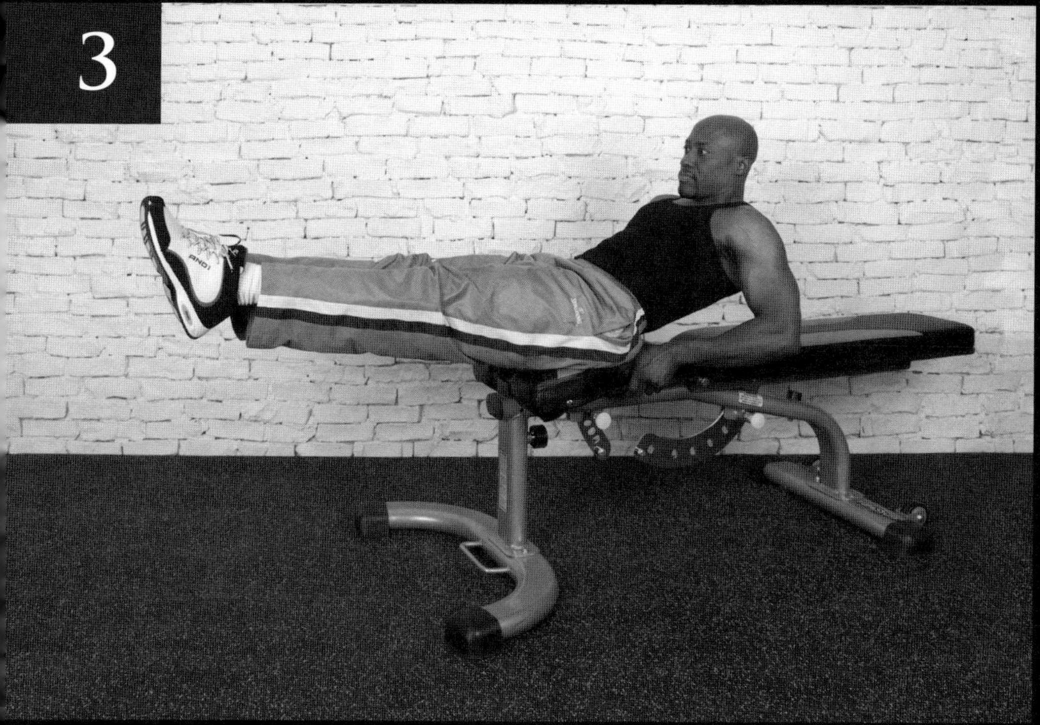

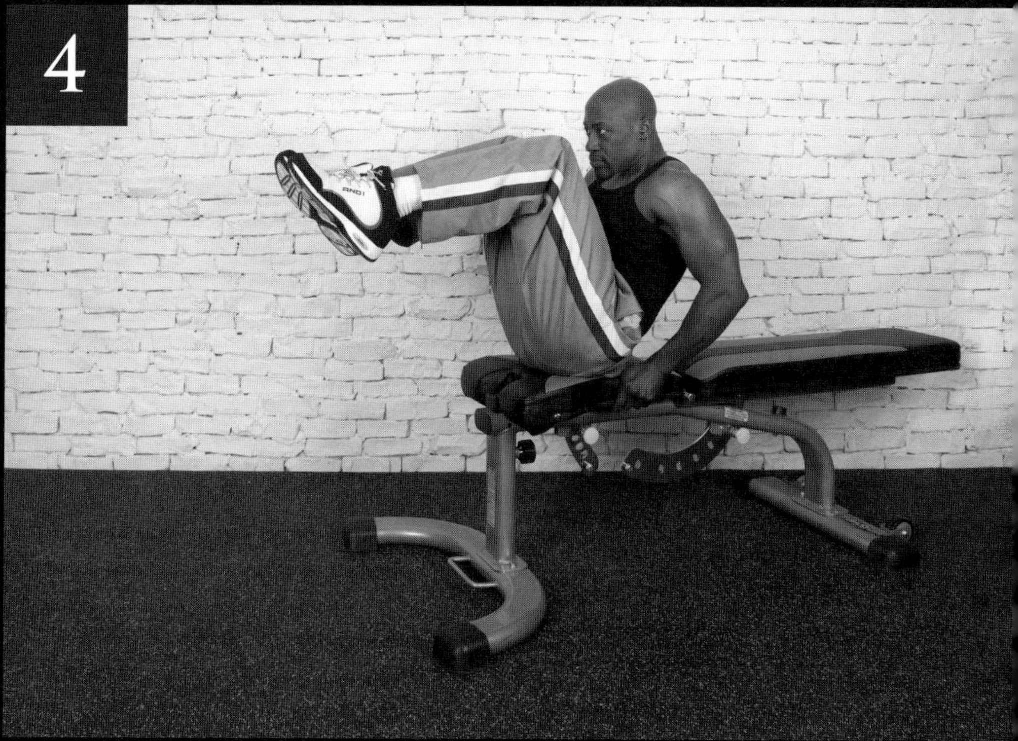

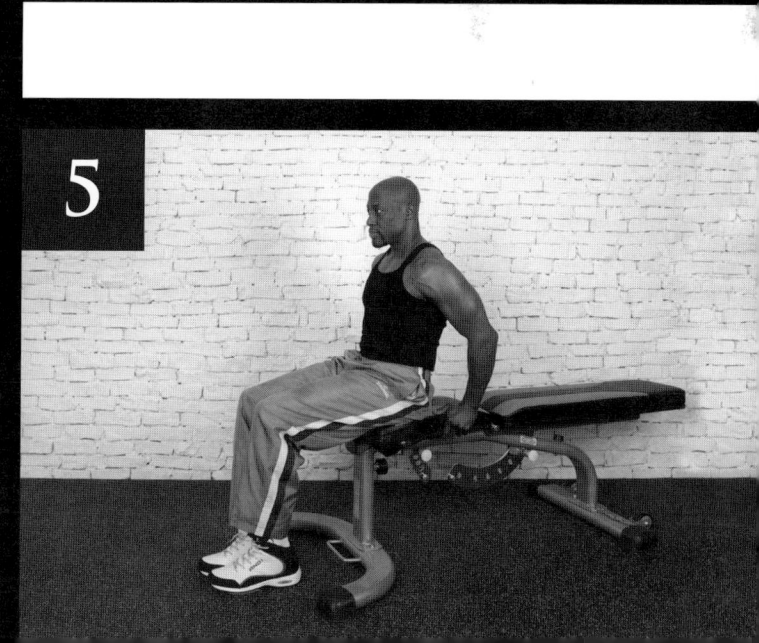

Combined V-Ups and Leg Lifts

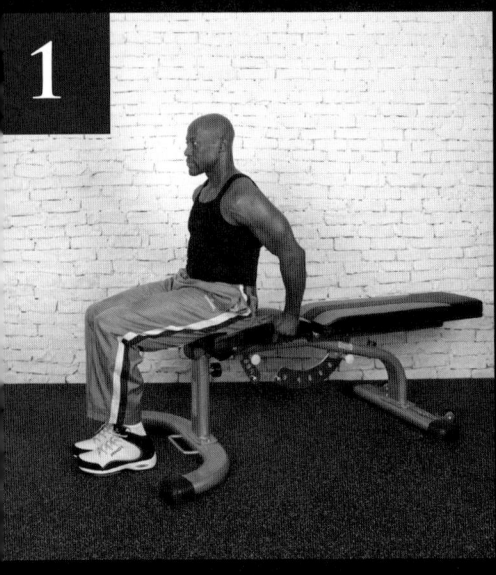

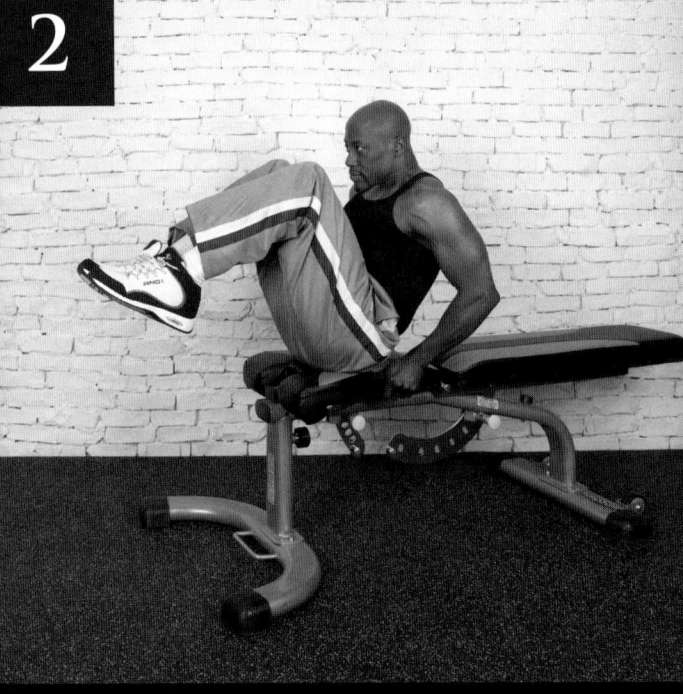

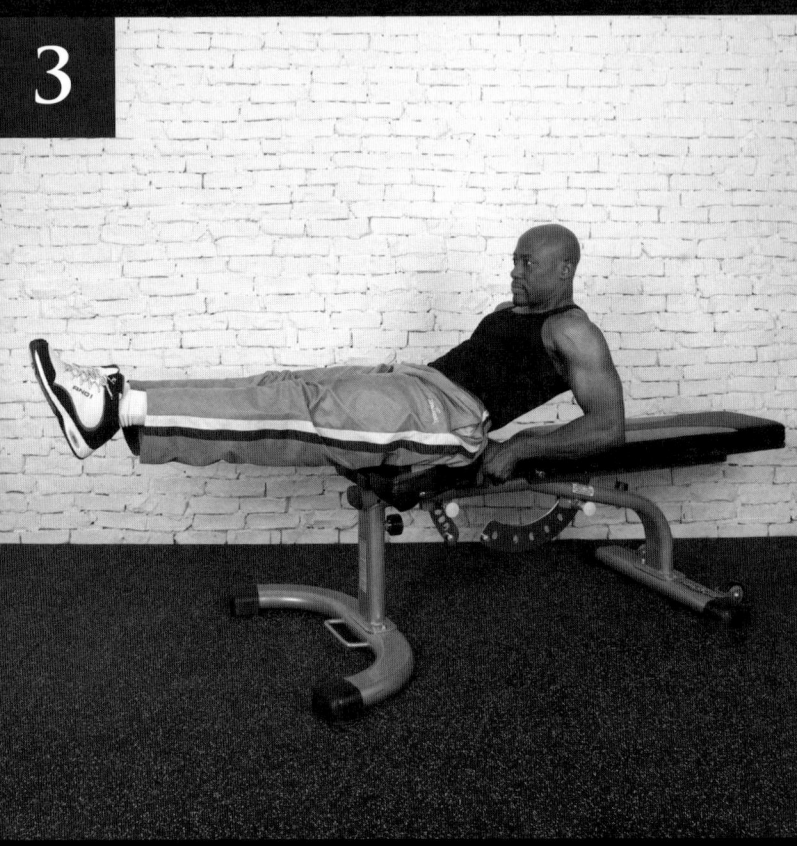

Sit at the edge of a bench or chair. Bring the knees up to the body. Extend the legs forward. Bring the extended legs back up toward the chest with the legs as straight as possible. Lower the legs in front straight. Bring the knees back up to the chest. Then, lower the legs and feet to the floor.

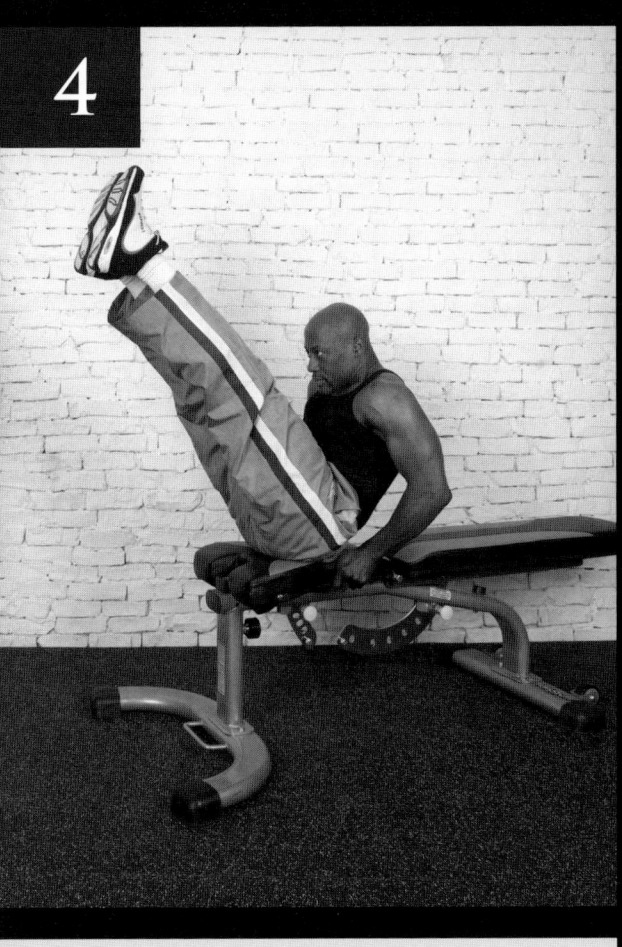

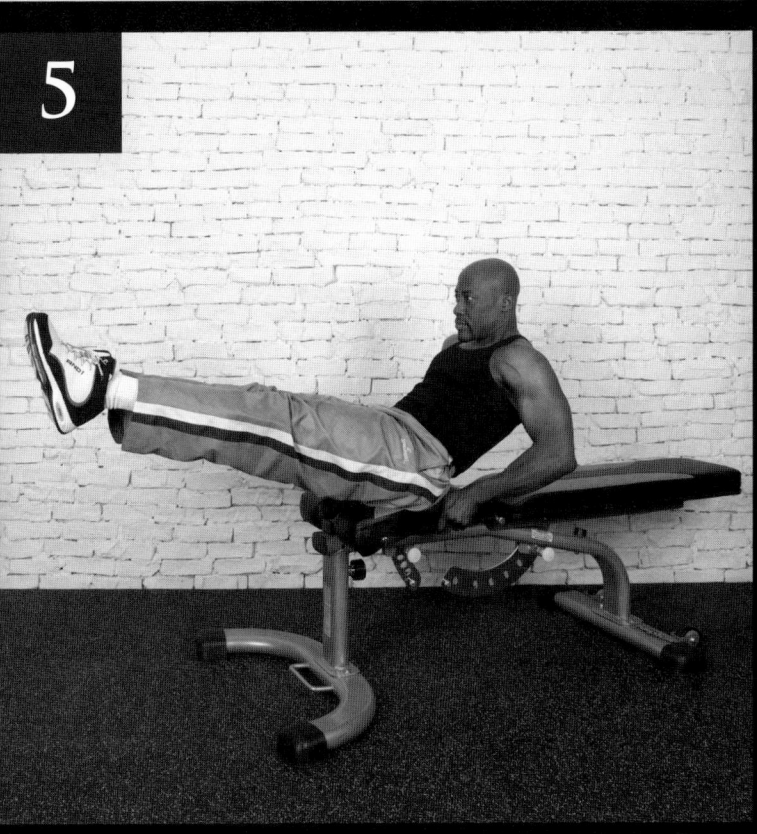

FIT TIP:
Hold this position for 15-30 seconds for 2 to 3 sets of 3 repetitions.

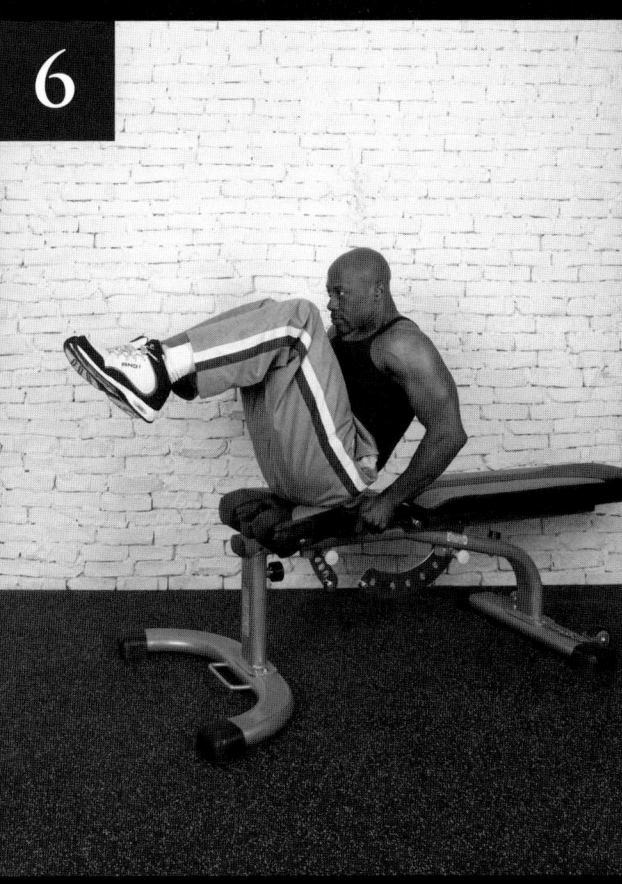

Recommended:
3 to 5 sets of
10 to 15 repetitions.

Overhead Leg Lift

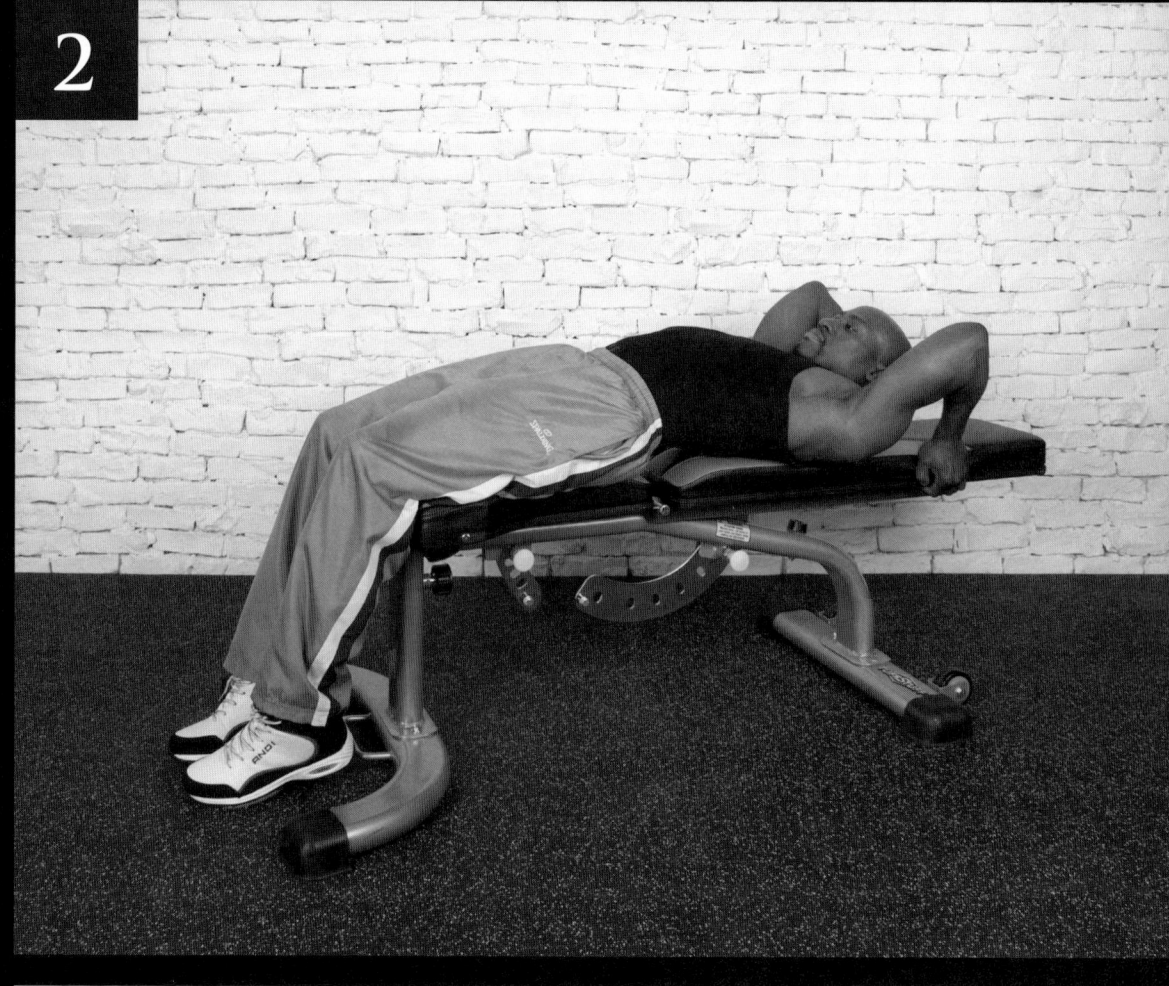

Sit at the edge of the exercise bench or chair. Lie backwards with the feet firmly on the floor. Bring your hands behind your head. Lift your knees up toward your chest keeping your back flat against the bench. Elevate your pelvis and legs overhead and gently bring your back off the chair with the knees bent. Then, slowly lower your back against the bench.

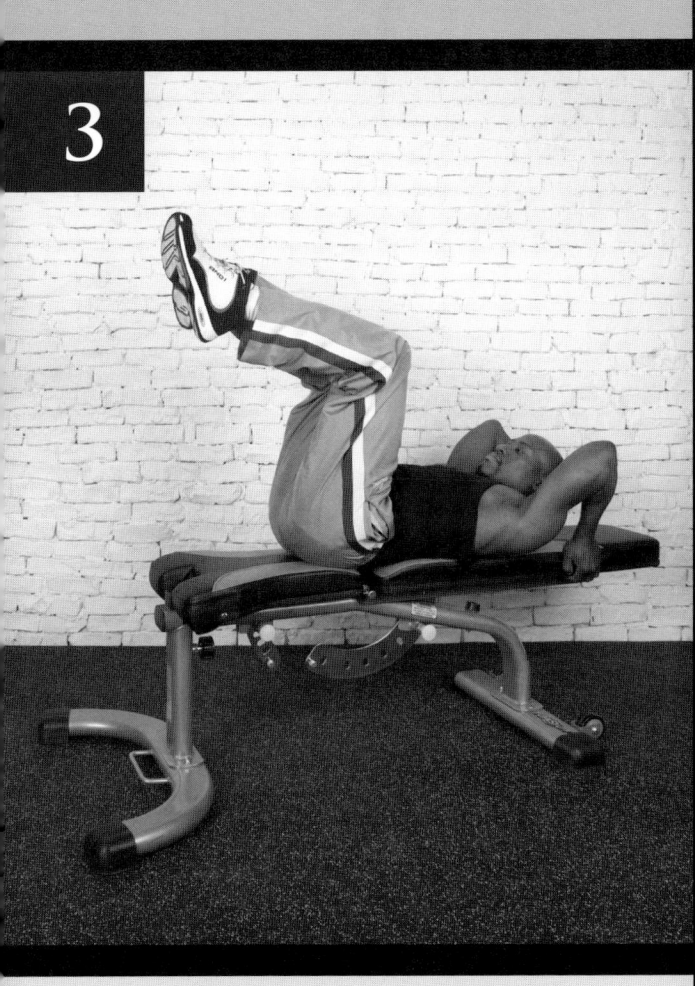

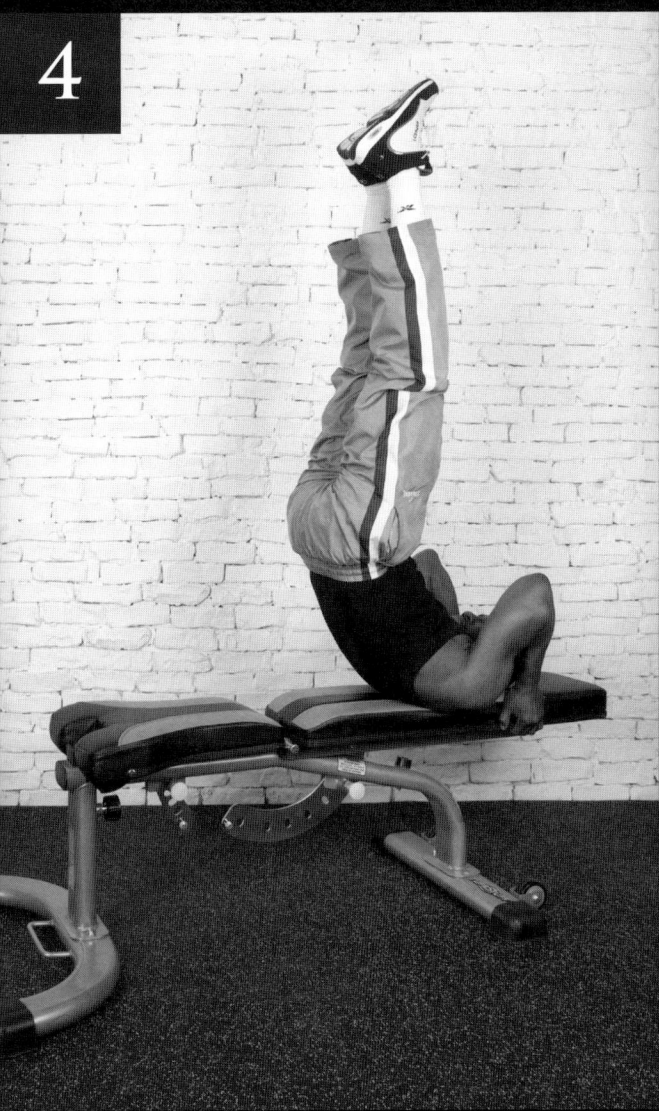

Recommended:
3 to 5 sets of
10 to 15 repetitions.

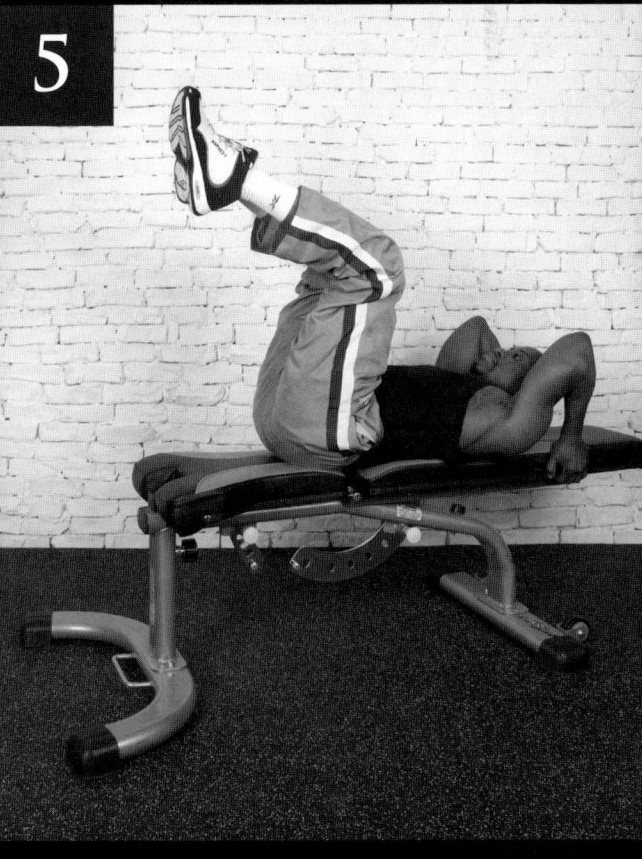

"Superman" Overhead Leg Lifts

Lie with your back against the bench, with your feet off the floor, with the knees flexed to 90 degrees. Put your hands behind your head holding onto the bench. Lift and extend your knees up above your chest and lift your pelvis and back upward off the bench.

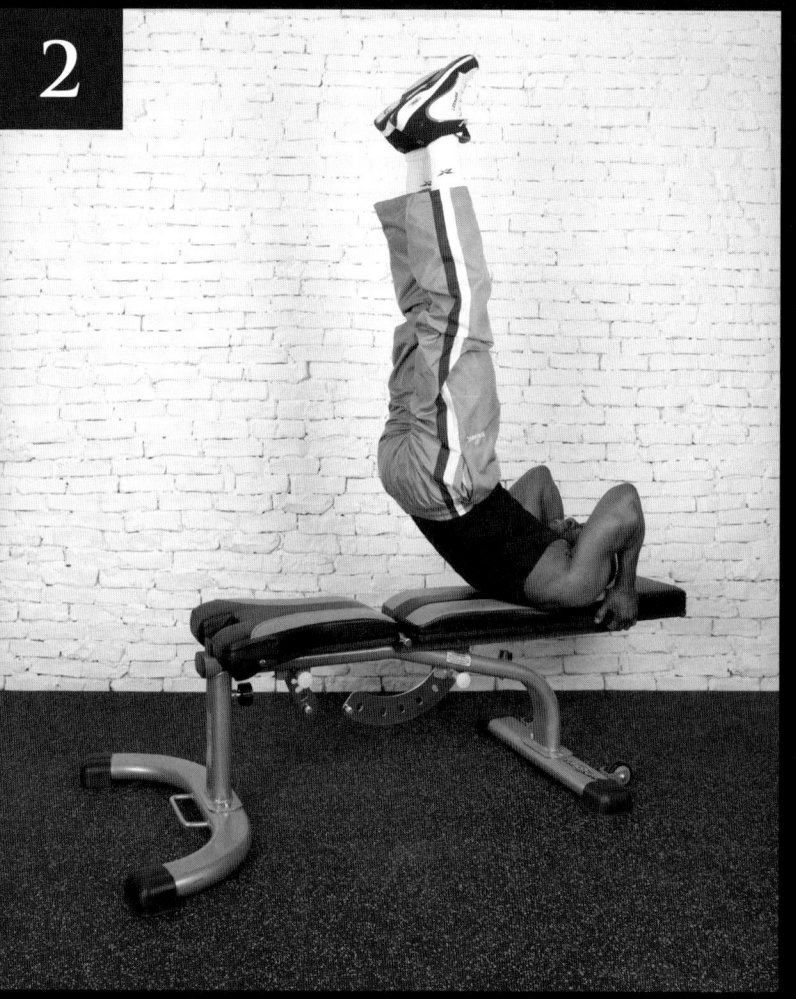

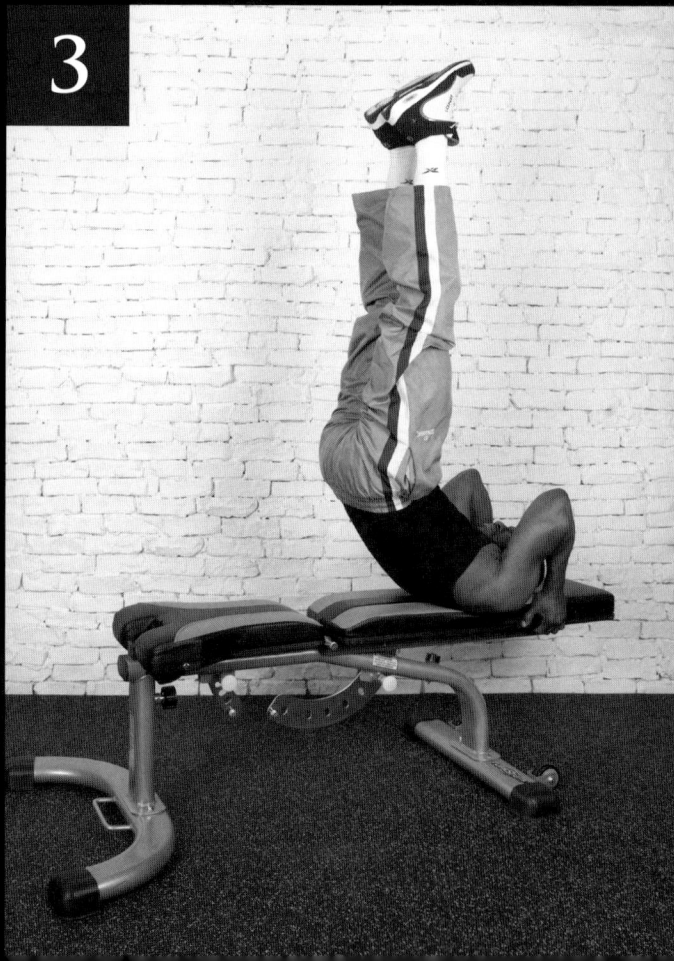

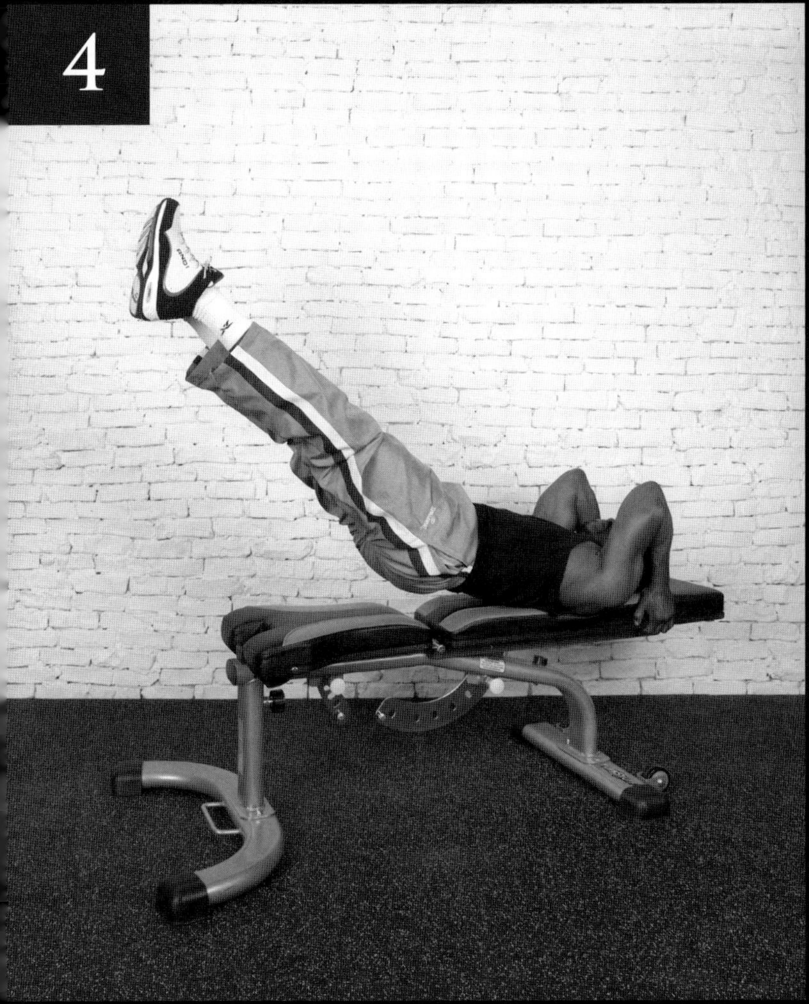

5

Recommended:
3 to 5 sets of
10 to 15 repetitions.

4

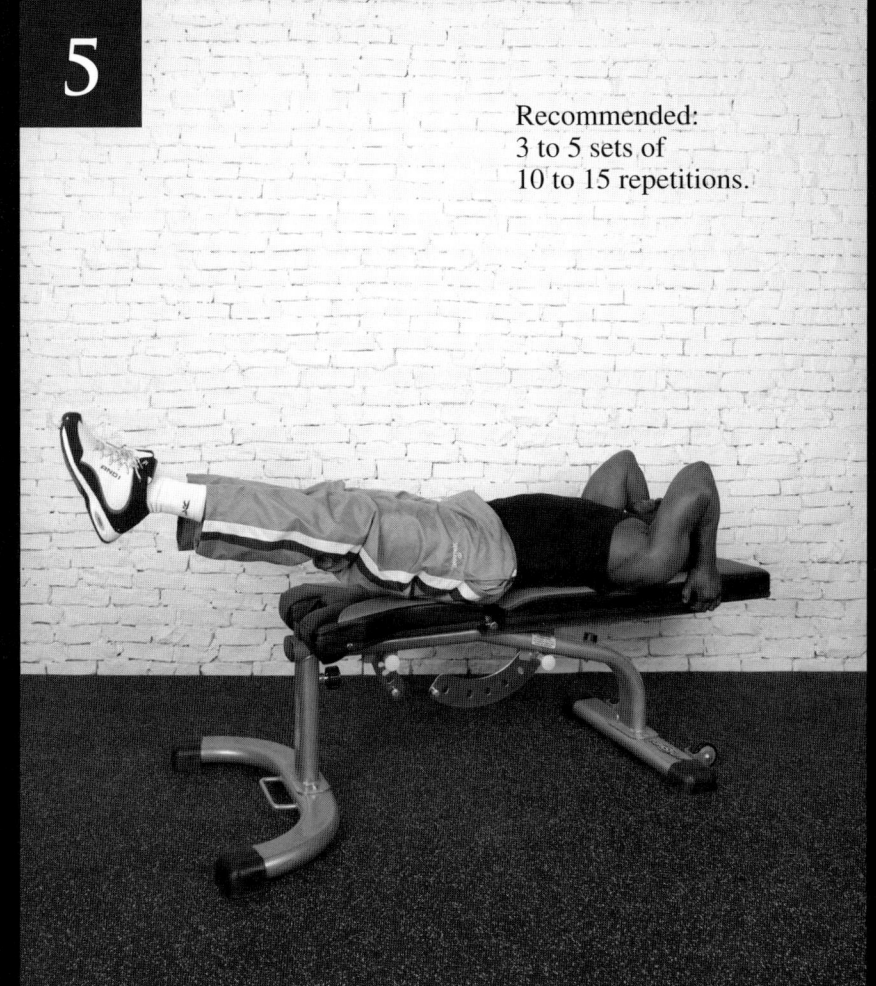

Slowly, lower your legs downward with your legs straight and back straight. Lower your body down to the bench and complete the exercise by bringing your feet to the floor.

6

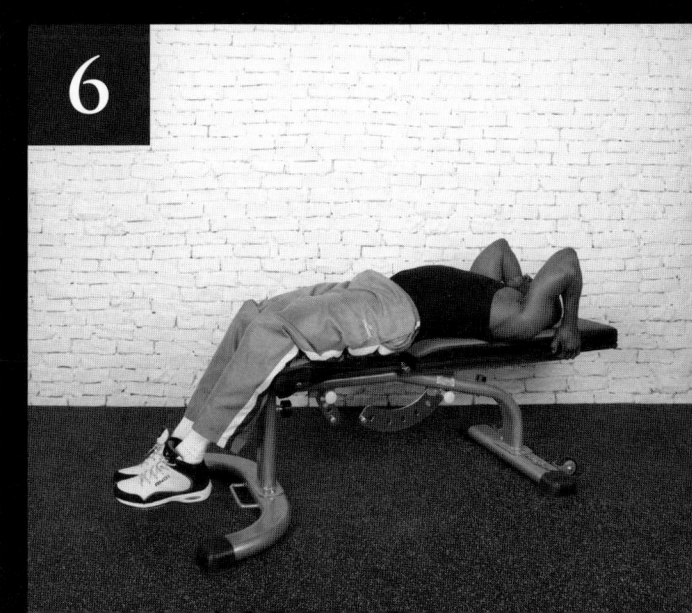

PLANK EXERCISE
Also Called The Elbow Bridge Plank Exercise

Start from a push-up position and then place both elbows on the floor. Hold the position for 15-30 seconds for 2 to 3 repetitions.

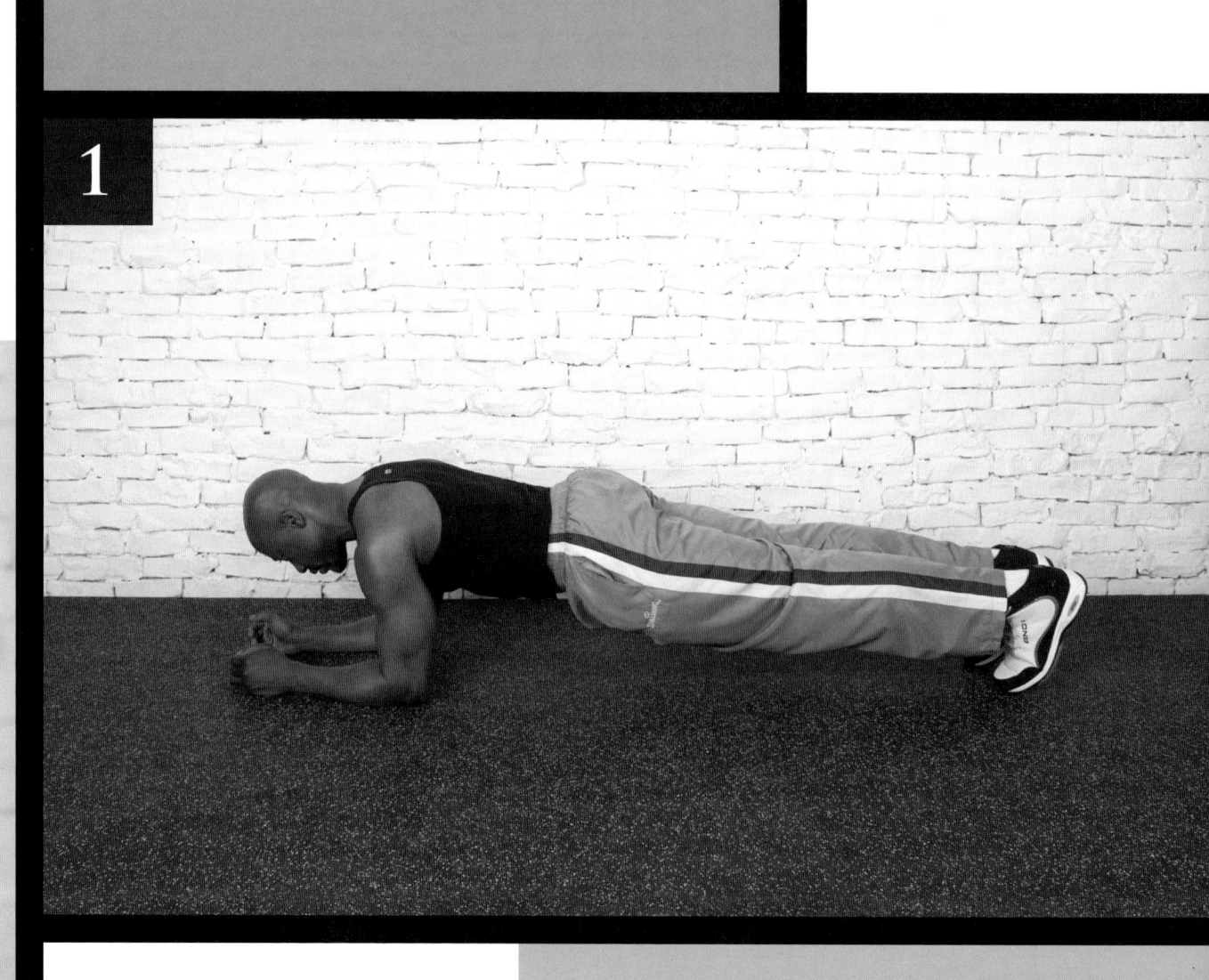

The Captain's Chair Core Position

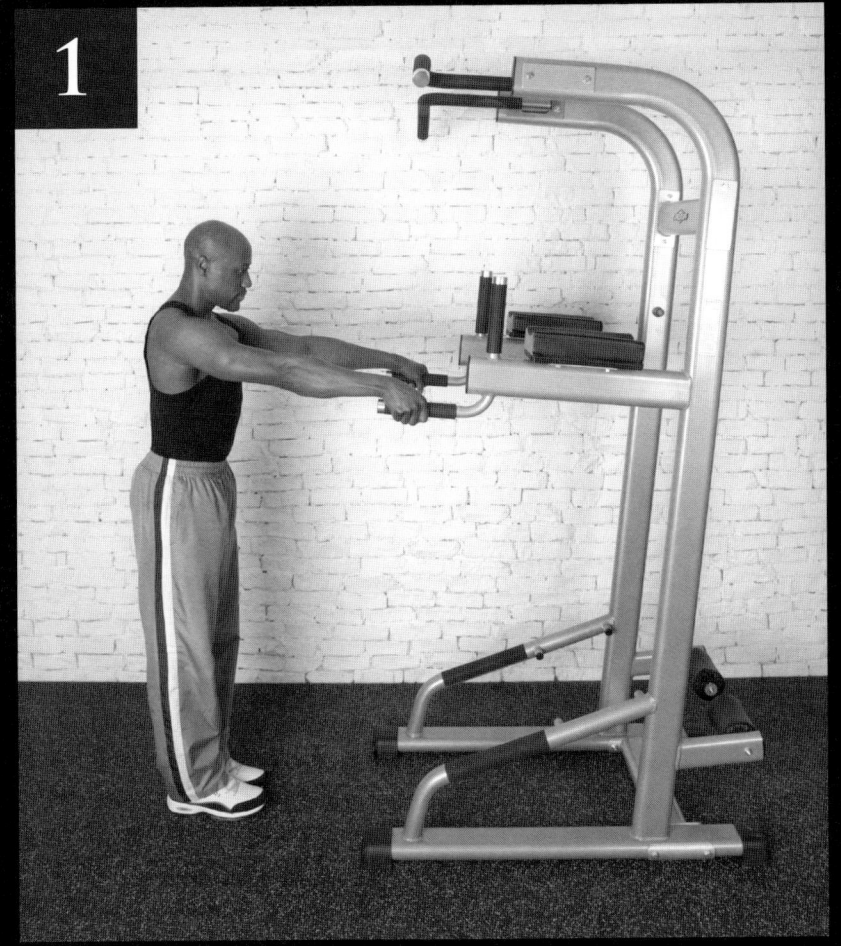

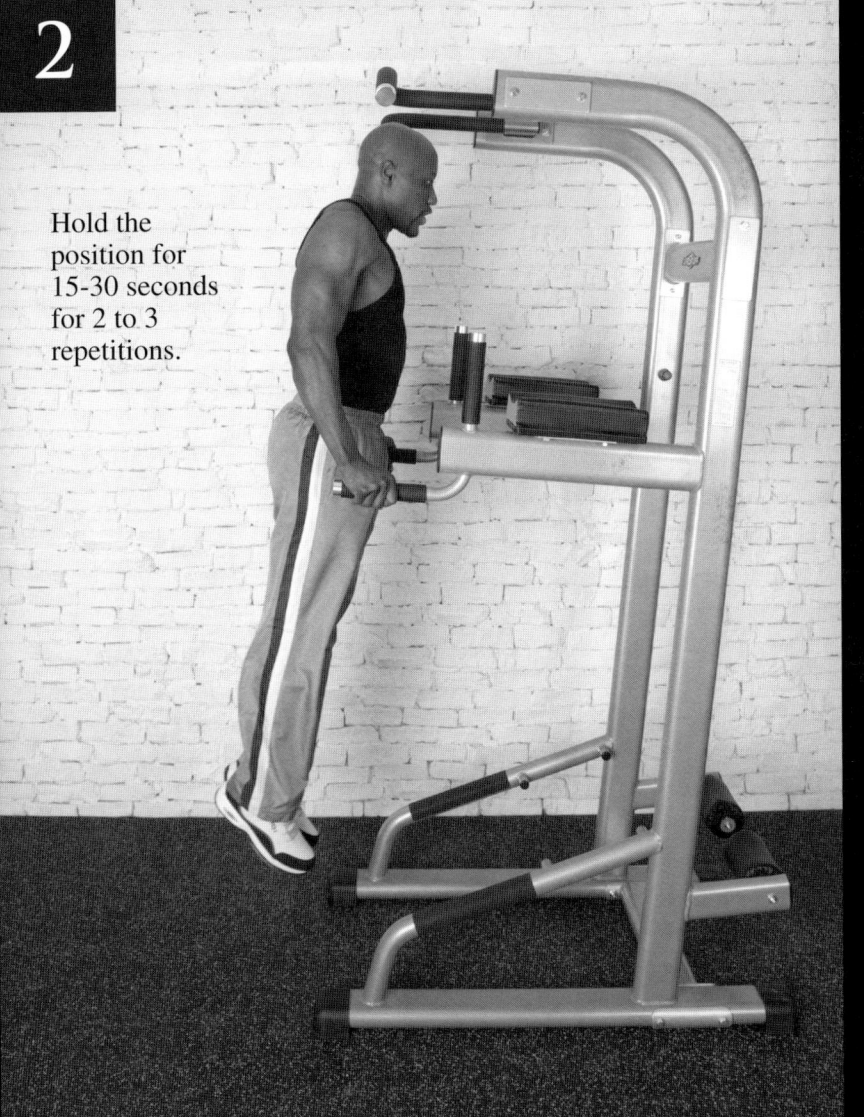

Hold the position for 15-30 seconds for 2 to 3 repetitions.

The Captain's Chair is mounted. While holding on to the chair handles, you are to elevate and lift your body and hold the arms in an extended position with no movement, with the abdominals tight, and no swaying in this position.

TRICEPS DIP
Using the Captain's Chair

This exercise is done from a starting Captain's Chair core position. The body is then lowered until the elbows are approximately 90 degrees.

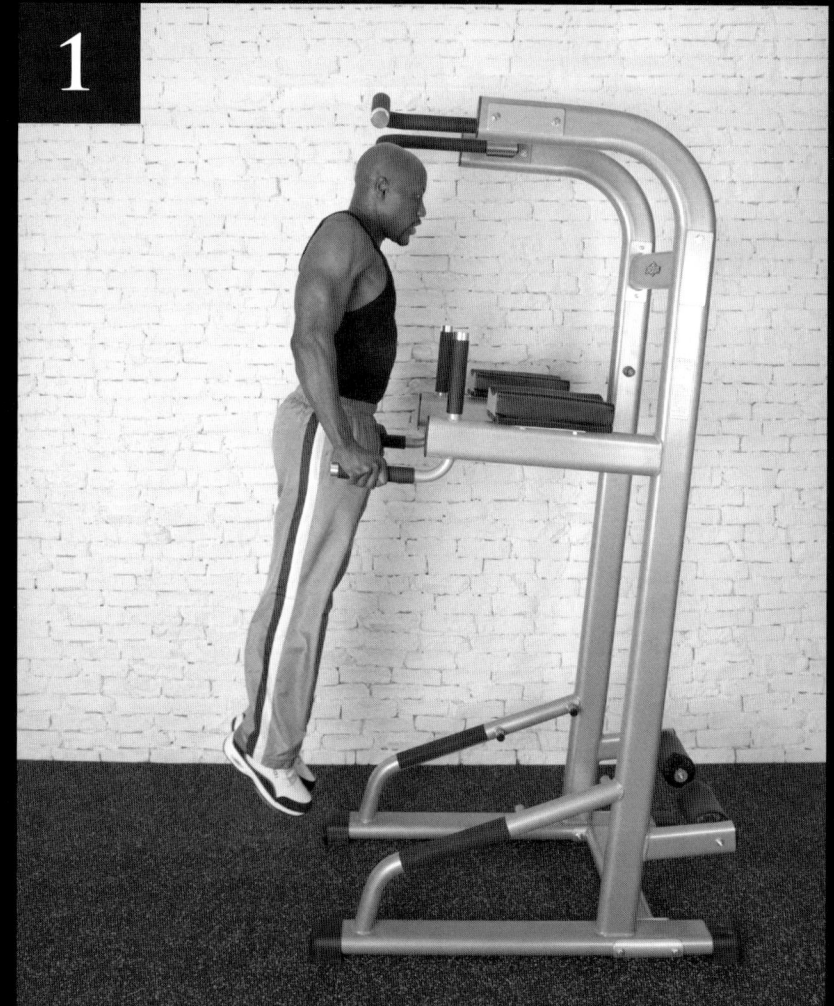
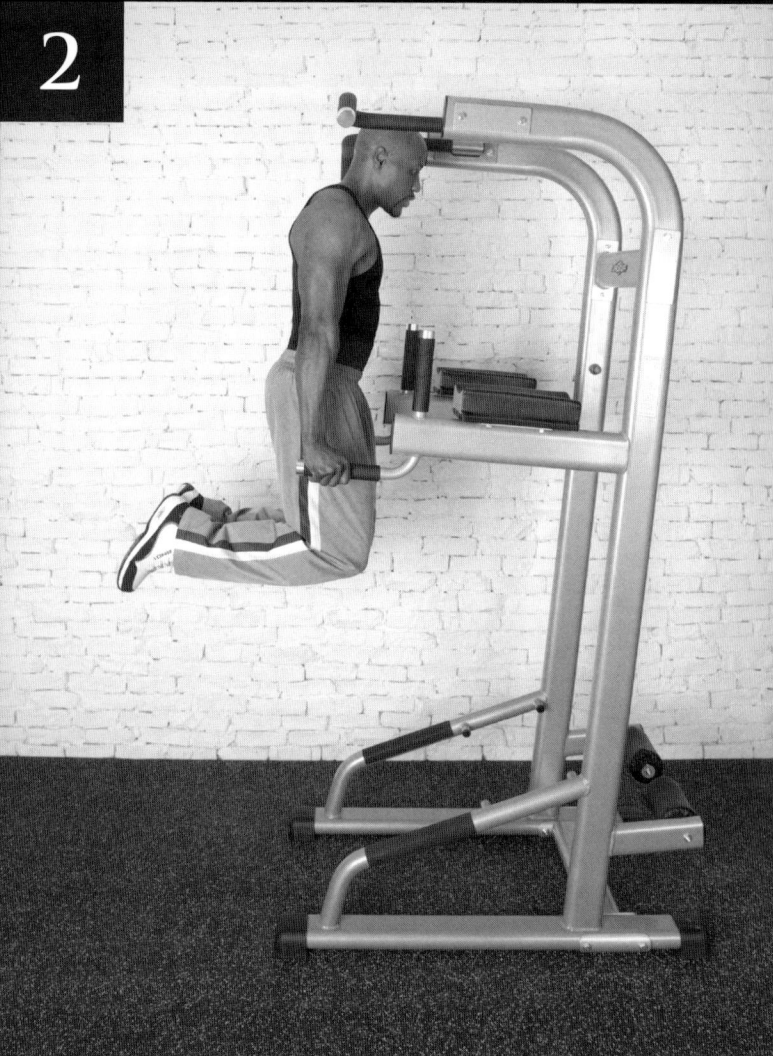

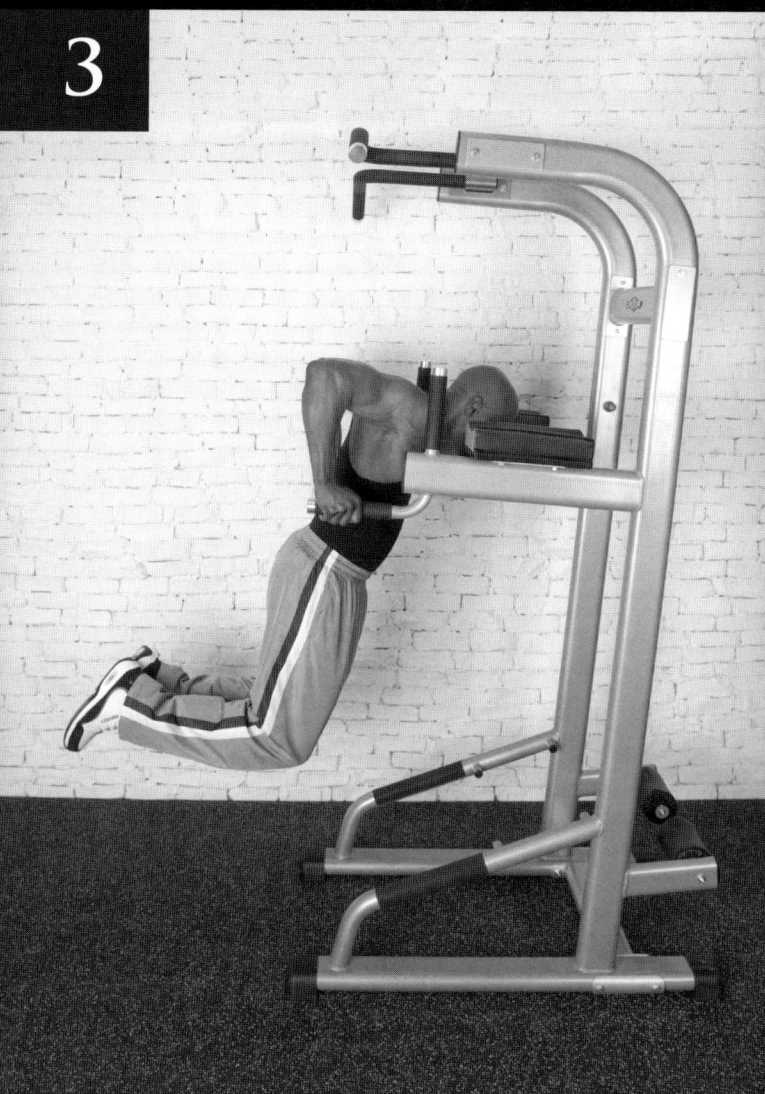

3

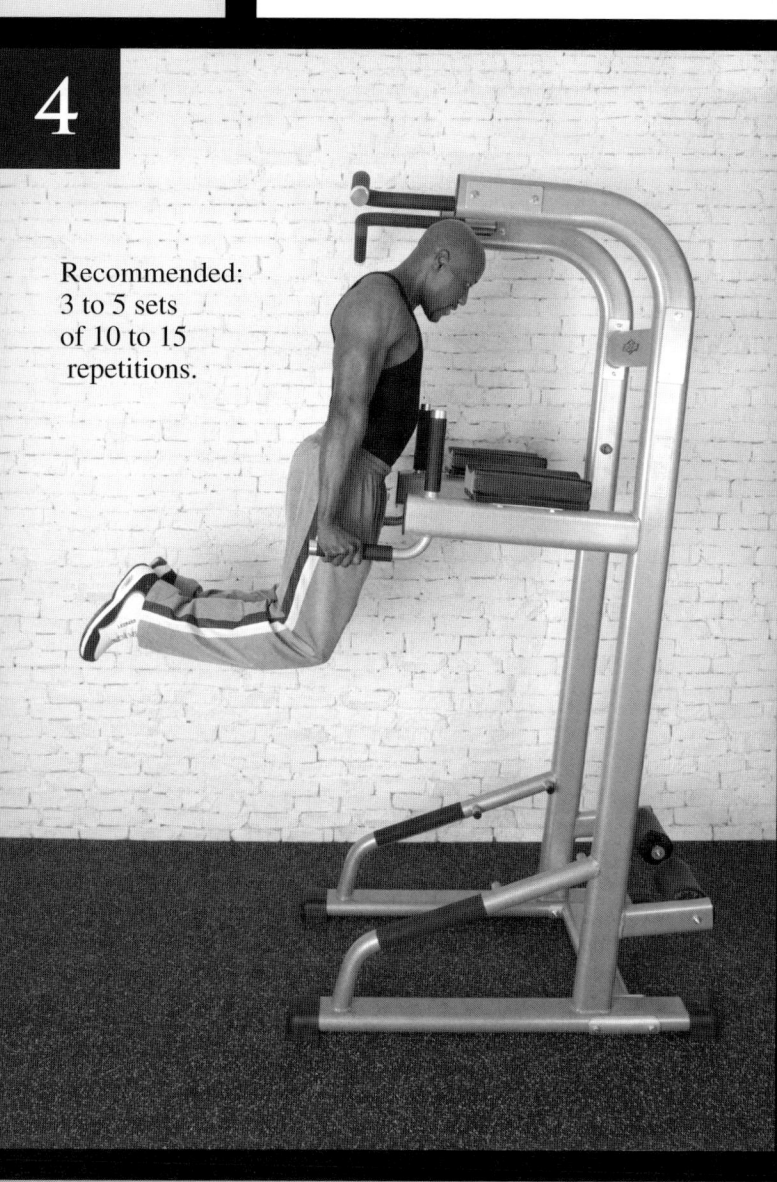

4

Recommended:
3 to 5 sets
of 10 to 15
repetitions.

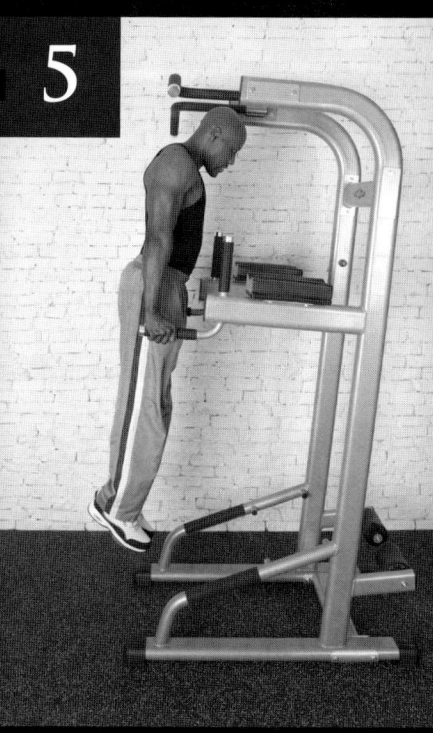

5

The body is then elevated by pushing downward on the handles of the Captain's Chair and elevating the body, completing the triceps dip. Swinging should be avoided.

KNEE LIFTS

Using the Captain's Chair

This exercise is done by first mounting the Captain's Chair and holding on to the arm posts and letting the forearms rest on the pads. The body should be suspended by holding on to the chair handles. The knees are then elevated and brought to the chest and held for 10 to 15 seconds and slowly brought down avoiding any swinging motion.

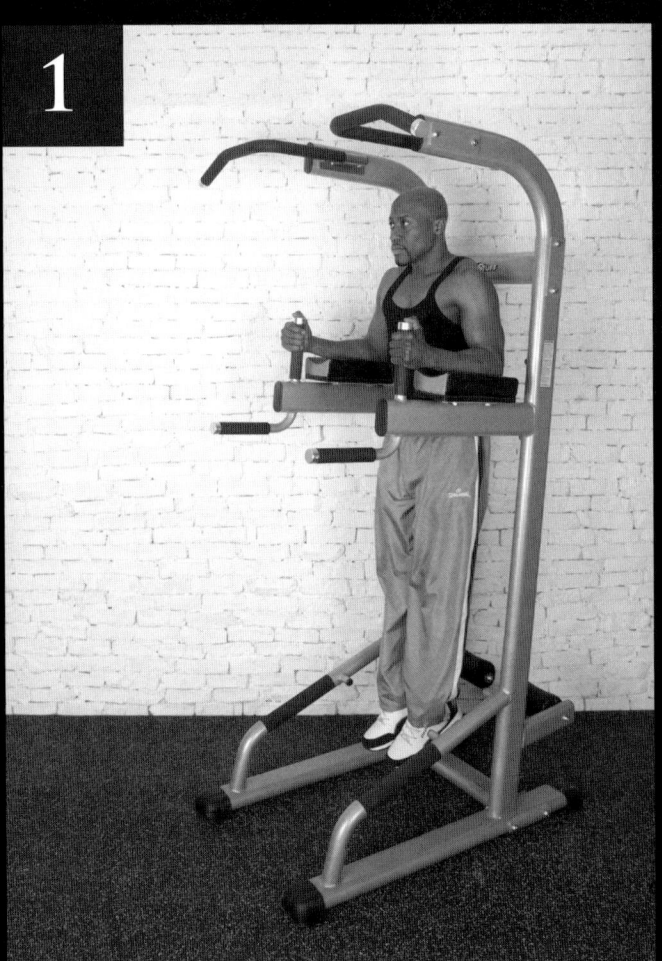

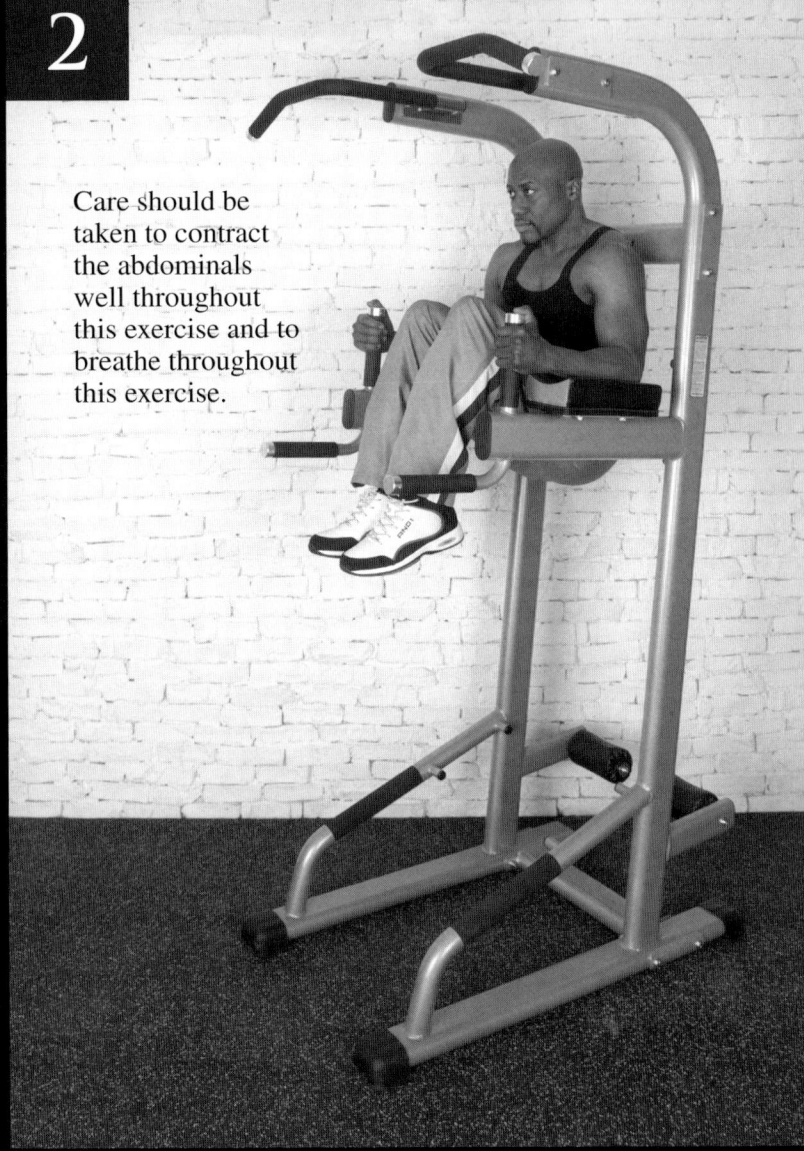

Care should be taken to contract the abdominals well throughout this exercise and to breathe throughout this exercise.

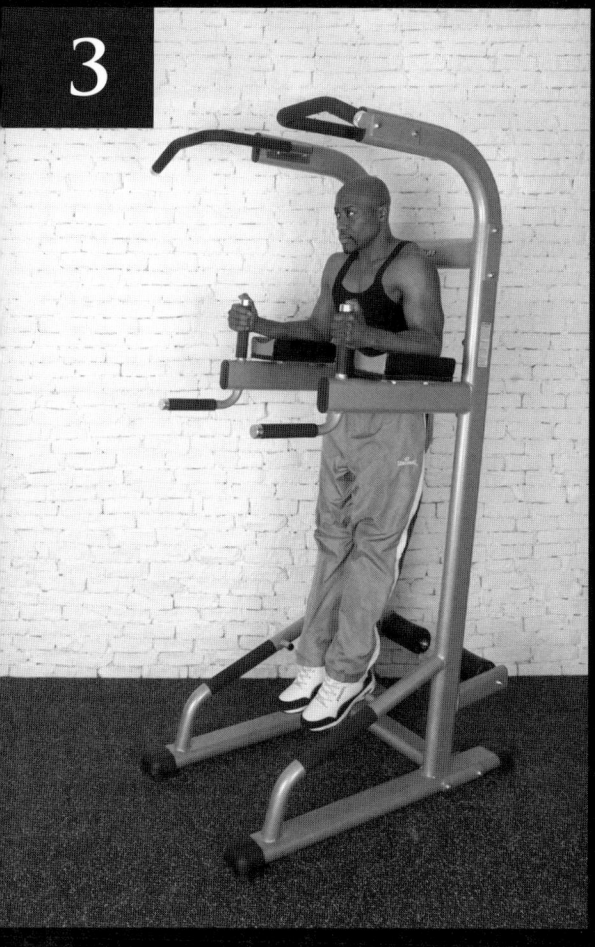

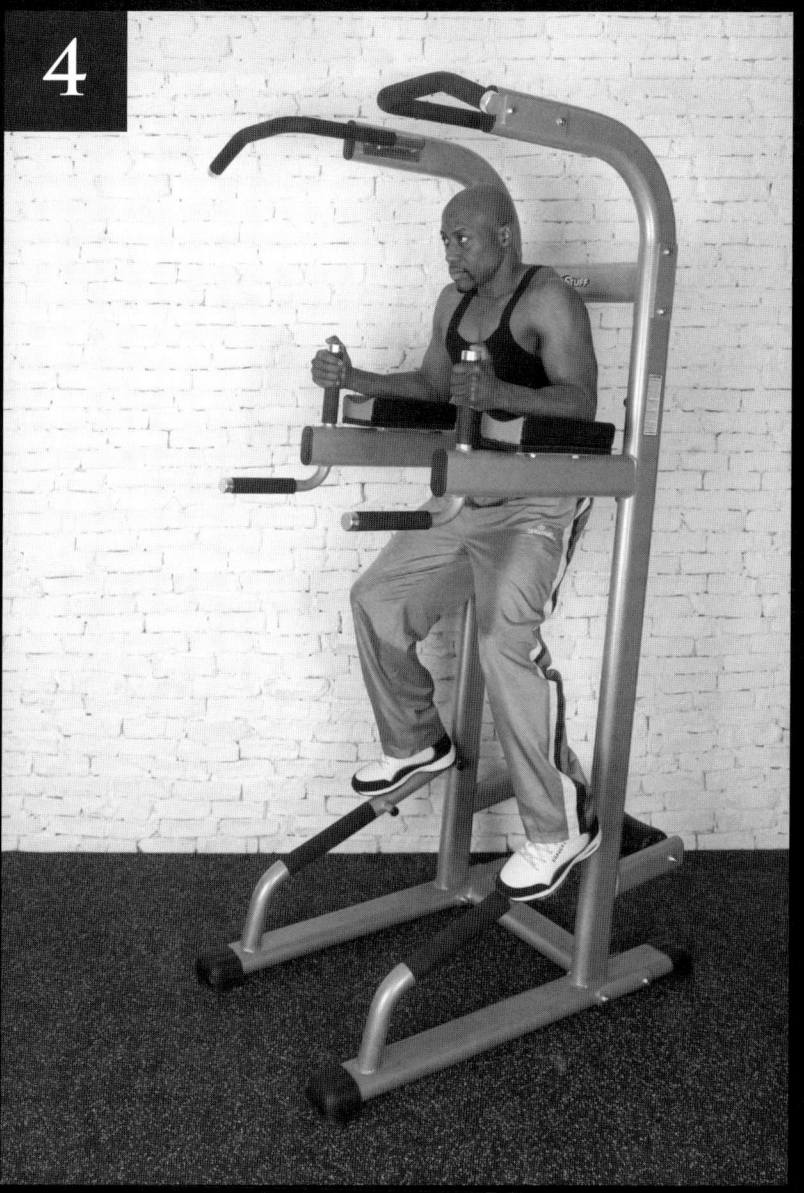

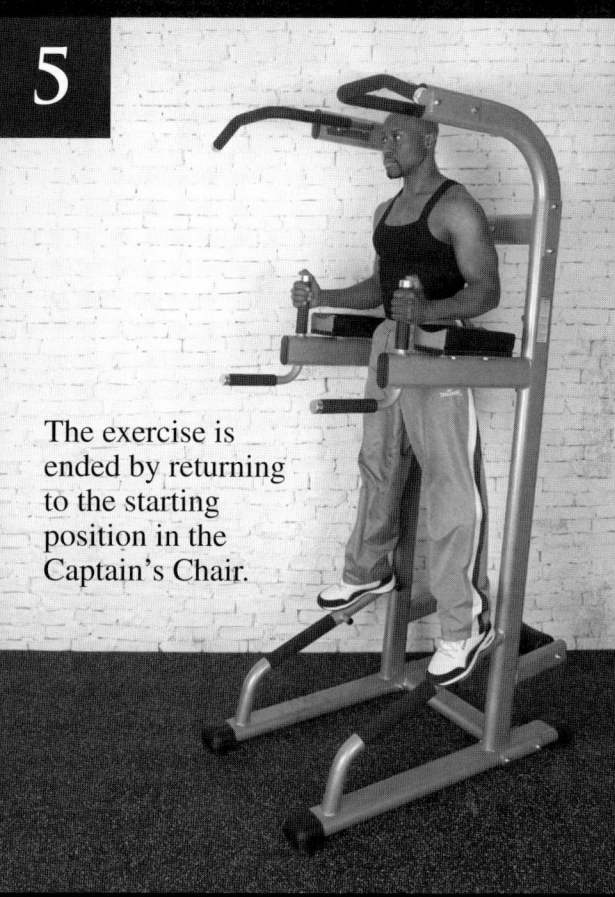

The exercise is ended by returning to the starting position in the Captain's Chair.

Recommended:
3 to 5 sets of
10 to 15 repetitions.

Combined Knee Lifts & Leg Extensions
Using the Captain's Chair

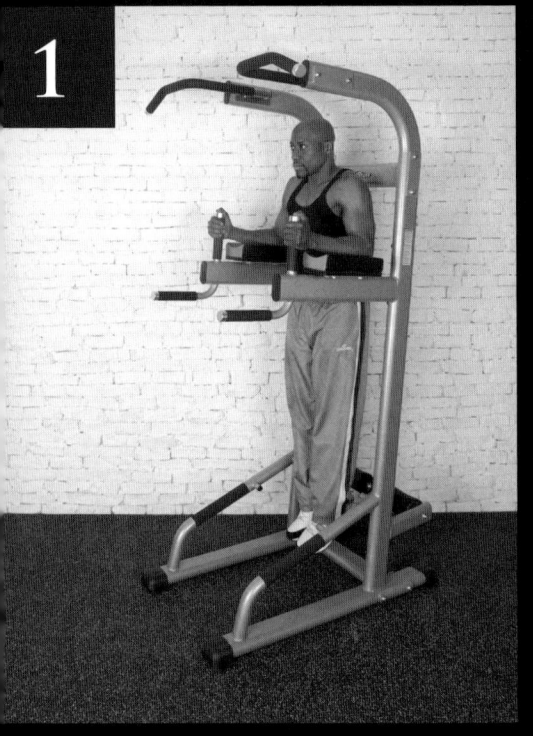

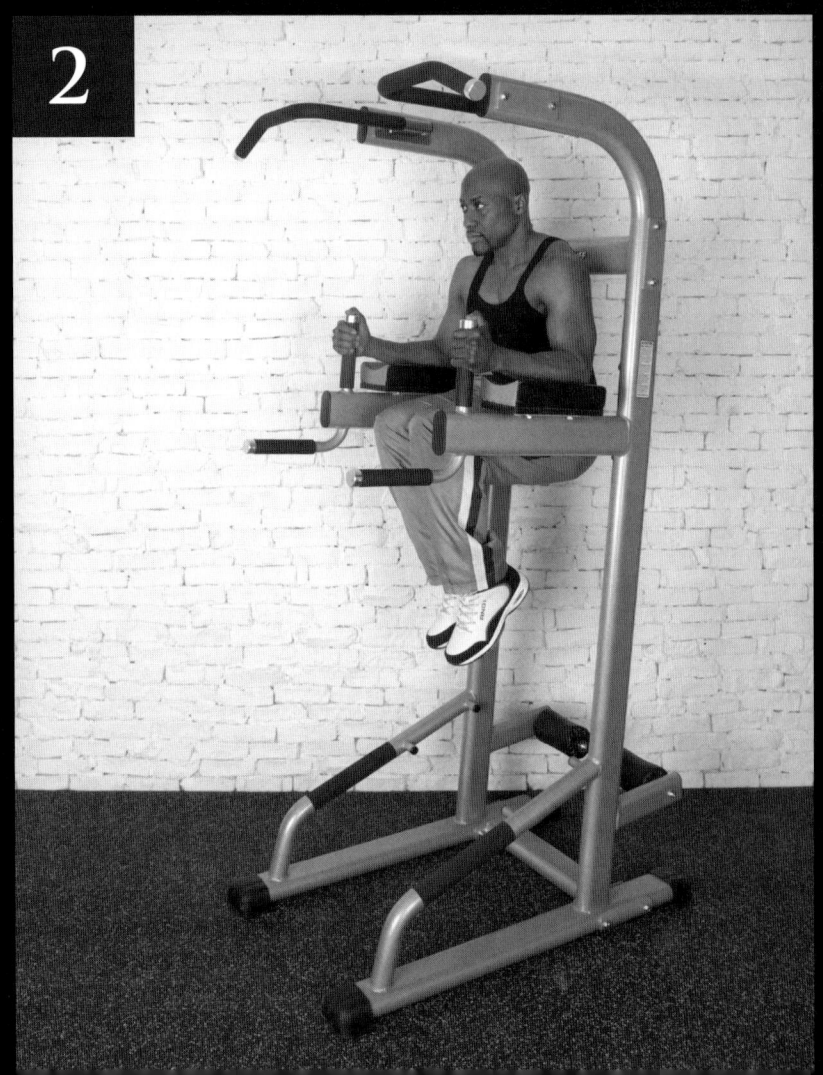

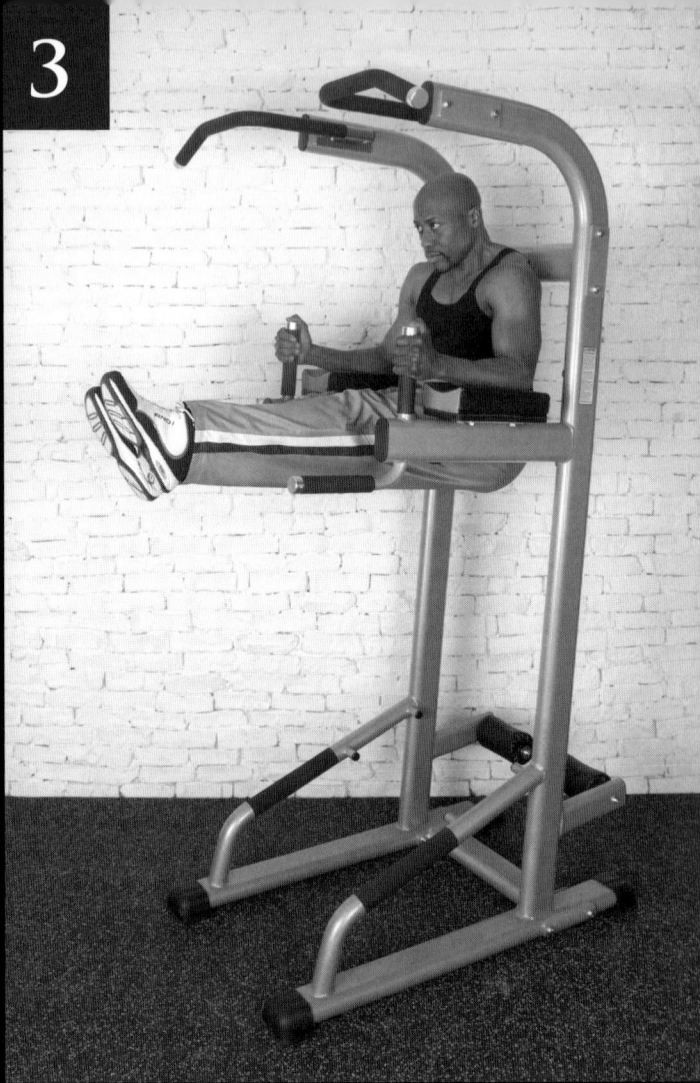

This is performed by starting in the Captain's Chair suspended position. The knees are then lifted upward to the abdomen and held at 90 degrees. The legs are slowly extended in front and held in an L-type position for 15 to 30 seconds. The knees are then bent and returned back to the suspended Captain's Chair position to dismount.

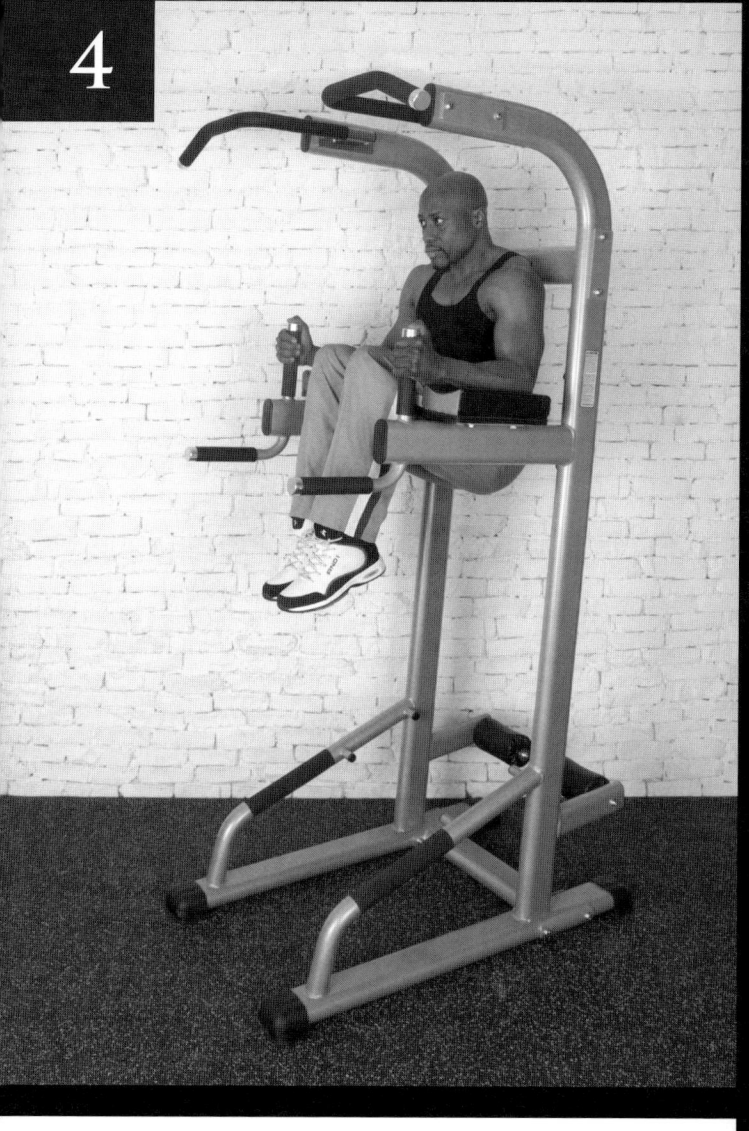

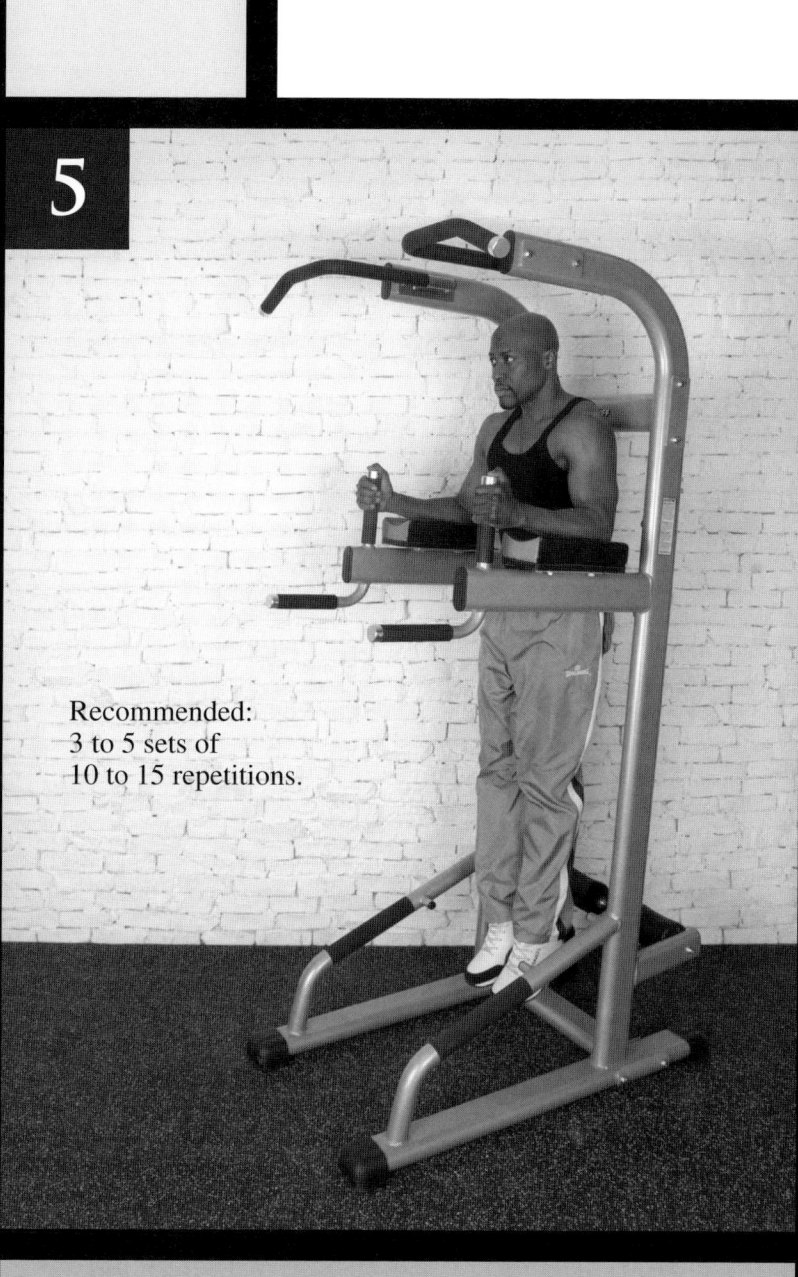

Recommended:
3 to 5 sets of
10 to 15 repetitions.

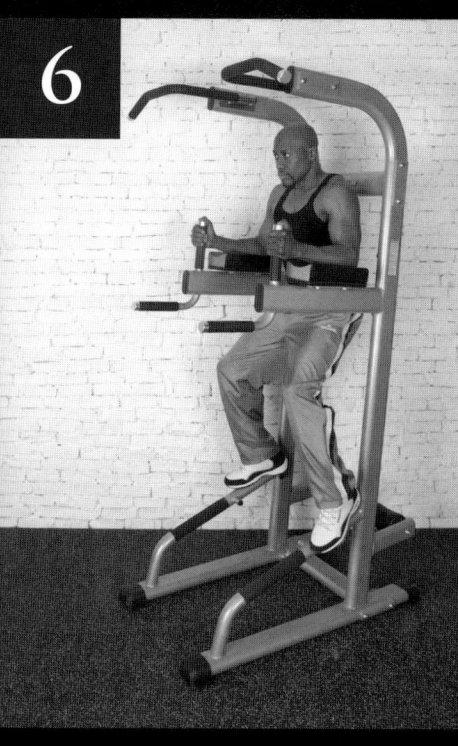

WIDE GRIP PULL-UP
Using the Captain's Chair

This exercise is done by mounting the pull-up bars with the arms wide apart. After holding on to the bars, the feet are lifted off the floor. The body is then pulled upward and slowly lowered downward.

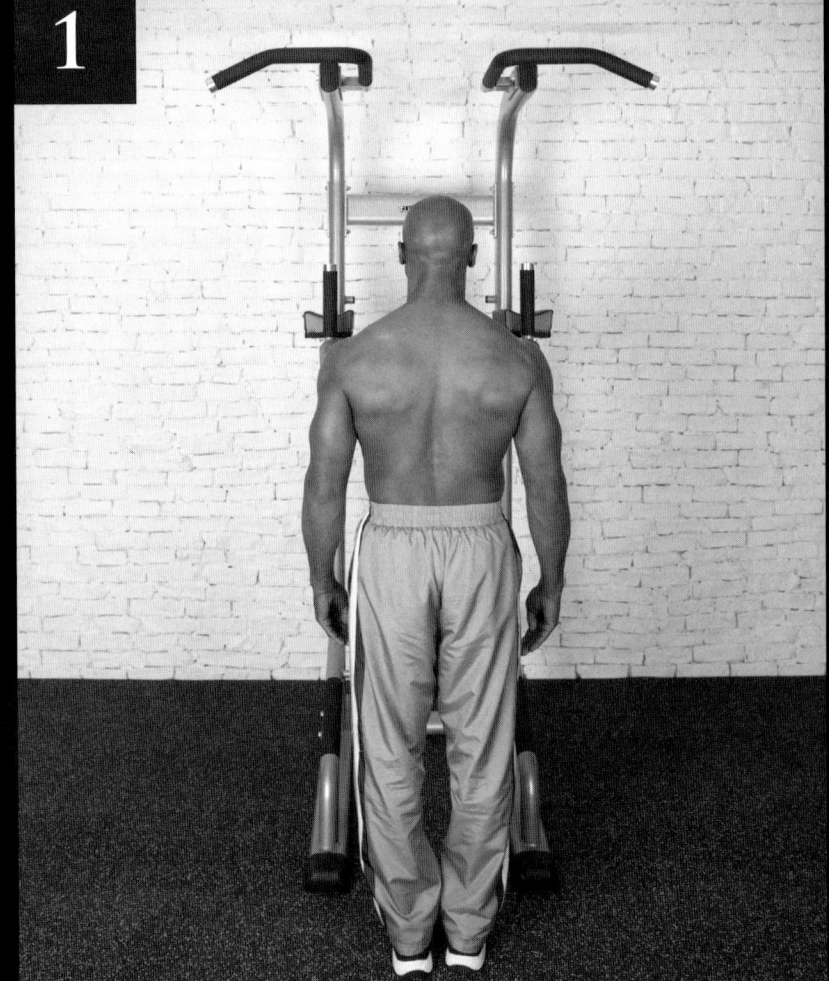

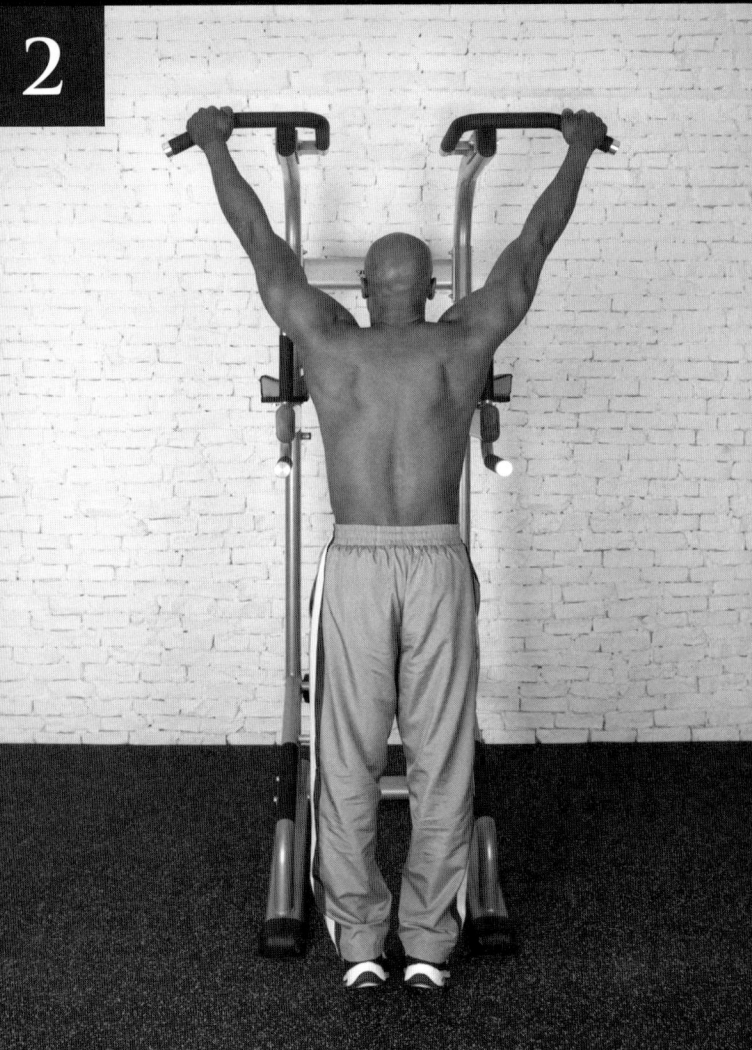

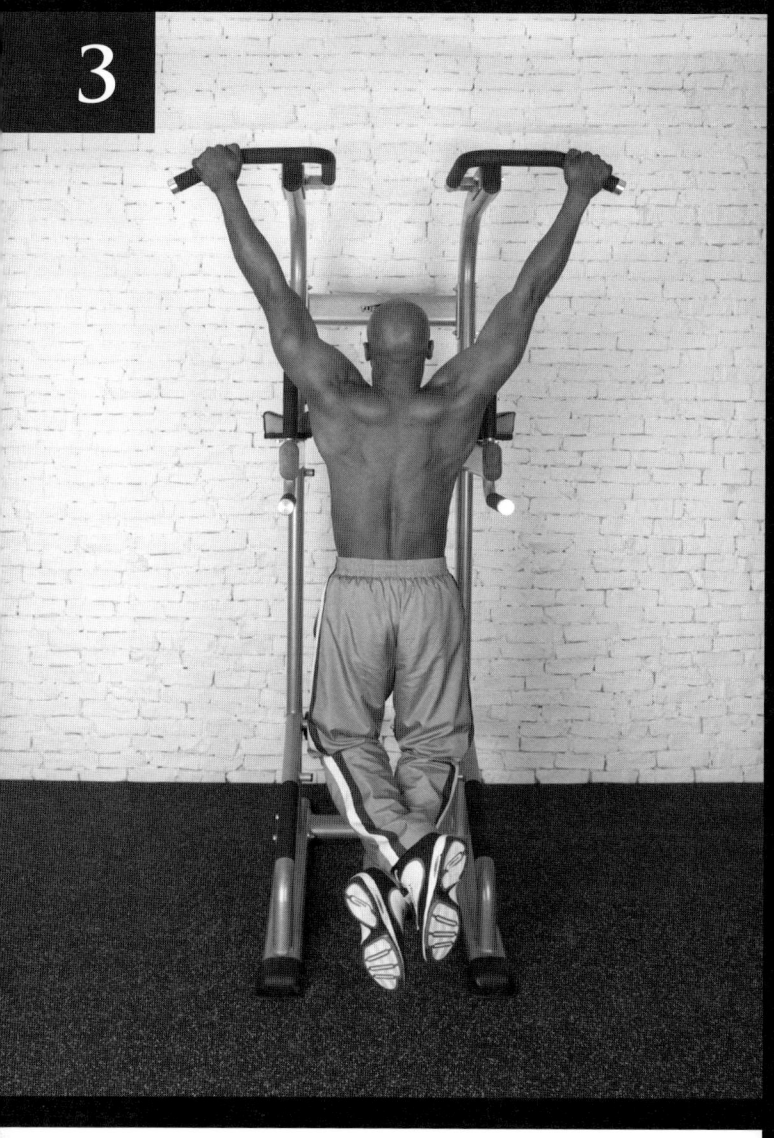
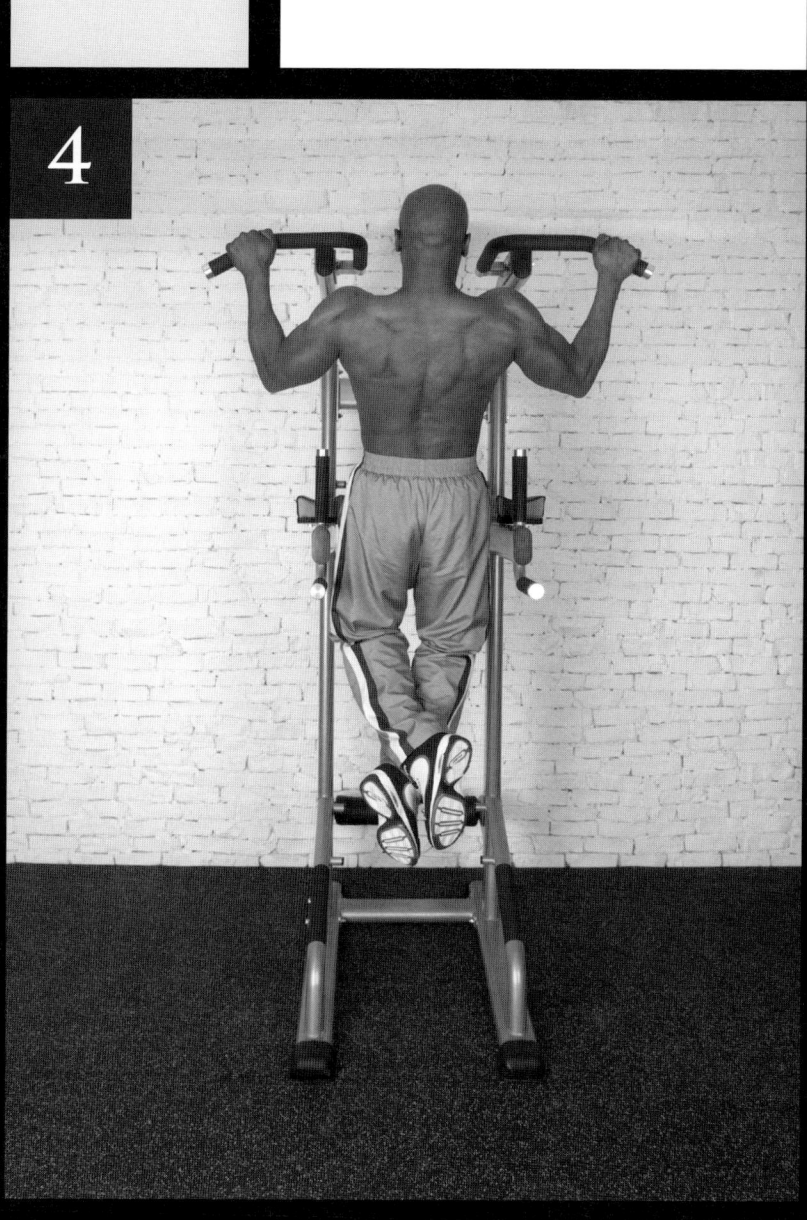
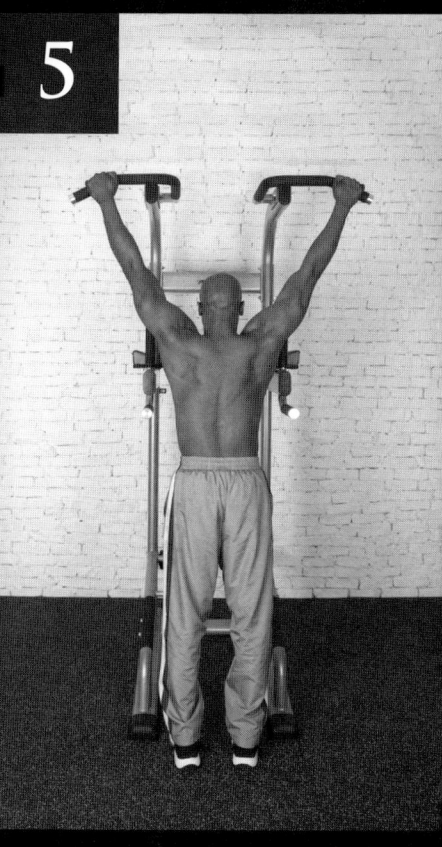

Recommended:
3 to 5 sets of
10 to 15 repetitions.

Derotation Straight Leg Lifts
Using the Captain's Chair

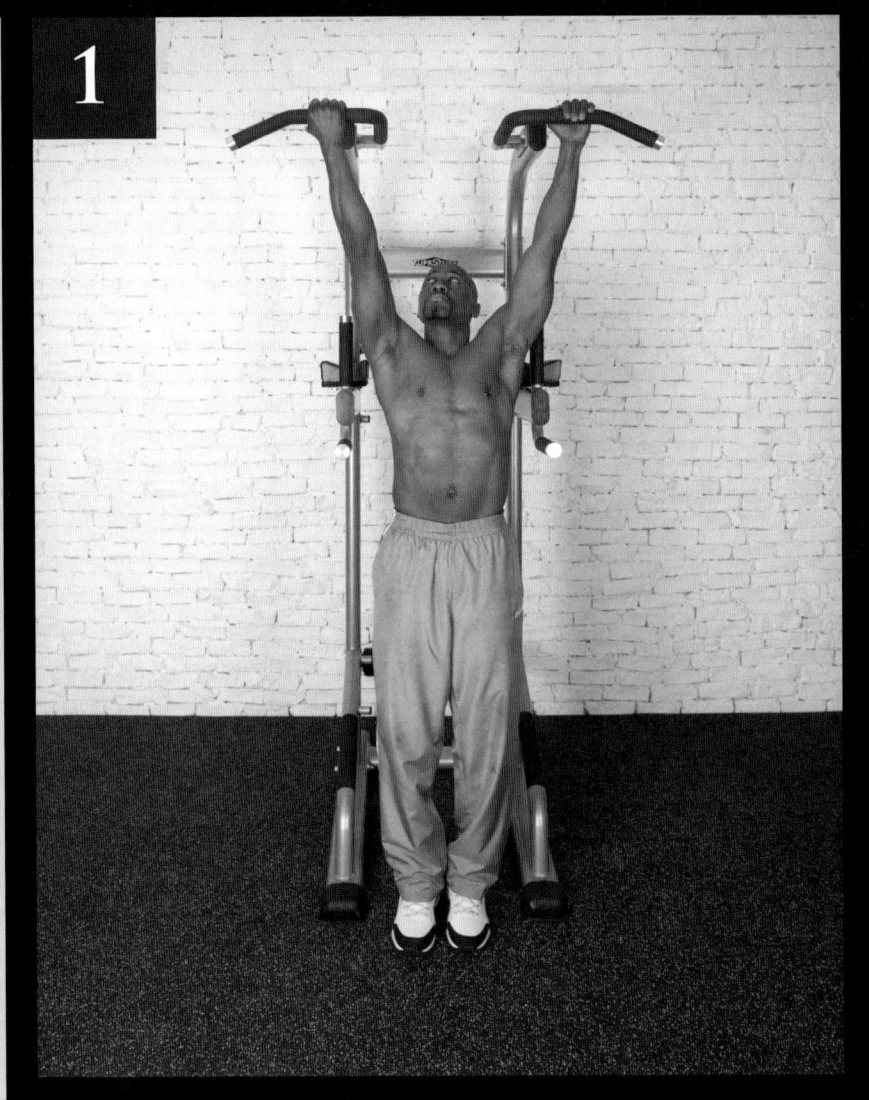

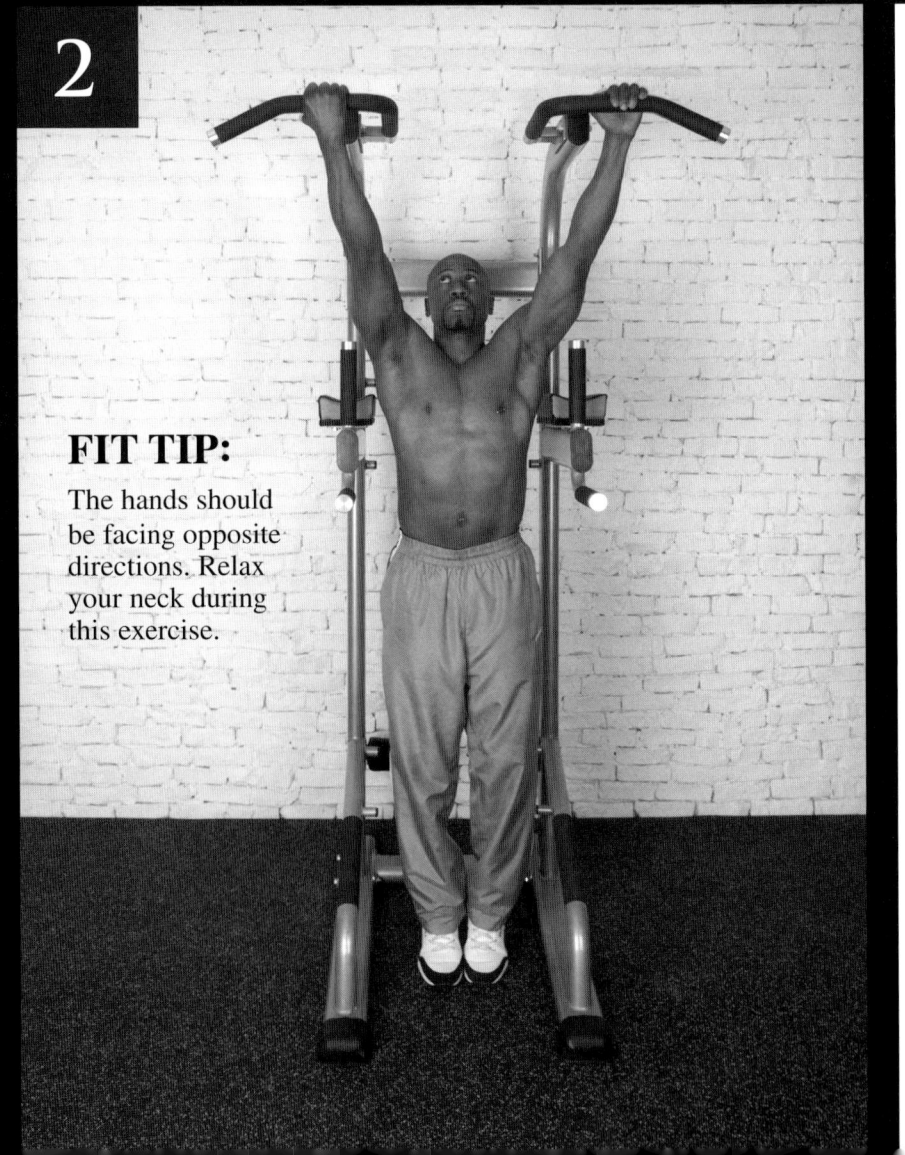

FIT TIP: The hands should be facing opposite directions. Relax your neck during this exercise.

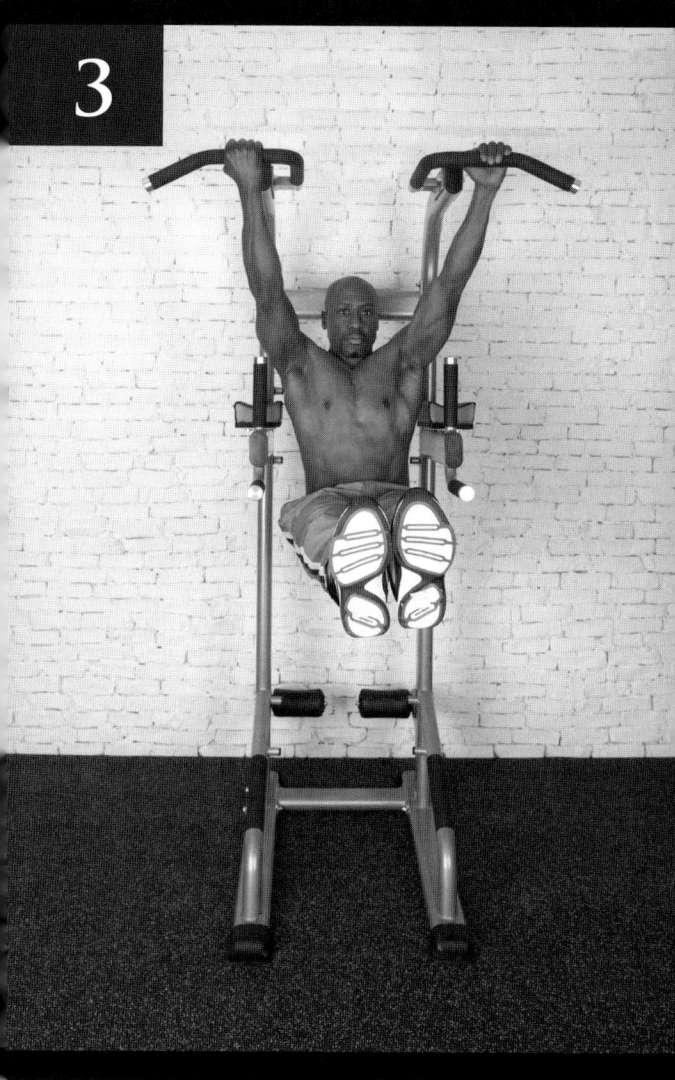

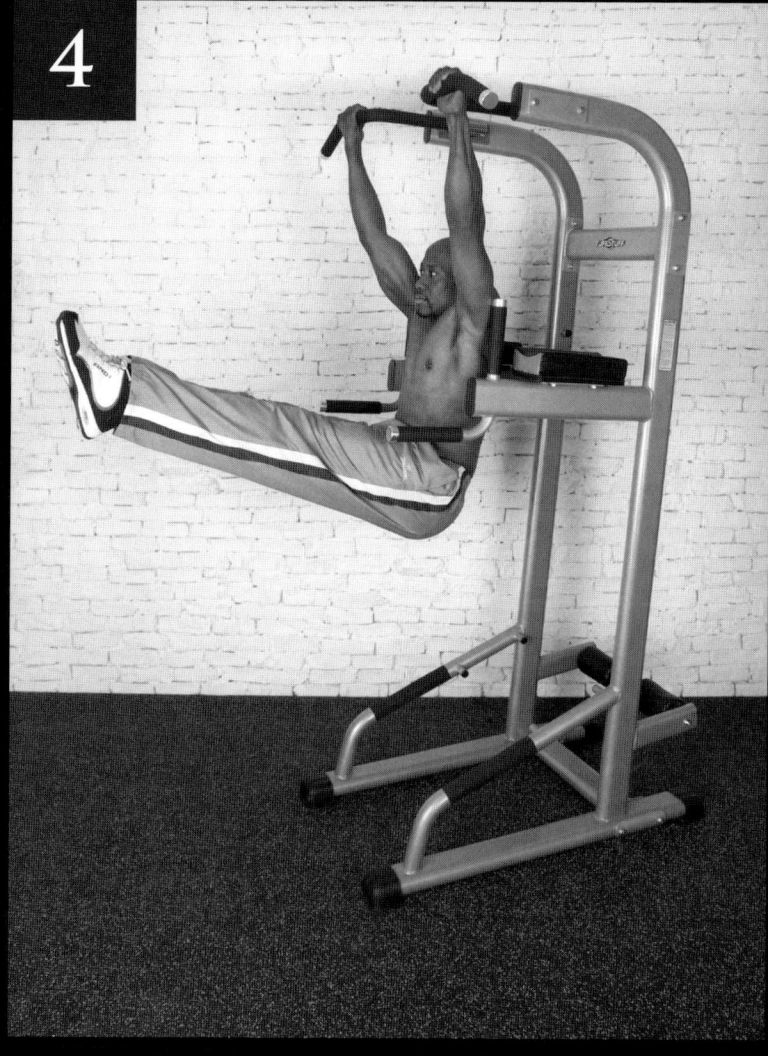

Recommended:
3 to 5 sets of
10 to 15 repetitions.

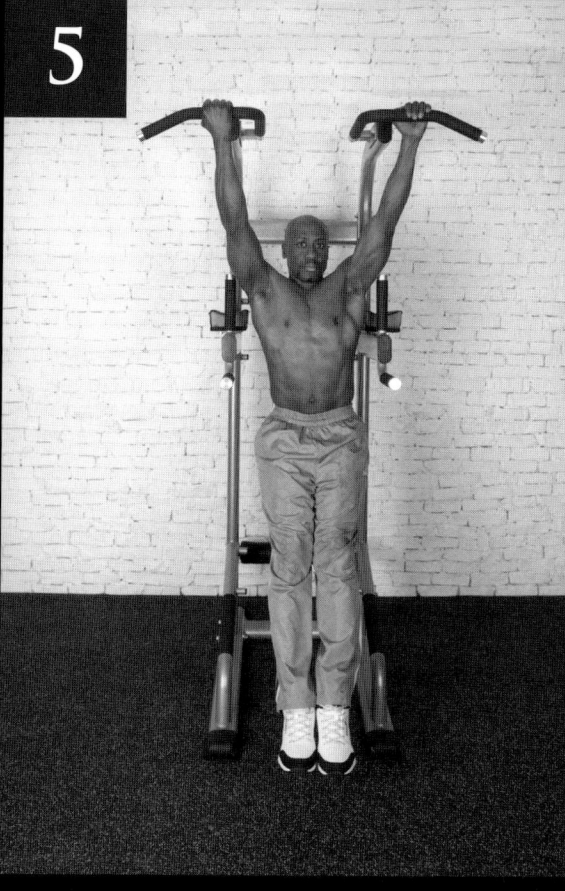

This exercise is done by mounting the Captain's Chair with one palm facing toward you and one palm facing outward. As you hold on to the bars, the legs are then elevated and suspended in front of you. This movement is held for 30 to 60 seconds. Next, lower your legs slowly downward. Avoid swinging during this exercise.

Side Leg Lifts

Using the Captain's Chair

This exercise is done by mounting the Captain's Chair from the side with one leg in front and one leg behind in a stride position. The leg that is in front should have that same arm against the elbow pad. The other arm should grasp the Captain's handlebar. The legs are then suspended and then lifted to the side, contracting the obliques, serratus, and abdominals.

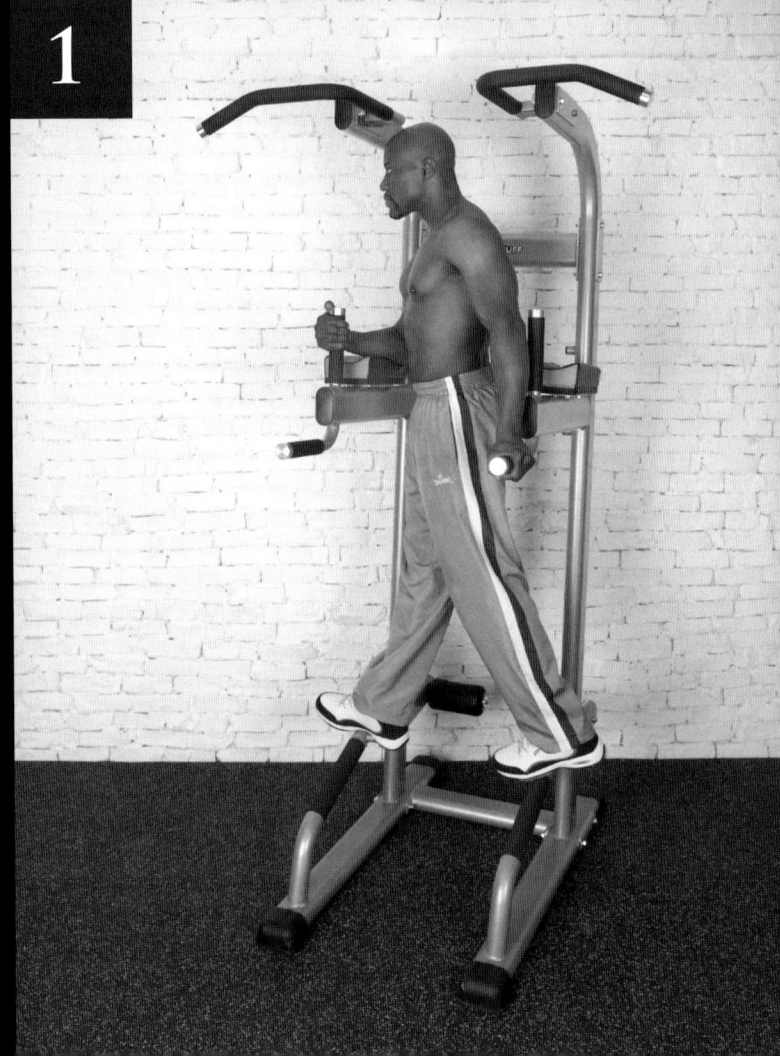

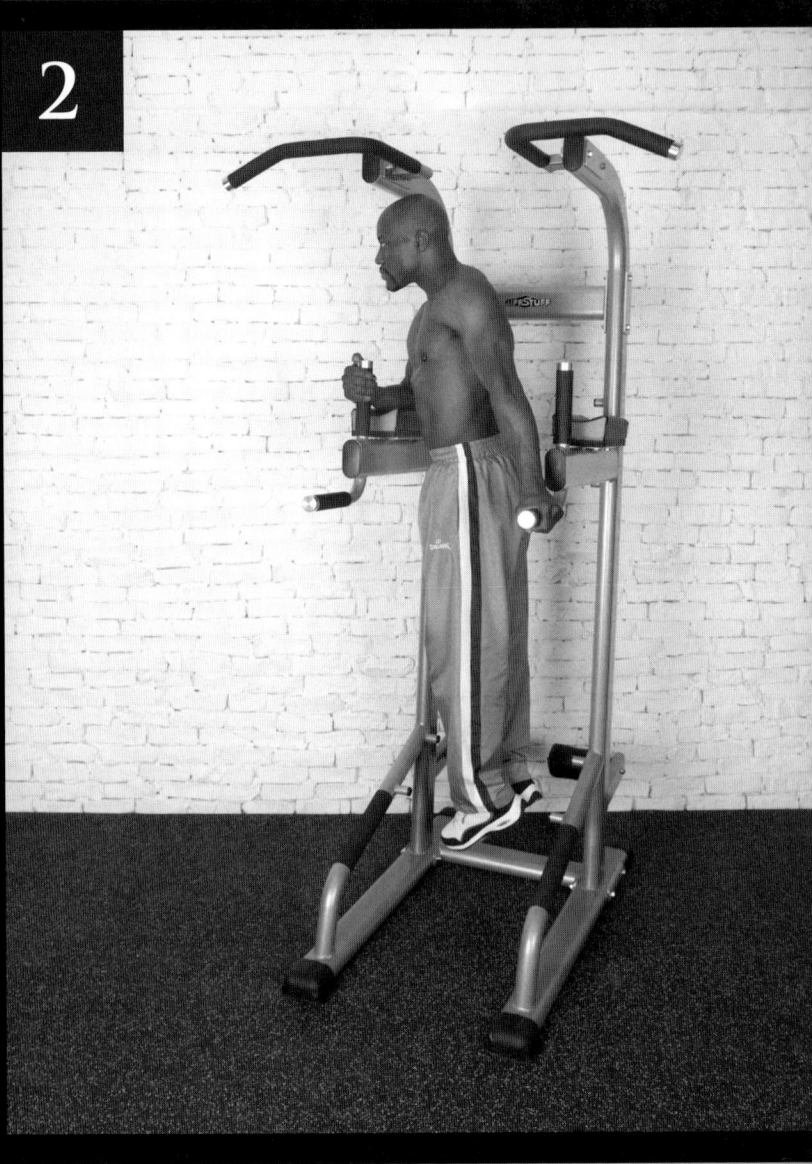

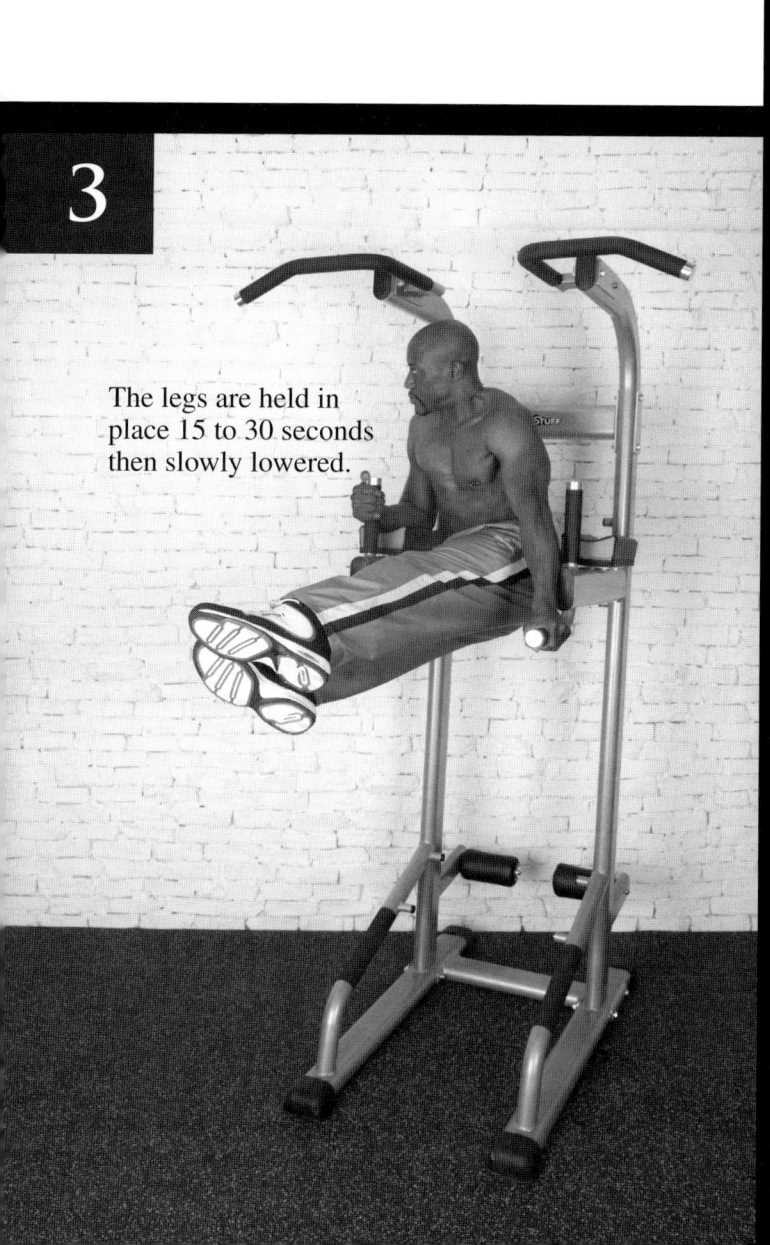

The legs are held in place 15 to 30 seconds then slowly lowered.

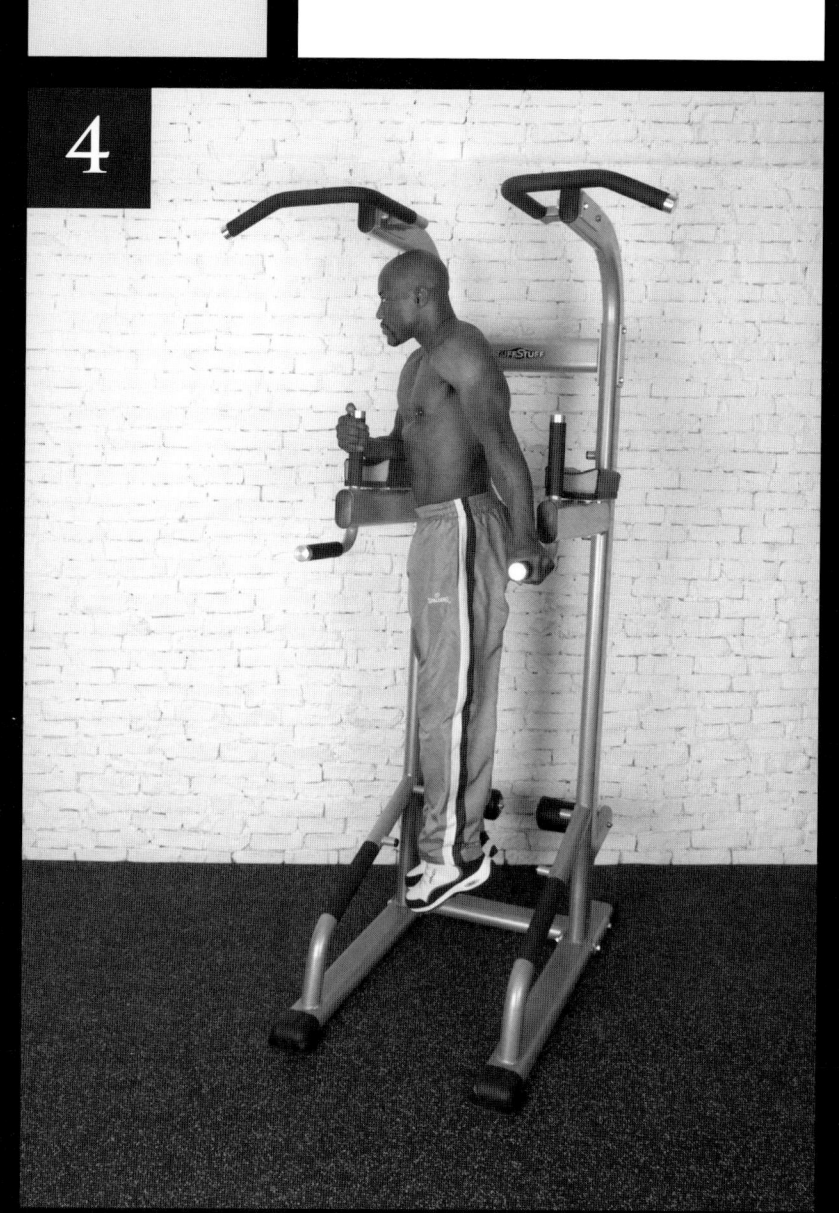

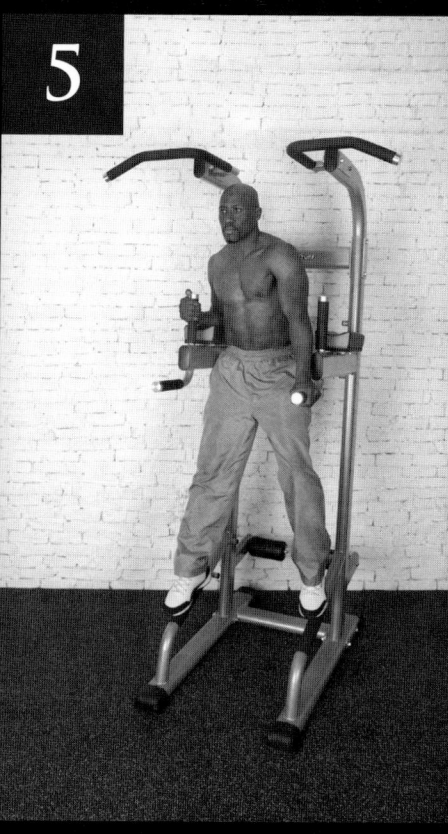

Recommended: 3 to 5 sets of 10 to 15 repetitions.

Flying Triceps Dip or "Superman" Dip

After you mount the Captain's Chair in the standard front suspended position, the elbows are flexed and the body is lowered with a steady cadence. After lowering the body to do the triceps dip, you are to push down on the handlebars of the Captain's Chair to elevate your body upward and then release the handlebars. You are to then recapture the handlebars, extend the legs and you dismount from the equipment.

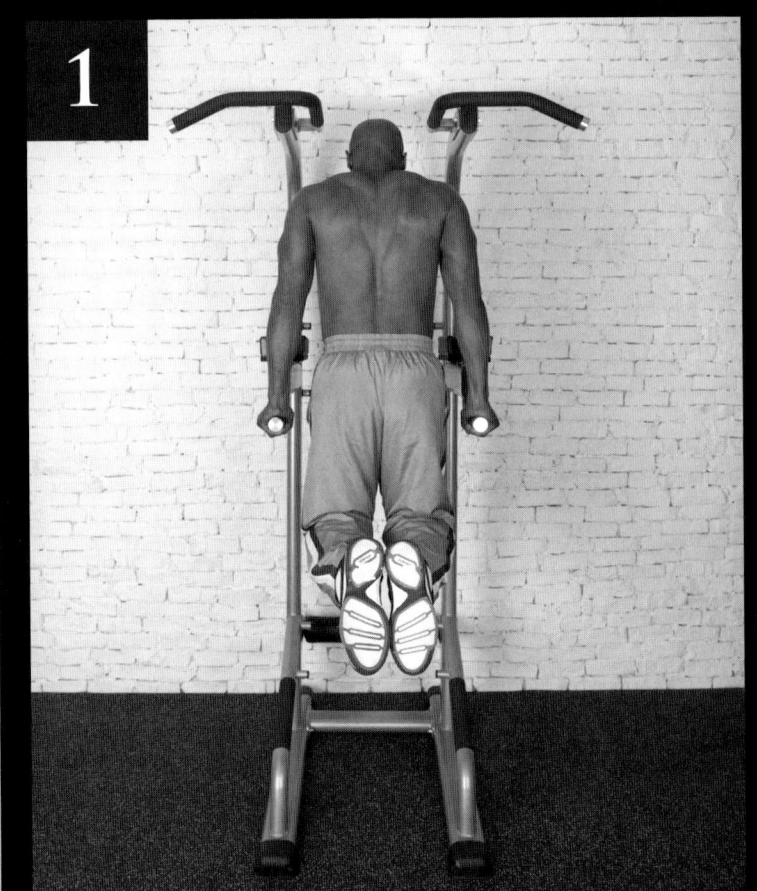

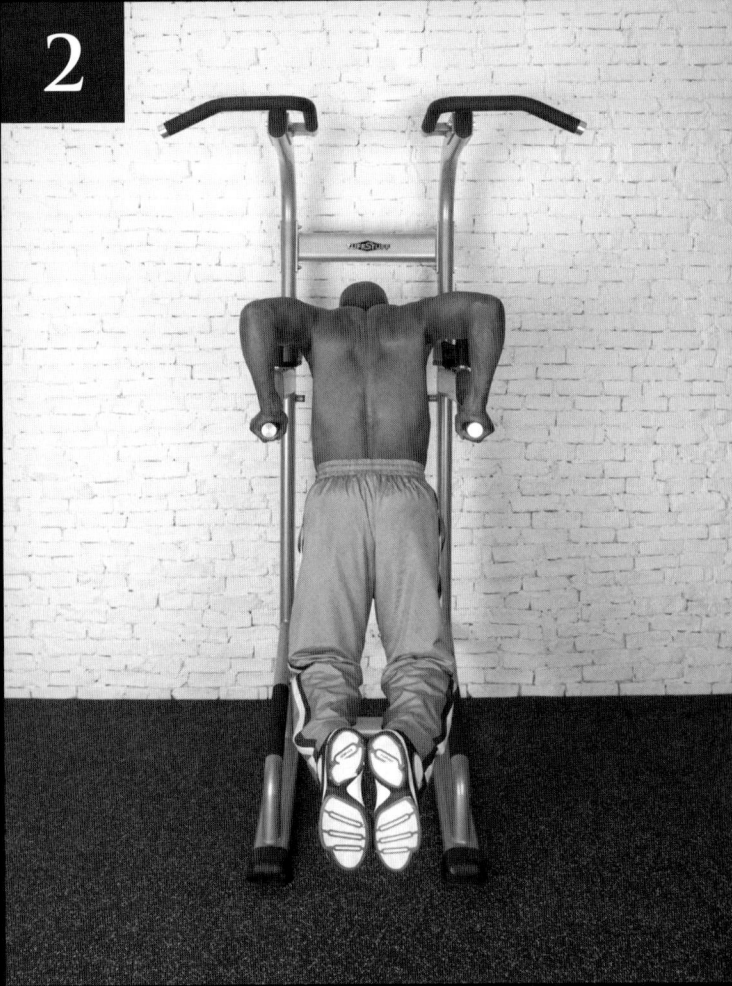

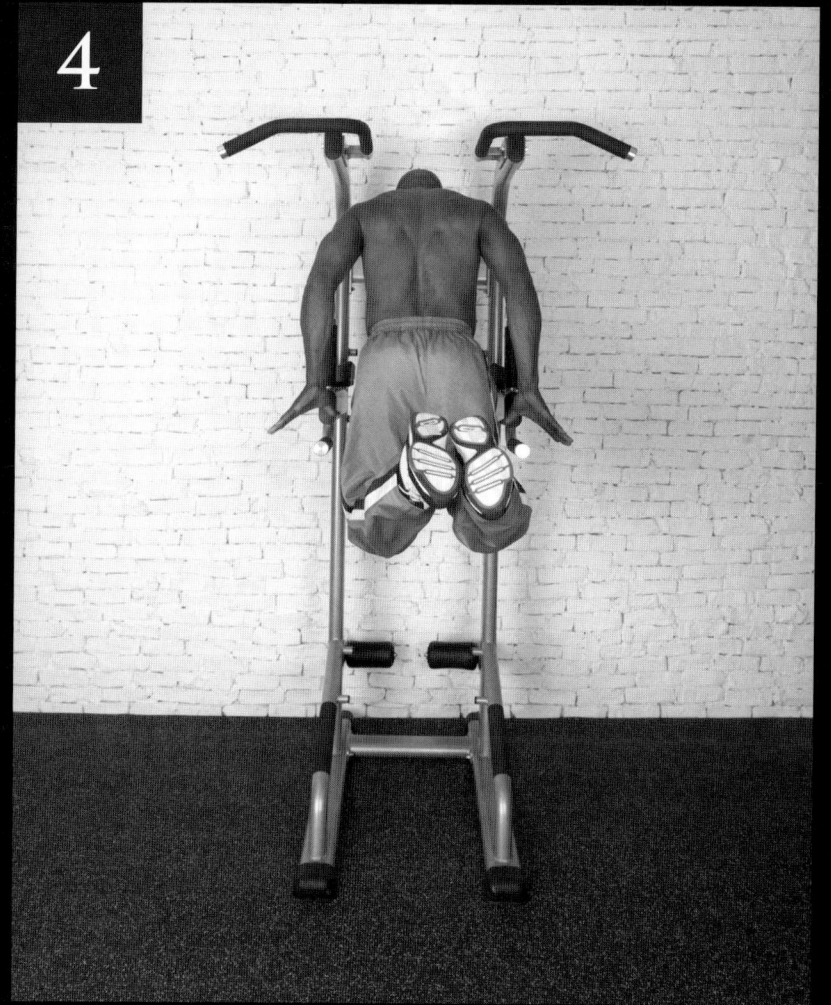

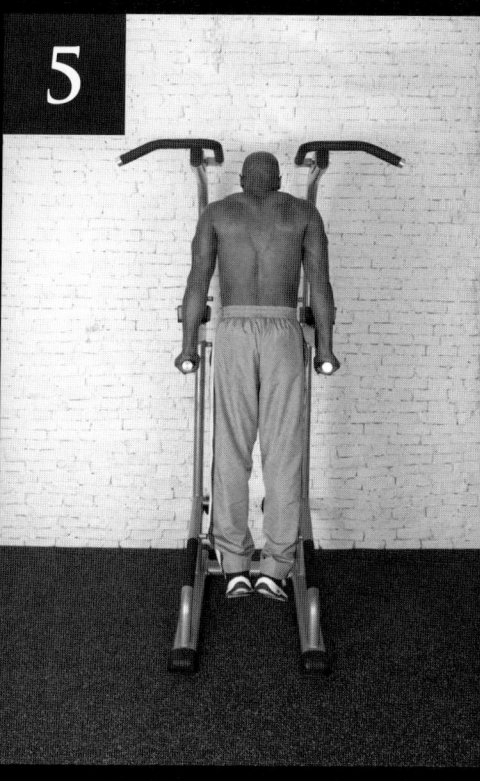

Recommended:
3 to 5 sets of
10 to 15 repetitions.

Care should be taken to have total control beginning the triceps dip before attempting to do a flyaway exercise from the Captain's Chair.

Roman Chair Sit-Up

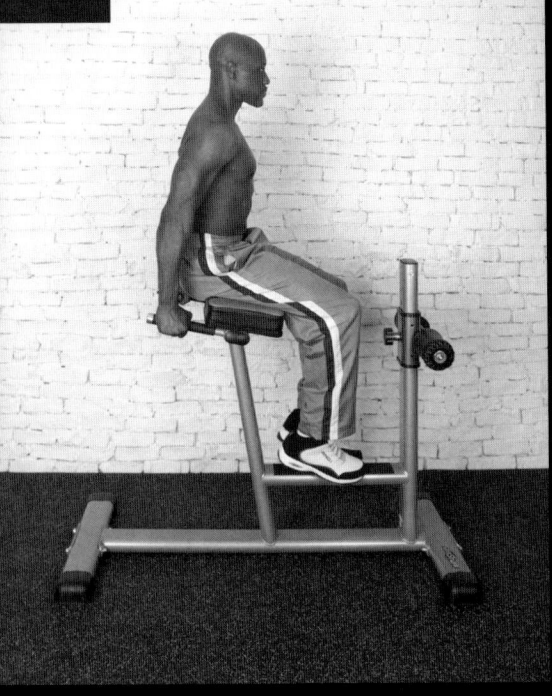

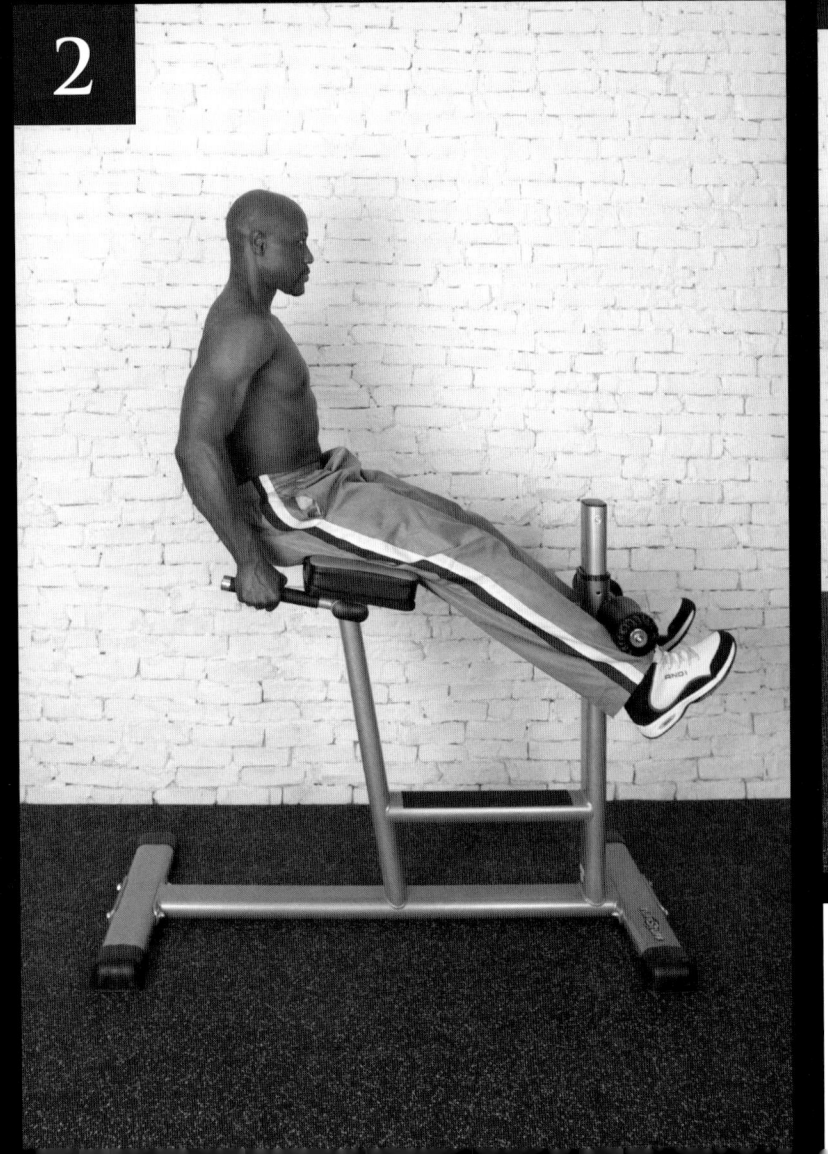

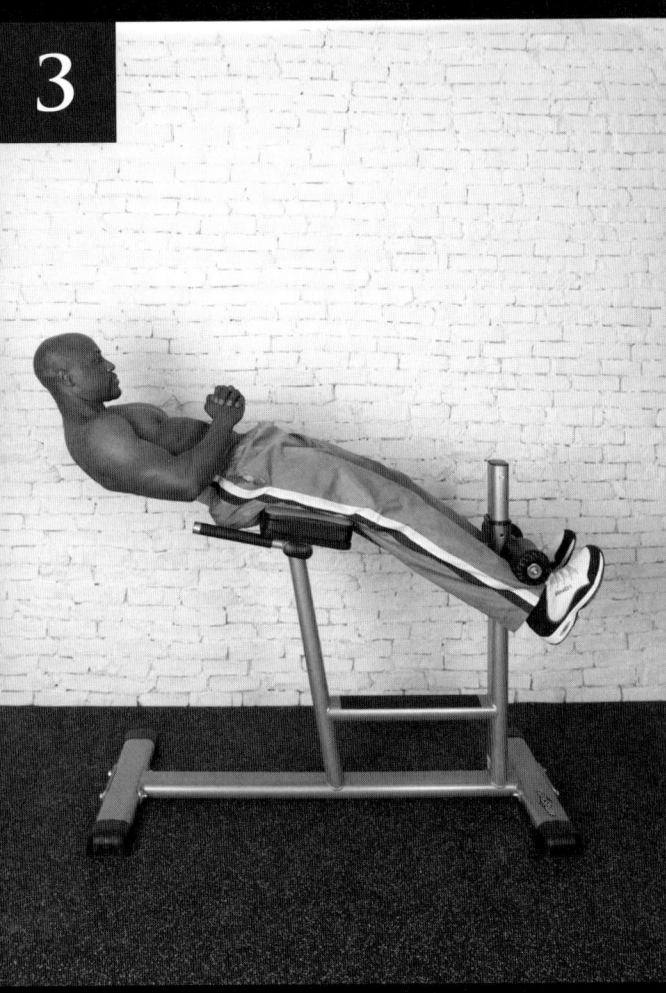

After mounting the Roman chair as seen, the legs should be extended under the ankle supports. Now lower your torso backwards slightly past 90 degrees and slowly lift up. This should be repeated by again letting your body go backwards and then lifting up again. This is ended by bringing the body completely up and supporting the body with your hands on the sides of the chair.

4

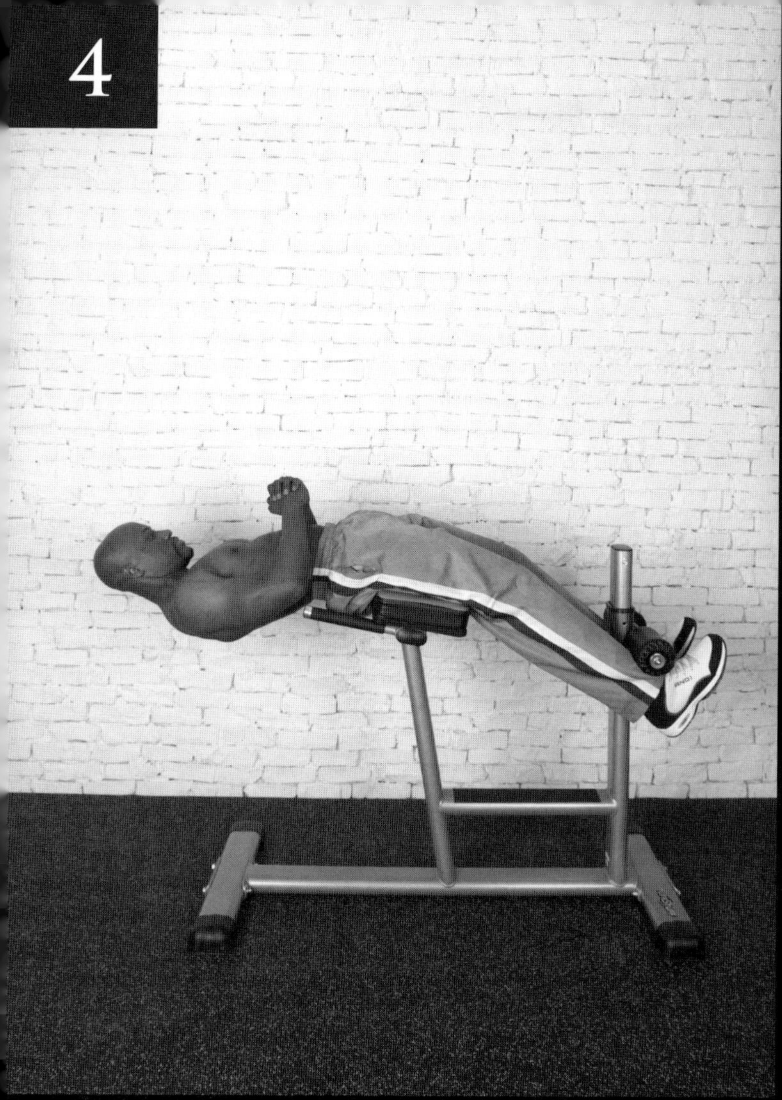

5

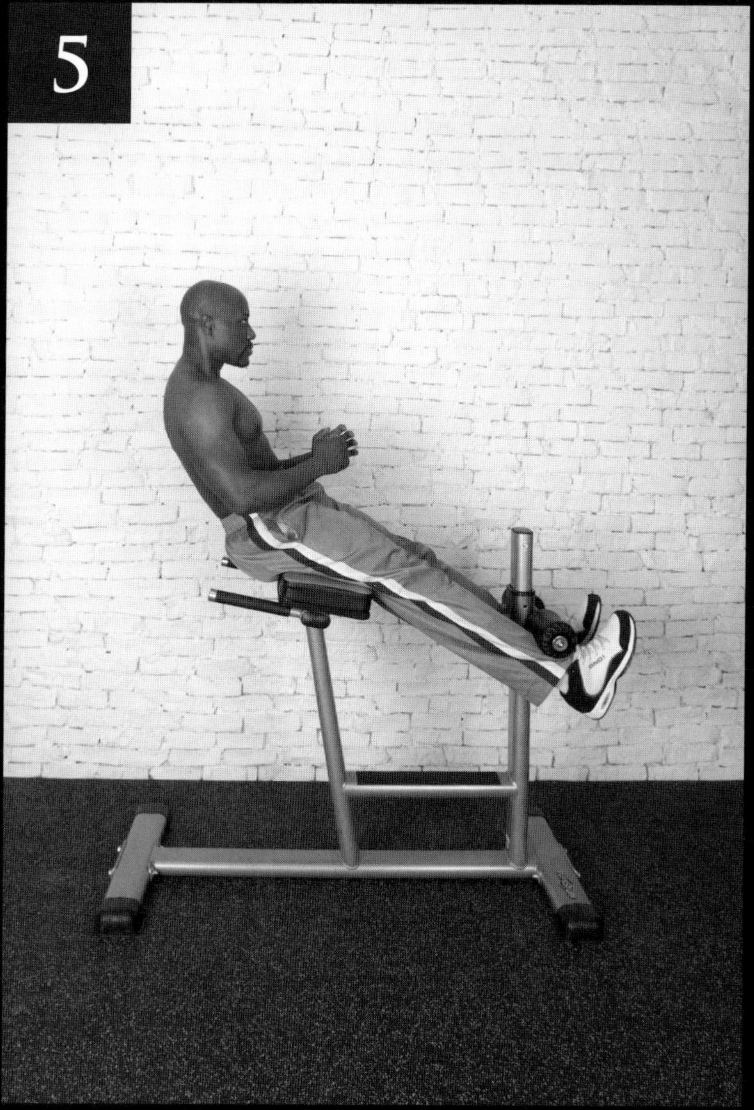

6

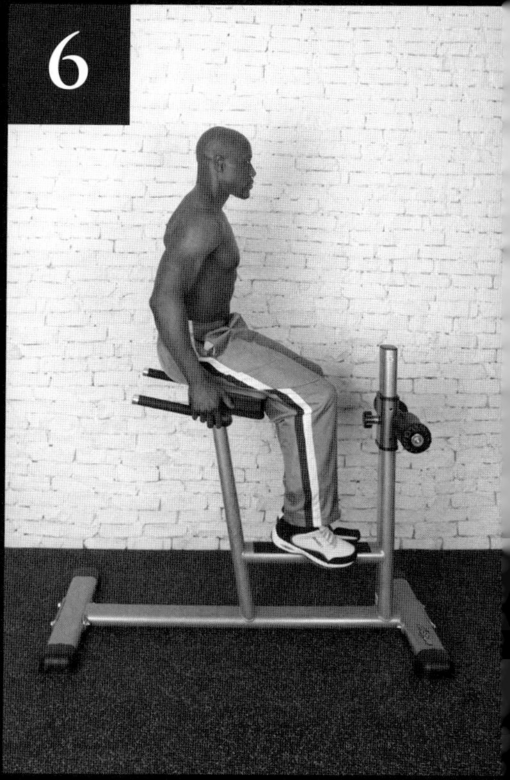

Recommended:
3 to 5 sets of
10 to 15 repetitions.

Side Roman Chair Sit-Up

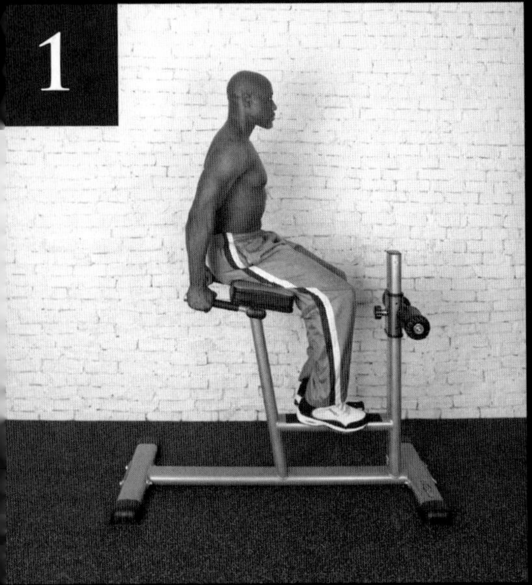

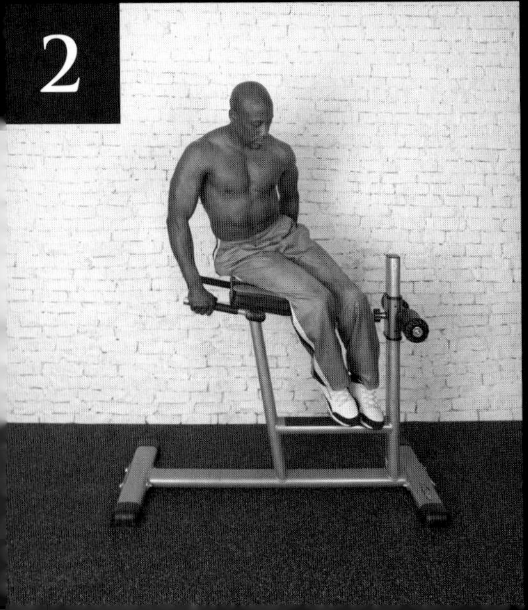

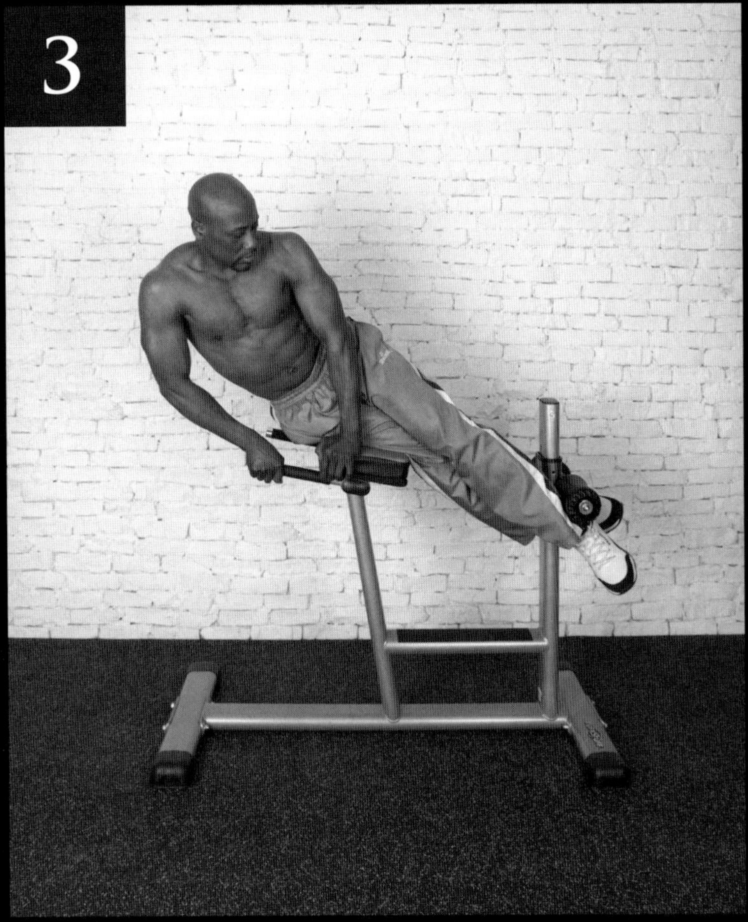

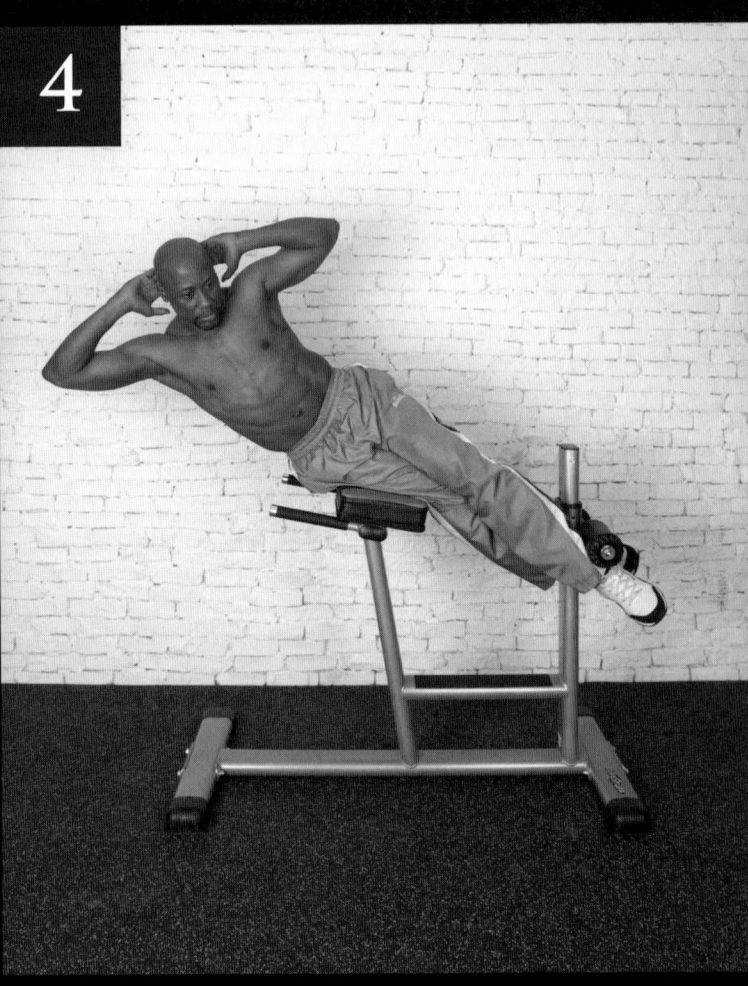

Mount the Roman chair from the side with the legs apart and crossed with the ankles resting against the ankle rest. The body should be lowered on the side with the hands behind the head, above or below the ears, with no pressure on the neck. The body should be lowered to the side in an oblique fashion and then lifted up in a controlled fashion.

5

Care should be taken to not arch the back during this exercise.

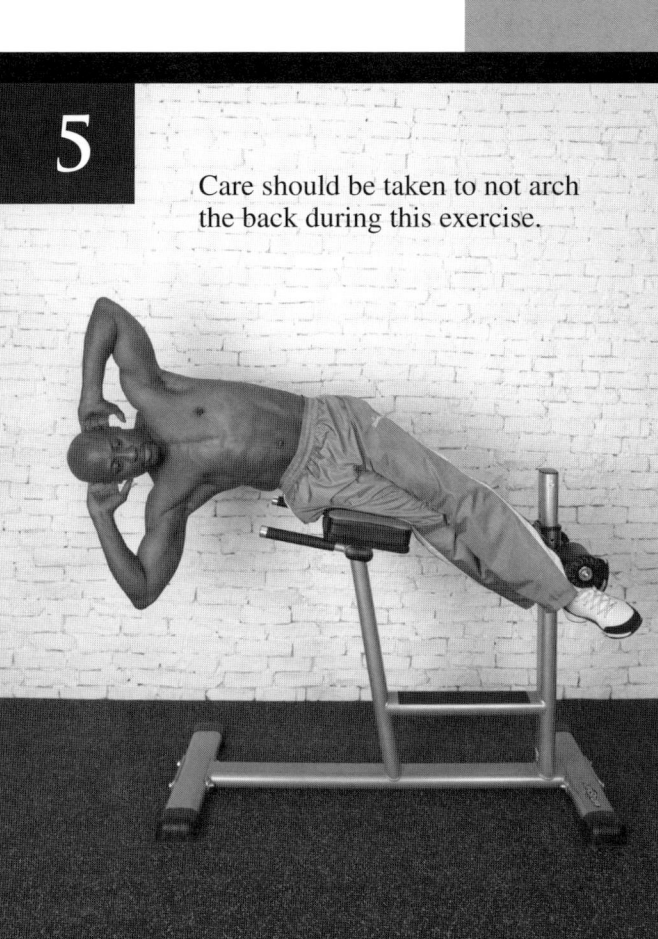

FIT TIP:

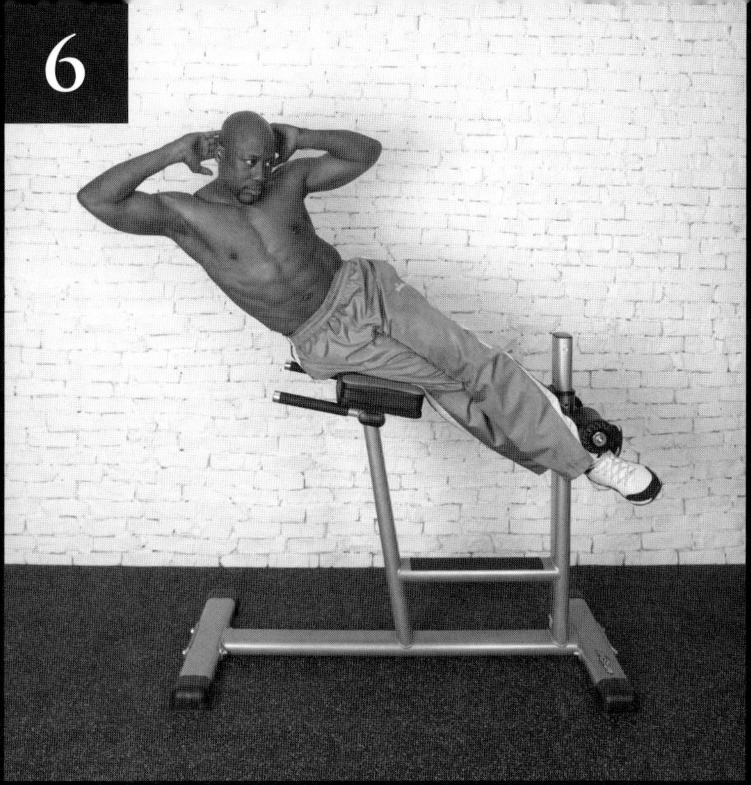

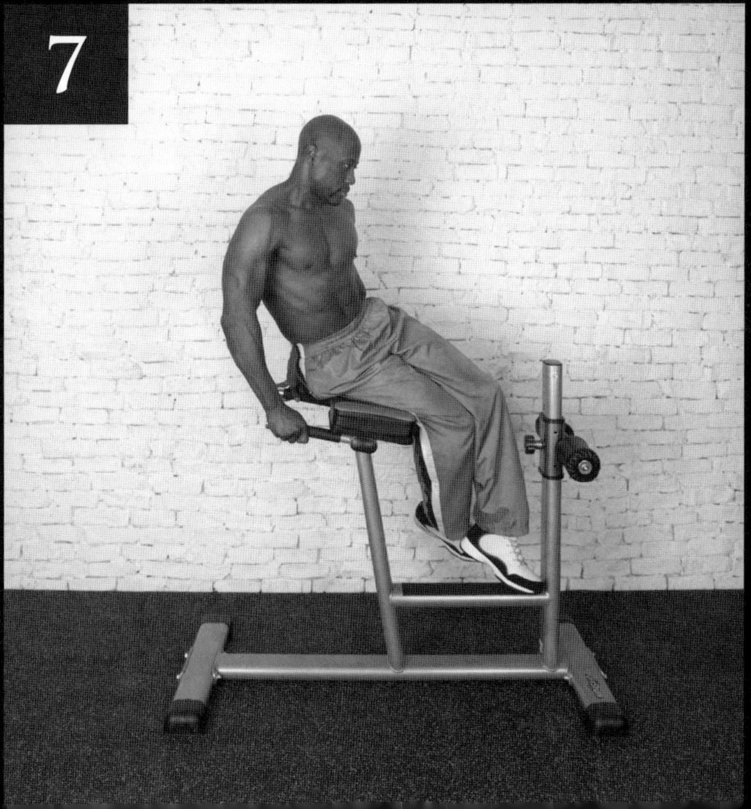

This exercise targets the obliques, serratus, and abdominals.

6

7

8

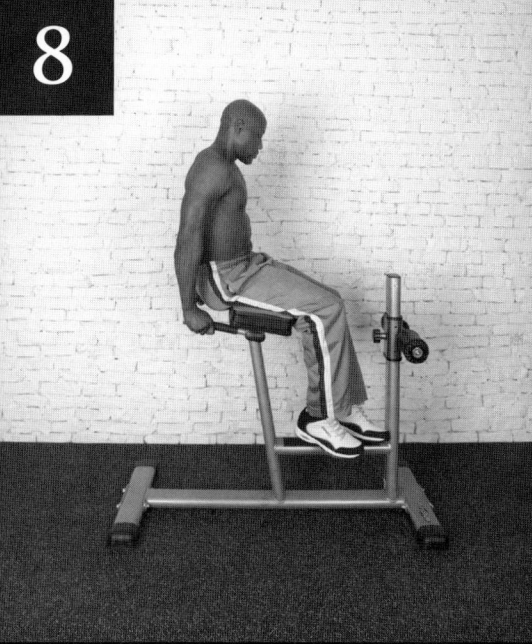

Recommended:
3 to 5 sets of
10 to 15 repetitions.

Roman Chair Back Extension Exercises

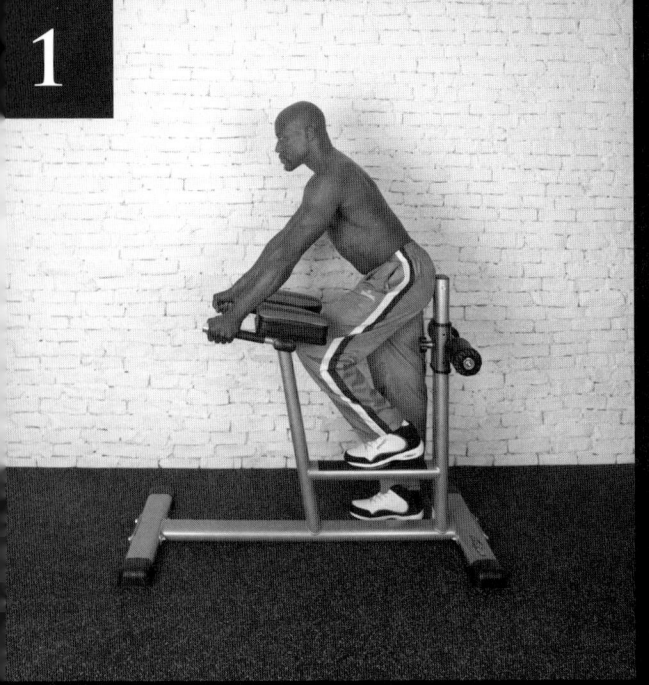

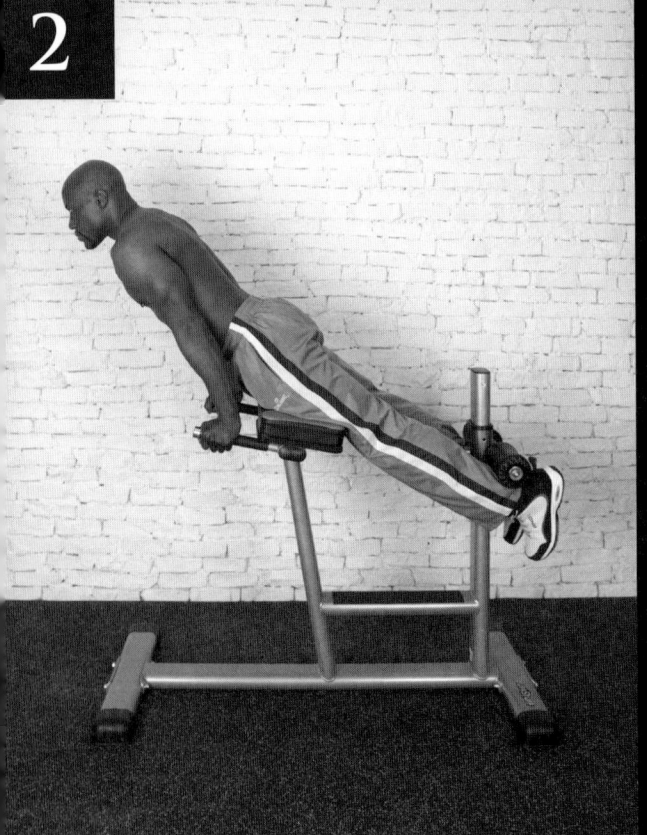

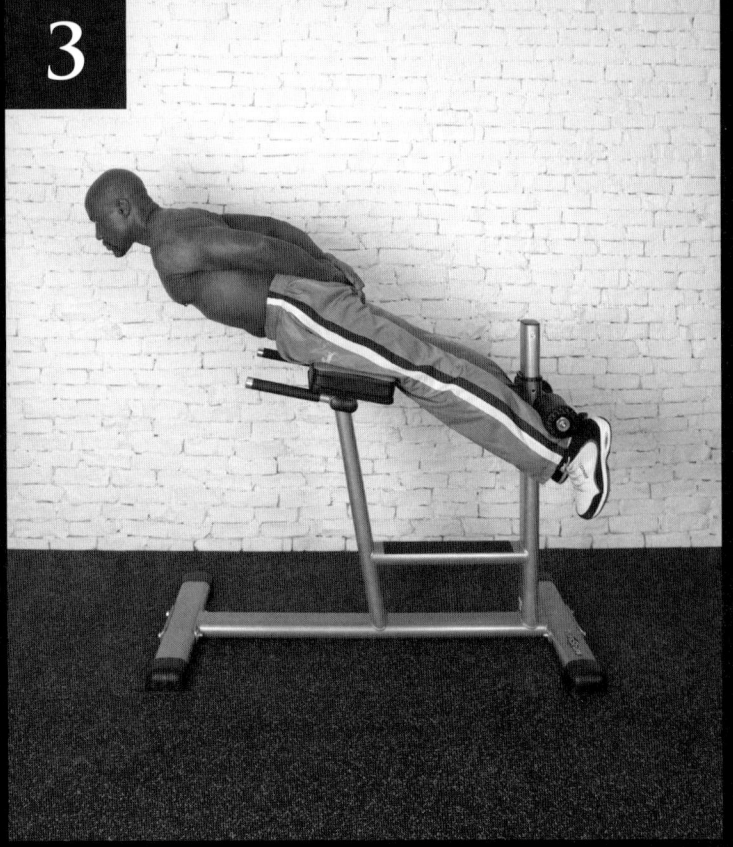

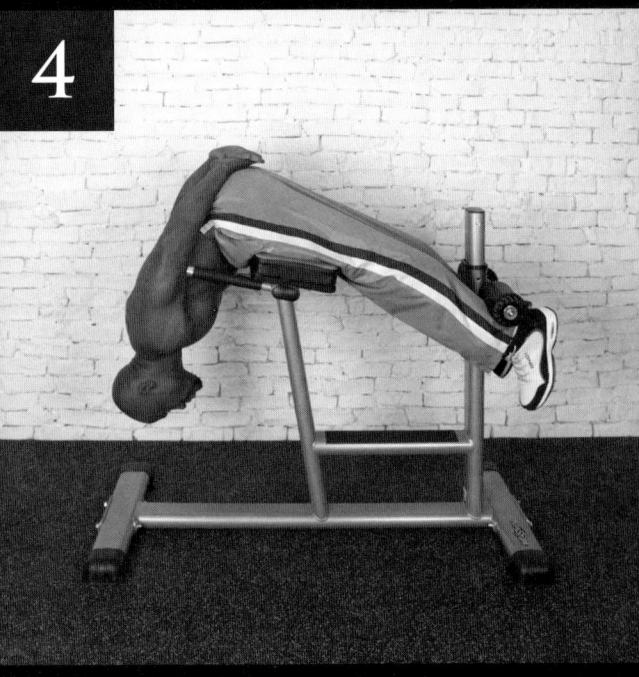

FIT TIP:
This exercise is to be done slowly.

The Roman chair should be mounted in a forward position, the back of the ankles against the ankle rest. The body should be tilted forward. Once suspended by the ankle rest, the hands can be placed behind the back or on the buttocks. The torso is then tilted forward and slowly lifted upright with the back hyperextended.

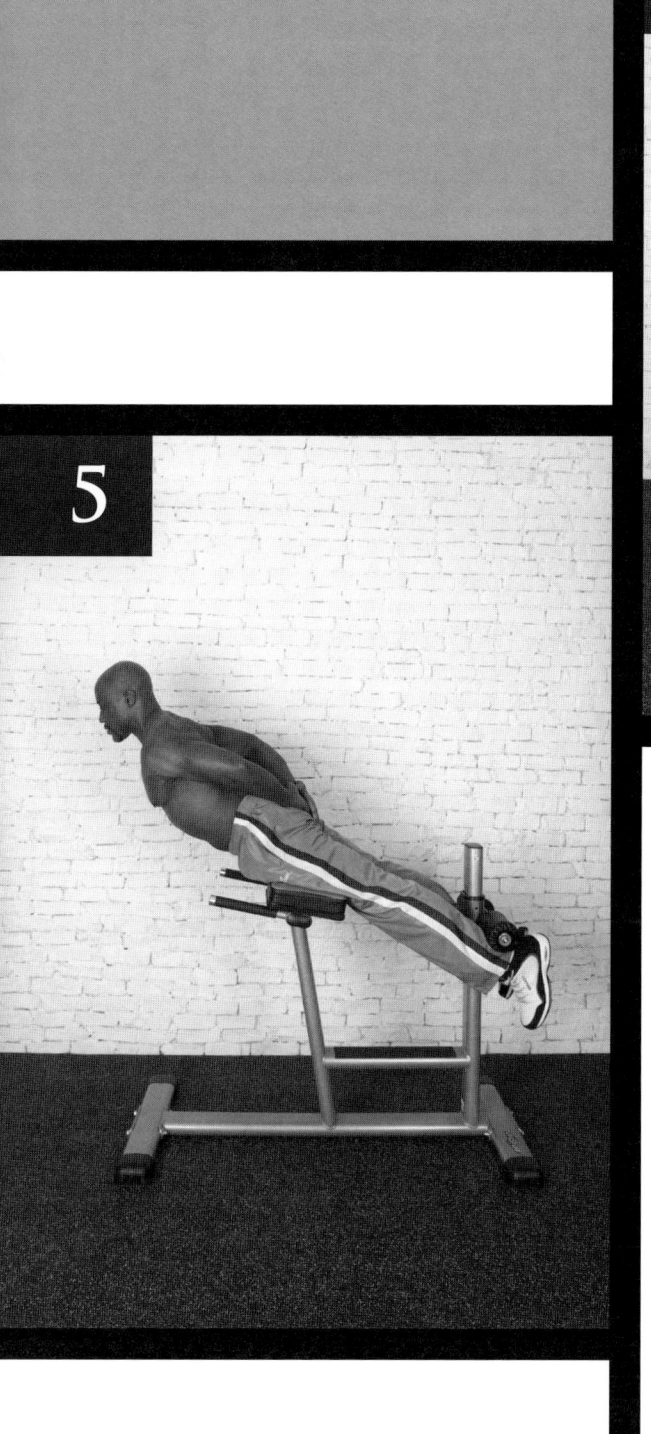

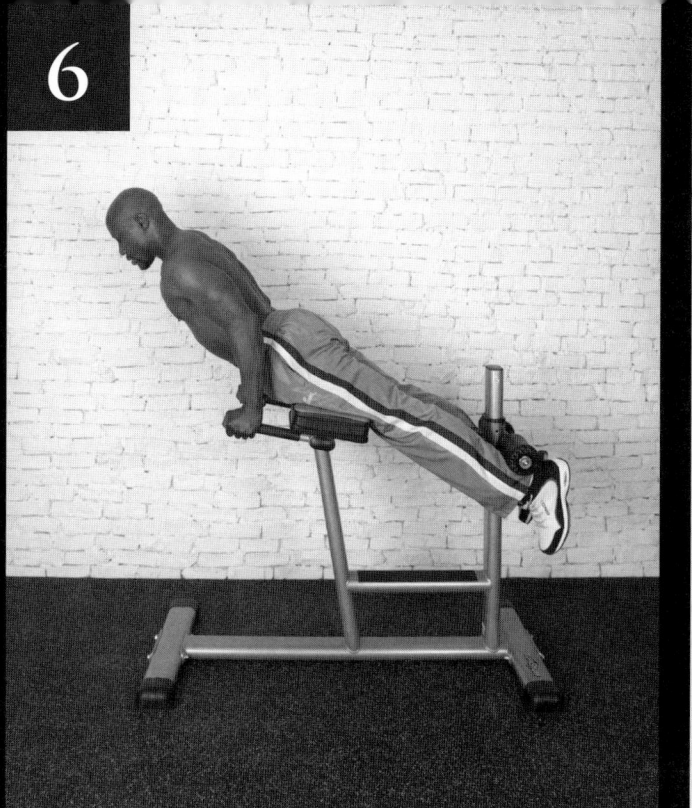

Recommended: 3 sets of 10 to 15 repetitions.

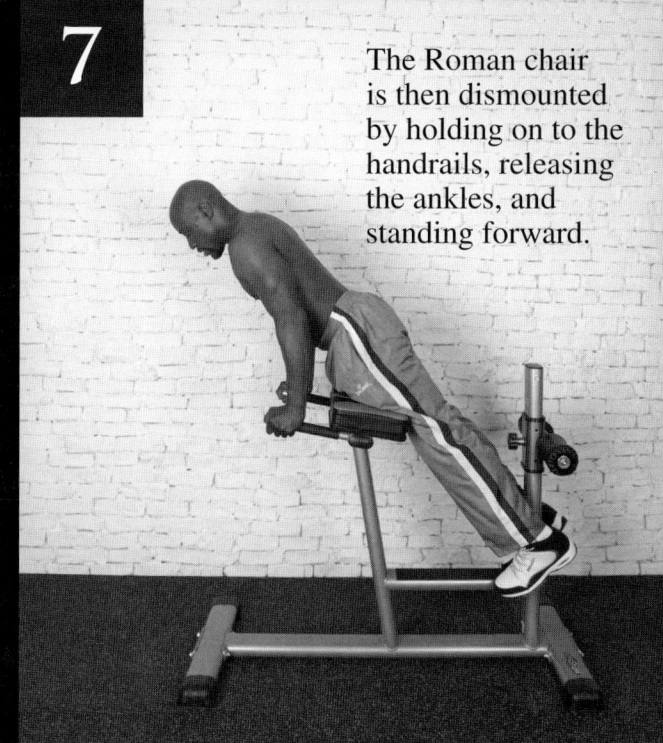

The Roman chair is then dismounted by holding on to the handrails, releasing the ankles, and standing forward.

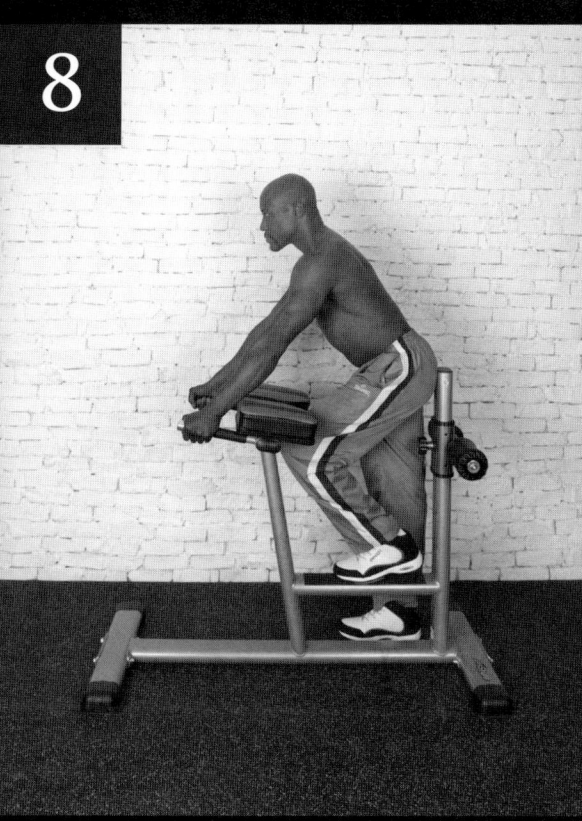

175

Straight Leg Raises
Using the Captain's Chair

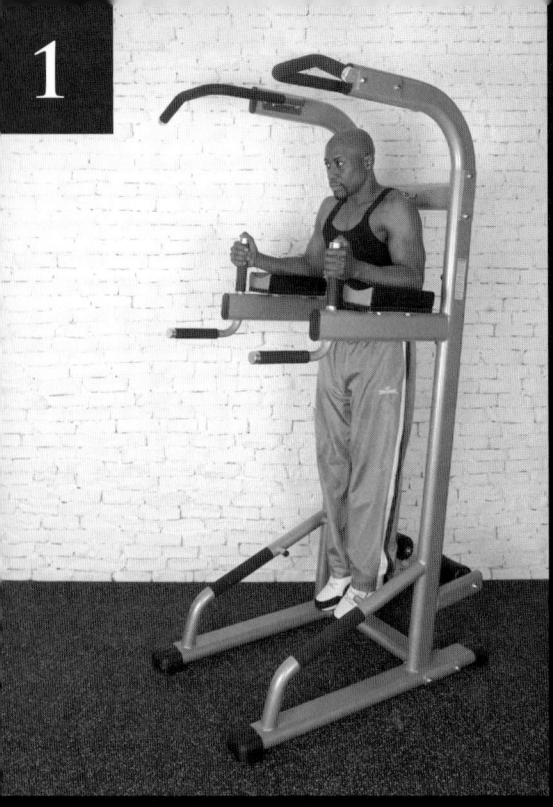

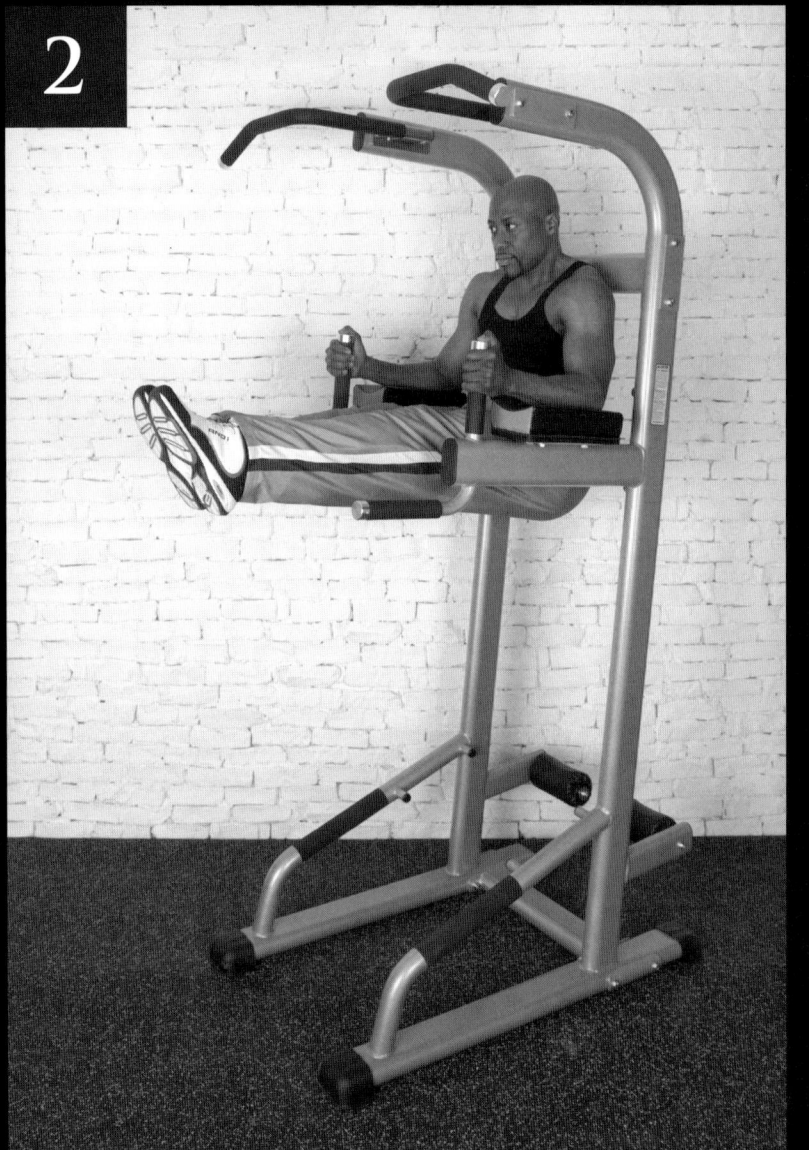

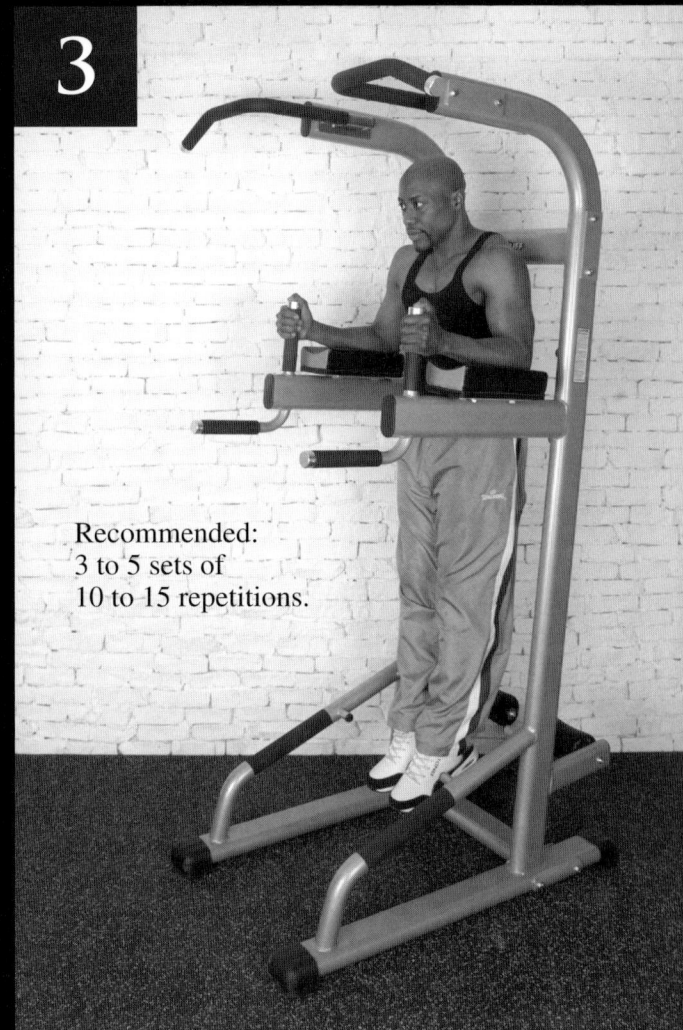

This exercise is done from the starting position of mounting the Captain's Chair. The legs are lifted in front with the knees straight and held for 10 to 30 seconds and then lowered downward. Do not sag or swing. The neck should also be relaxed throughout this exercise.

Recommended:
3 to 5 sets of
10 to 15 repetitions.

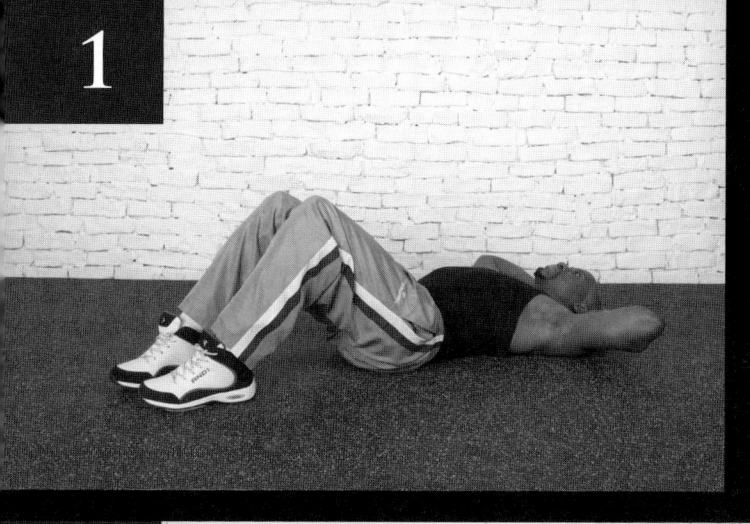

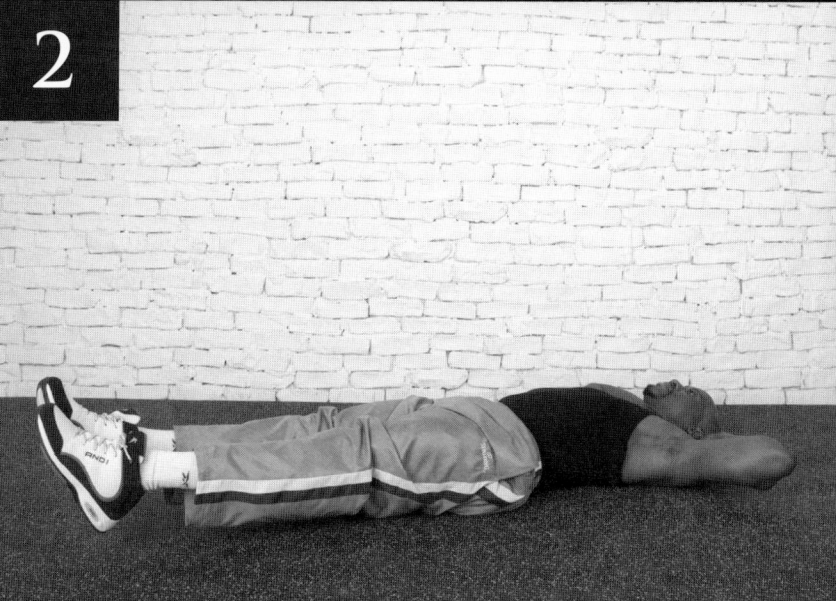

SIX-INCH CRUNCHES

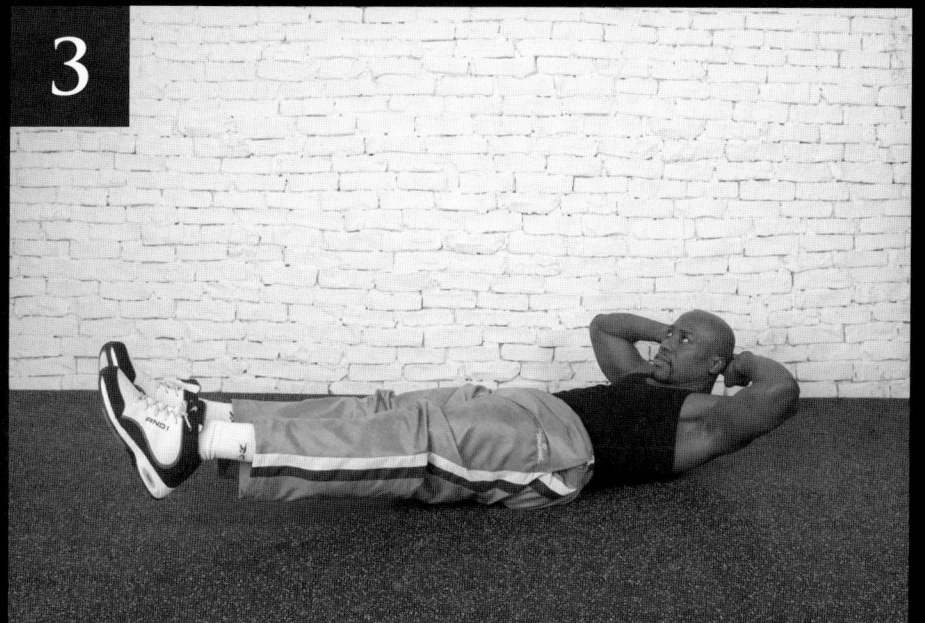

Starting from the regular sit-up position, the legs are then elevated approximately 6 inches off the ground; the hands are behind the head in a regular standard abdominal crunch position. The shoulders are then elevated, and the chin is also lifted upward. Care should be taken to focus the eyes upward. The chin is not to be tucked down onto the chest. The legs should stay elevated.

FIT TIP:

Recommended: 3 to 5 sets of 10 to 15 repetitions.

A variation of this can be done with the hands tucked under the pelvis and lower back for greater support.

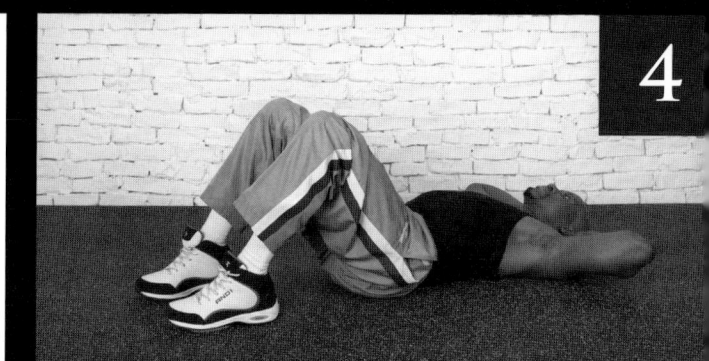

BICYCLE CRUNCH

Recommended:
3 to 5 sets of
10 to 15 repetitions.

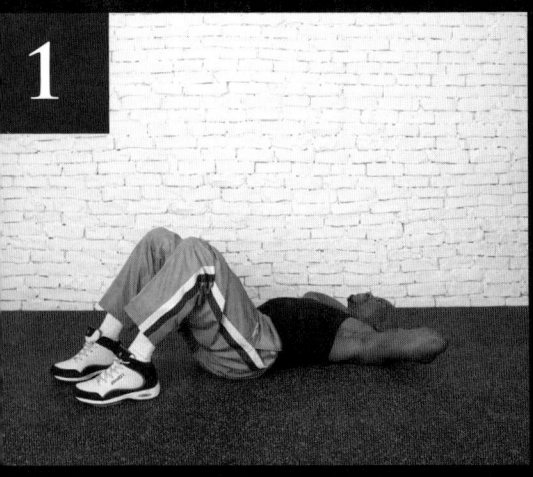

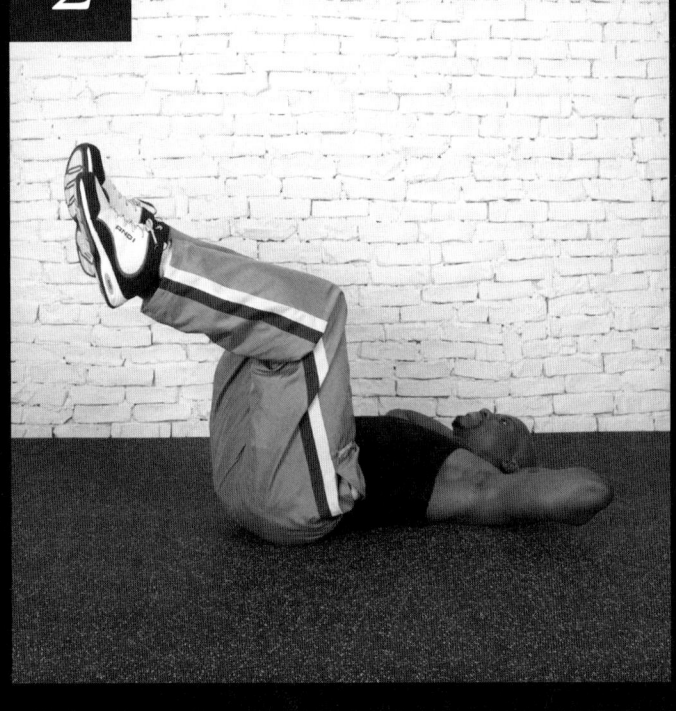

This exercise is done by starting in a standard sit-up position with the legs elevated for a bicycle-type maneuver. The opposite elbow should be brought forward and toward the opposing knee and thigh, and this should be done in a sequence going from right to left in the cycling-type position. The exercise should be done without putting any strain on the neck and without pulling the neck forward.

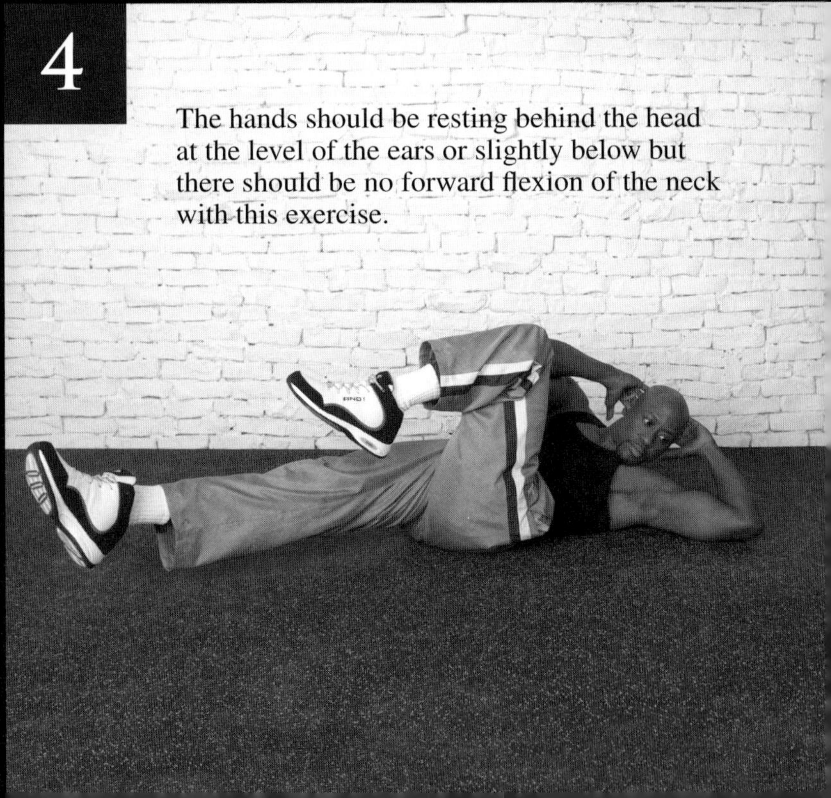

The hands should be resting behind the head at the level of the ears or slightly below but there should be no forward flexion of the neck with this exercise.

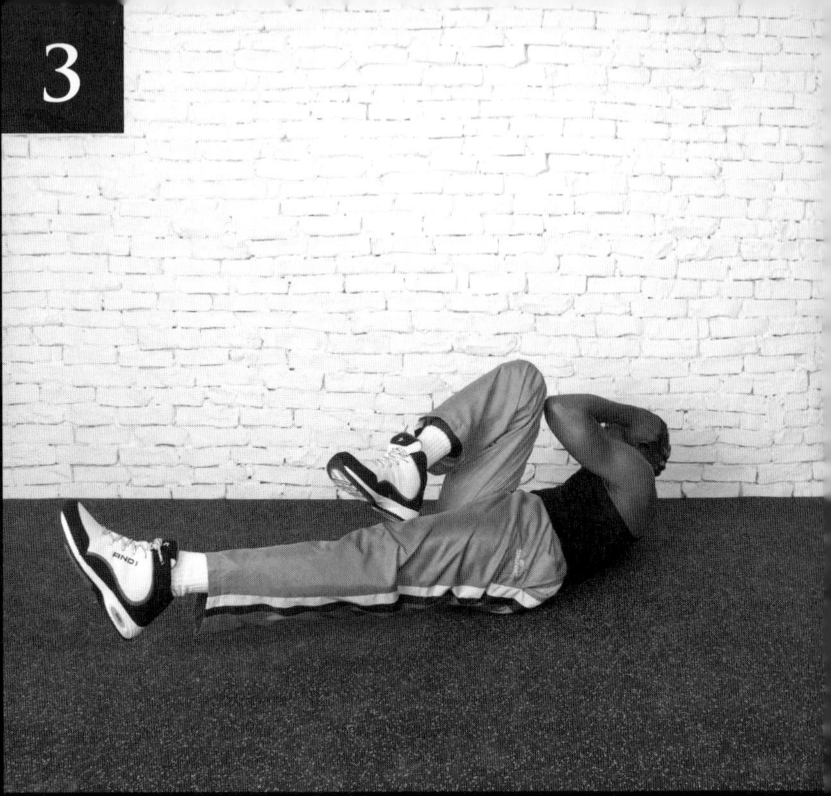

Straight Leg V-Up Crunch

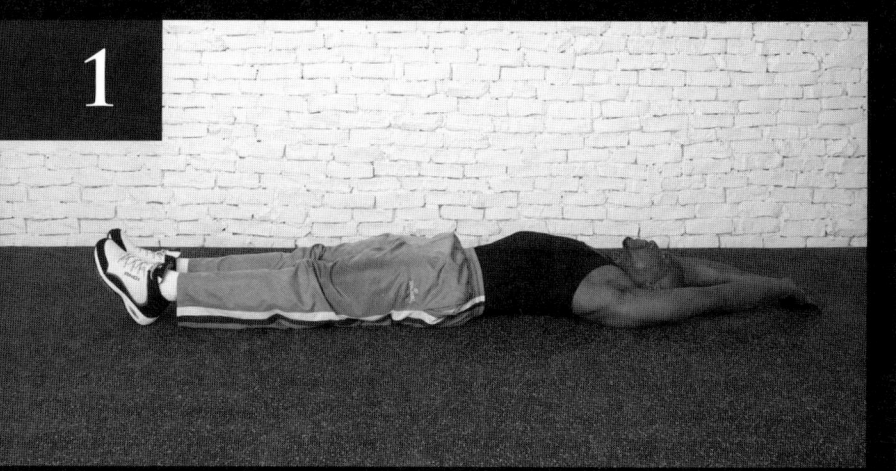

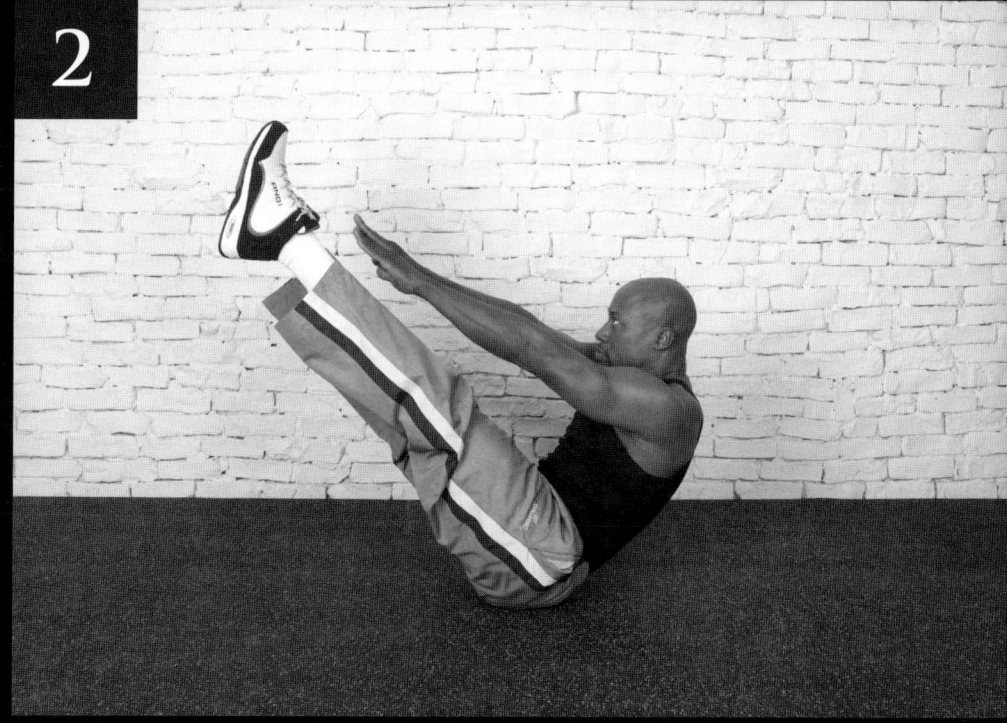

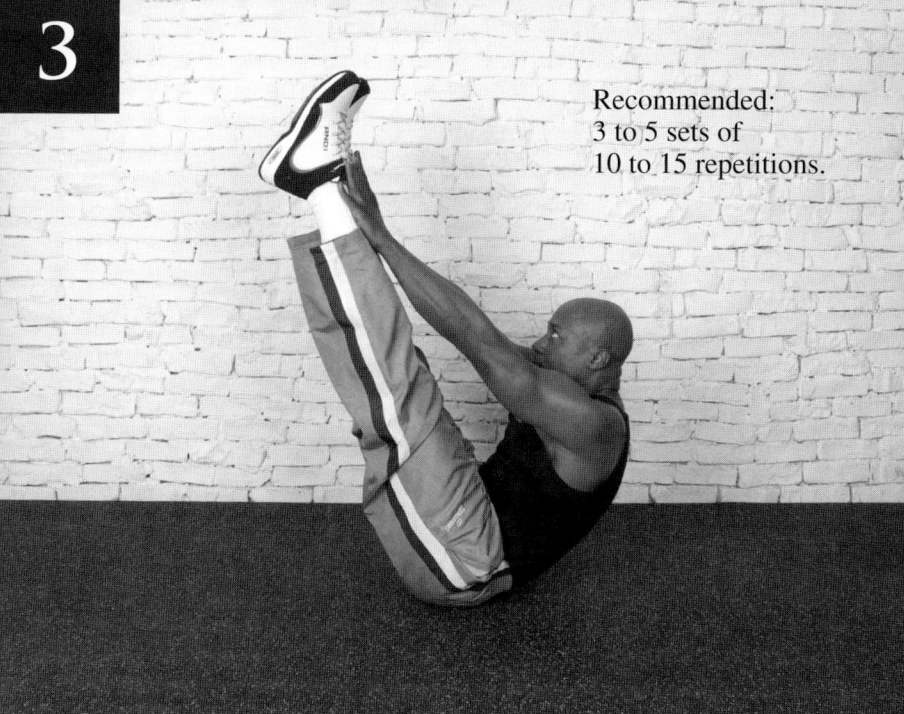

Recommended:
3 to 5 sets of
10 to 15 repetitions.

These are performed lying flat on your back, hands above your head, palms up. Bring the feet up straight and bring the arms toward the feet with the arms straight, attempting to touch the toes with the fingers in a very harmonious, synchronous, single motion. This should be done with the neck relaxed.

LATERAL SIDE CRUNCH
With Elevated Knees

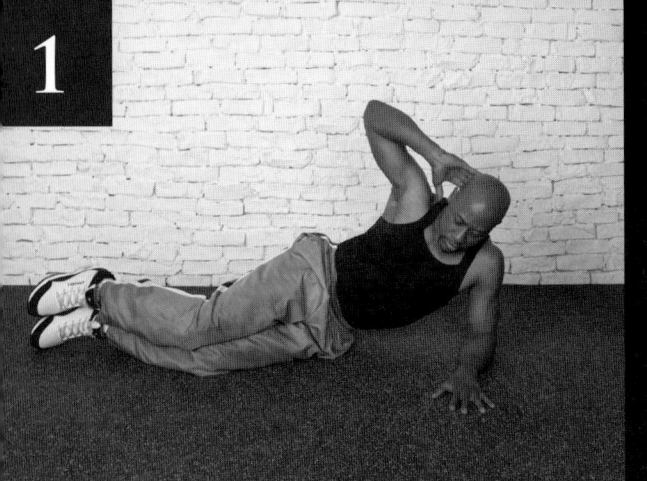

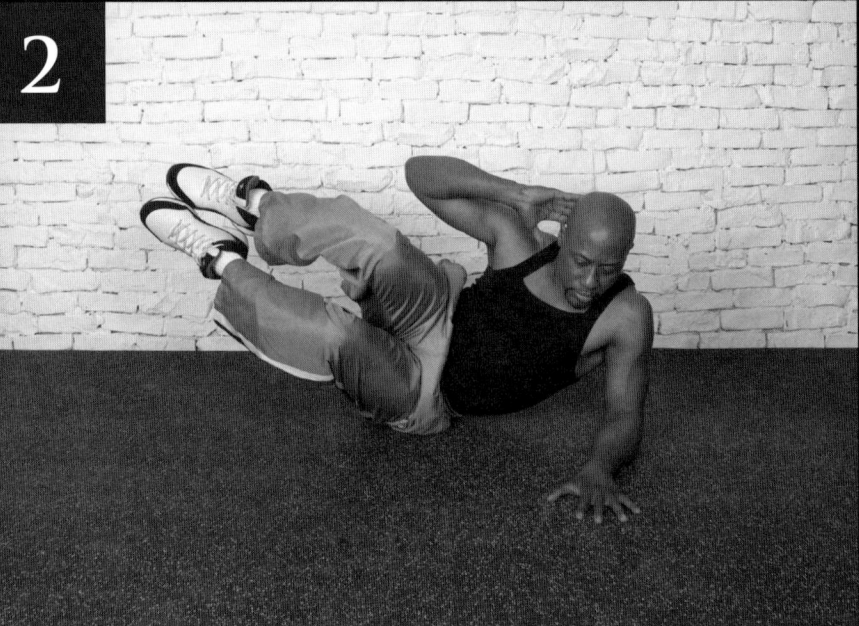

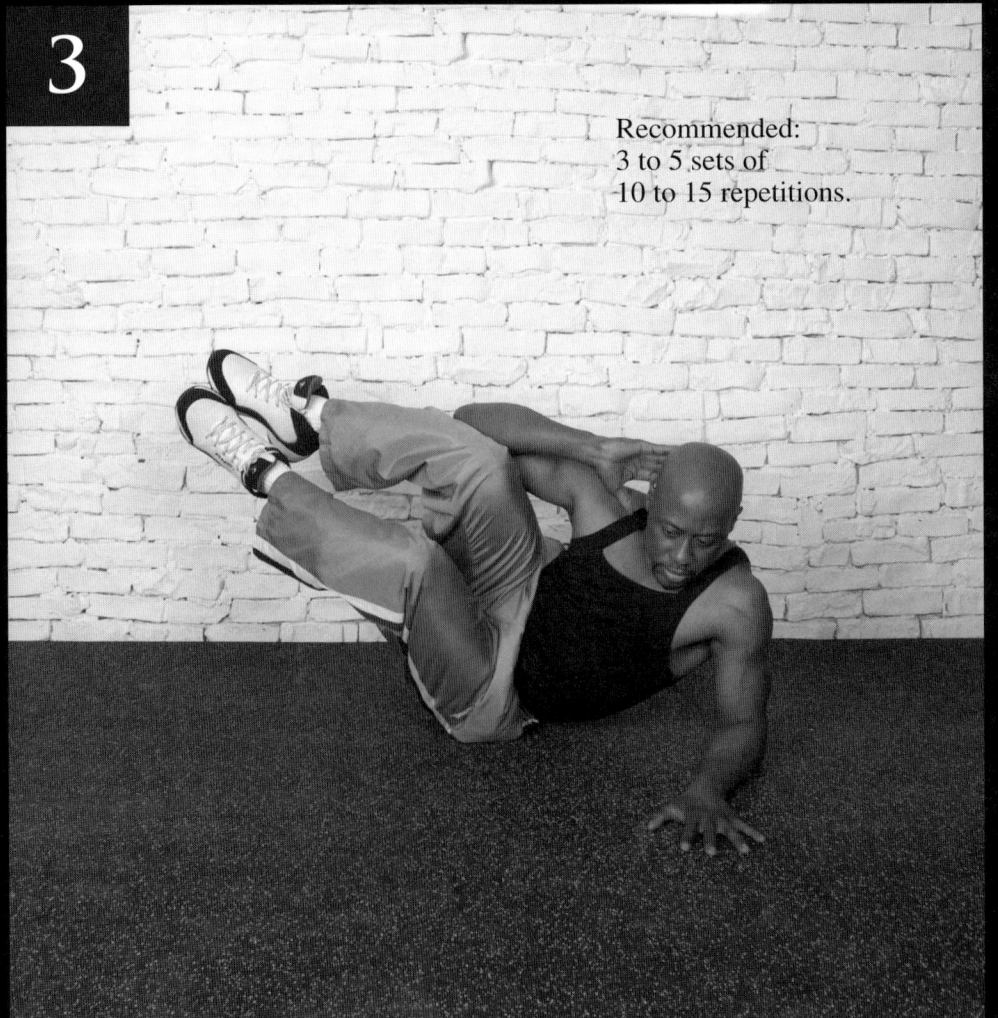

Recommended:
3 to 5 sets of
10 to 15 repetitions.

The exercise is executed by lying on your side, balanced on one elbow as illustrated. The knees are then brought to the elbow with the hand behind the head, and the body is crunched to the side.

Standing Front Abdominal Curl and Knee Lift

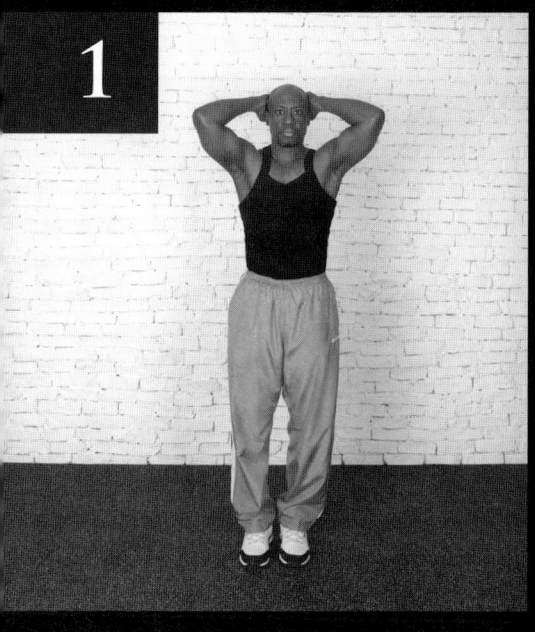

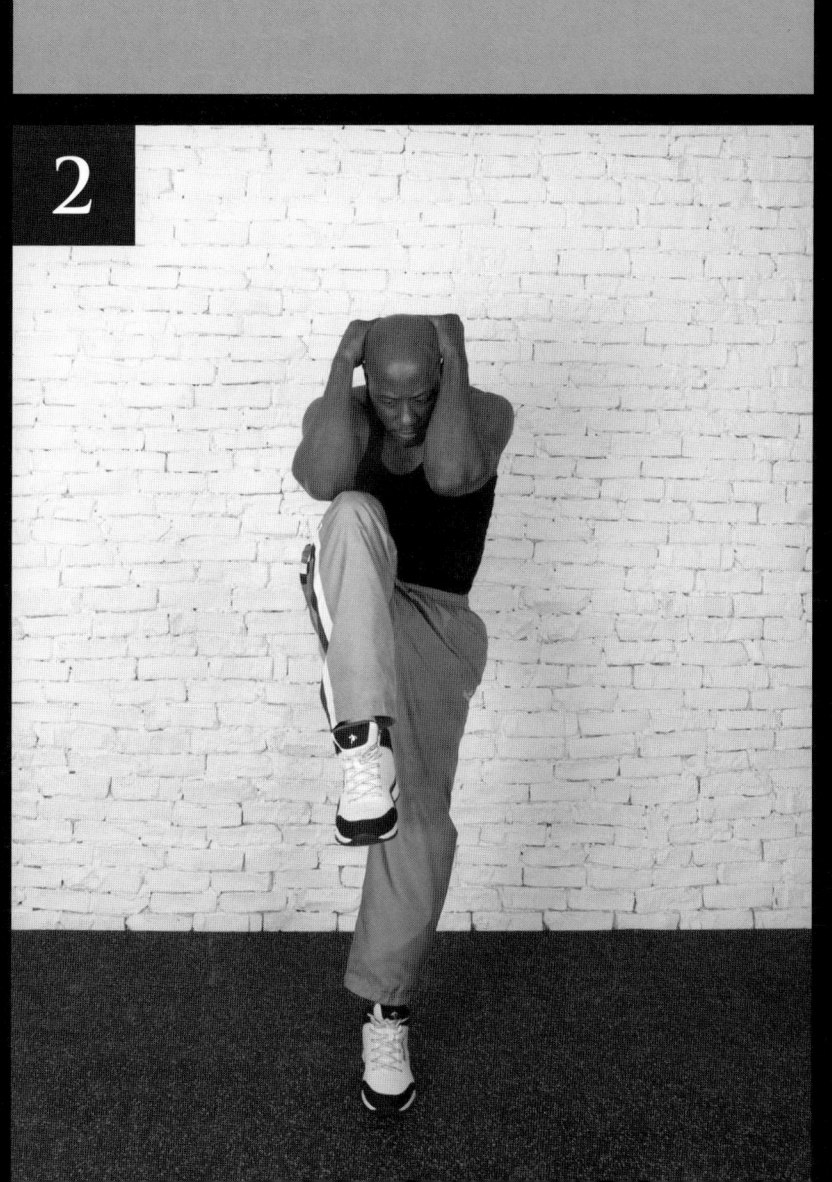

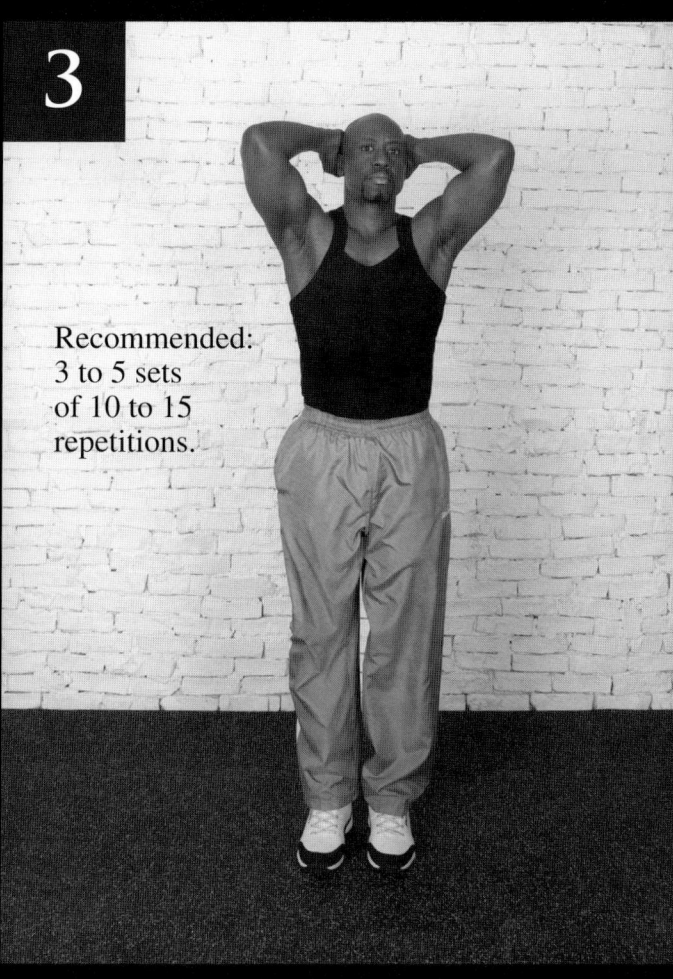

Recommended: 3 to 5 sets of 10 to 15 repetitions.

This exercise is done by standing with the feet together, and the hands behind the head. Lift the knee up high and crunch forward toward that knee. Balance on the opposing leg. The neck should not be flexed forward forcefully by the hands.

Standing Lateral Side Crunch and Knee Lift

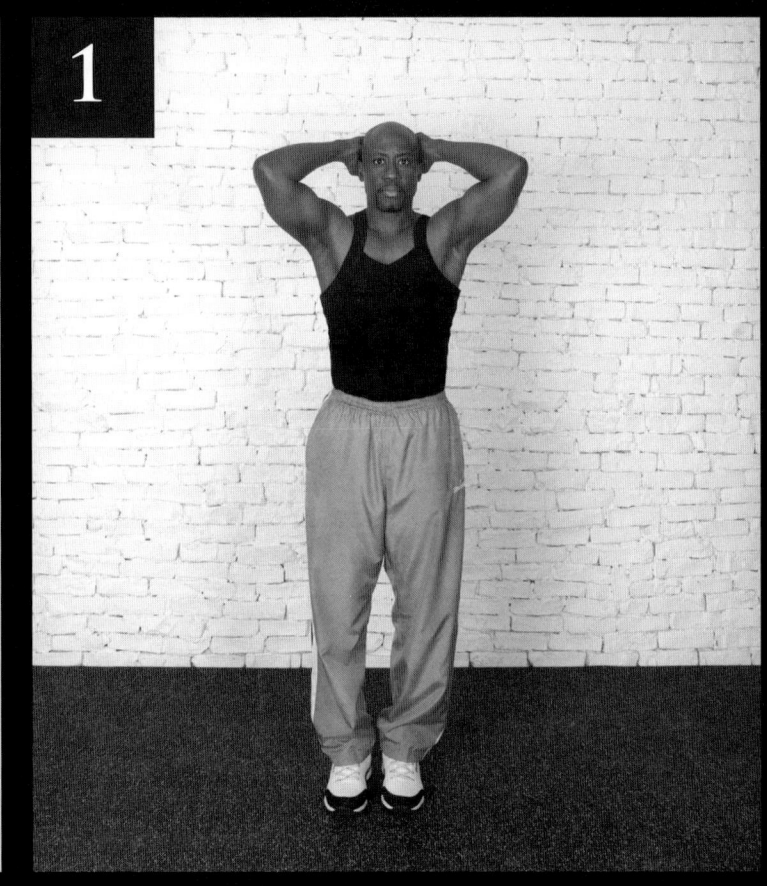

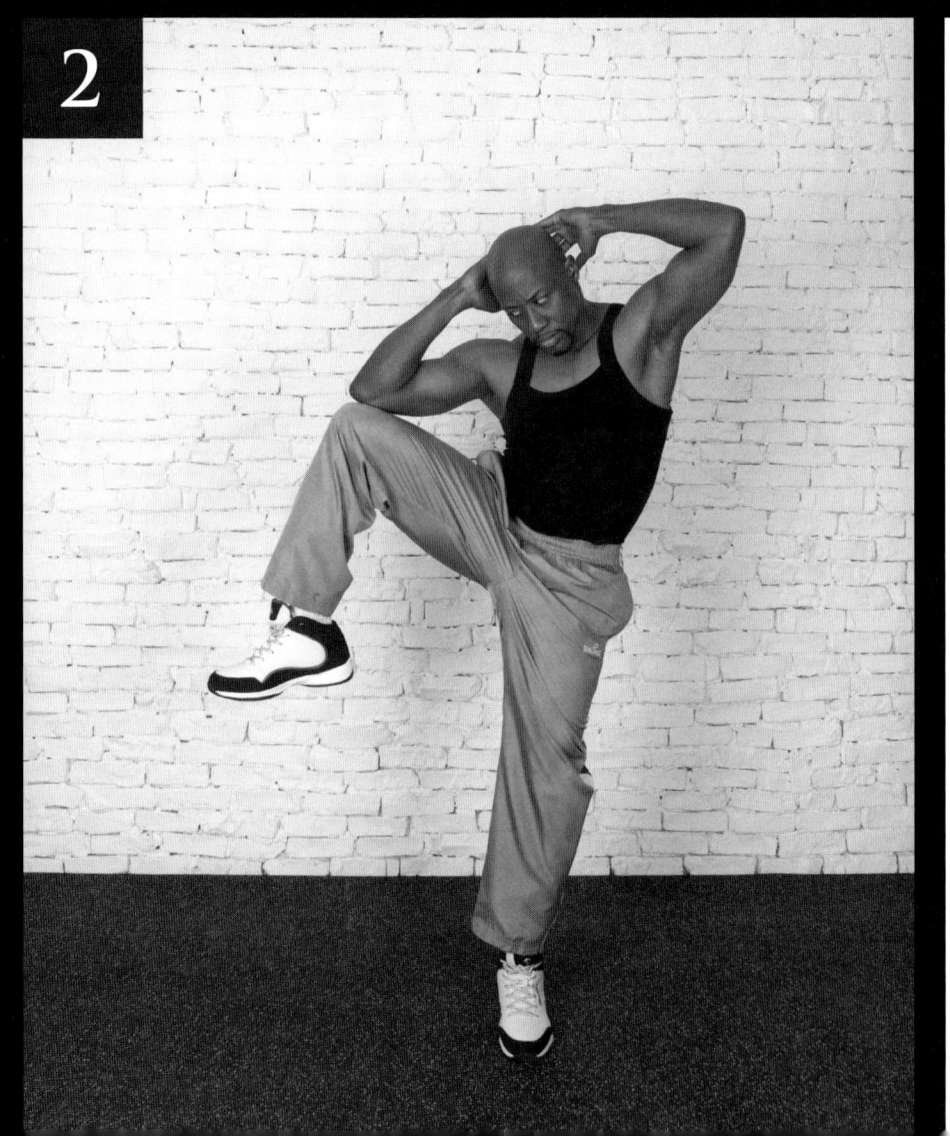

The exercise is done by starting in the neutral position with the hands behind the head, the elbows flexed. Lift up one leg and bend over to the side with that elevated leg. Balance on the leg, which is planted on the floor, while crunching toward the knee.

STANDING FORWARD ABDOMINAL CRUNCH

With Straight Leg Elevated

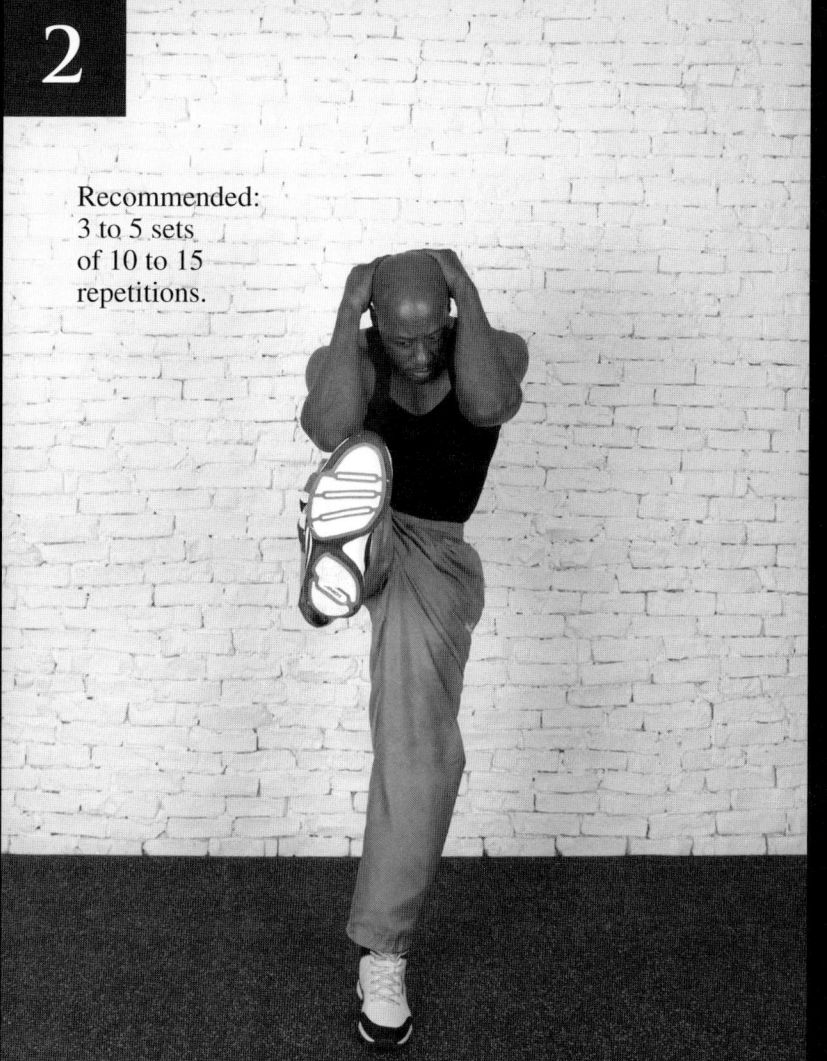

Recommended: 3 to 5 sets of 10 to 15 repetitions.

The exercise is done by starting in the standard standing position, feet approximately shoulder width, hands behind the head, the straight leg is elevated, the elbow on the side of the elevated leg is brought toward the knee, and the torso is curled toward the thigh.

FIT TIP:
Relax your neck for this exercise.

LATERAL SIDE CRUNCH
With Lateral Straight Leg Raise

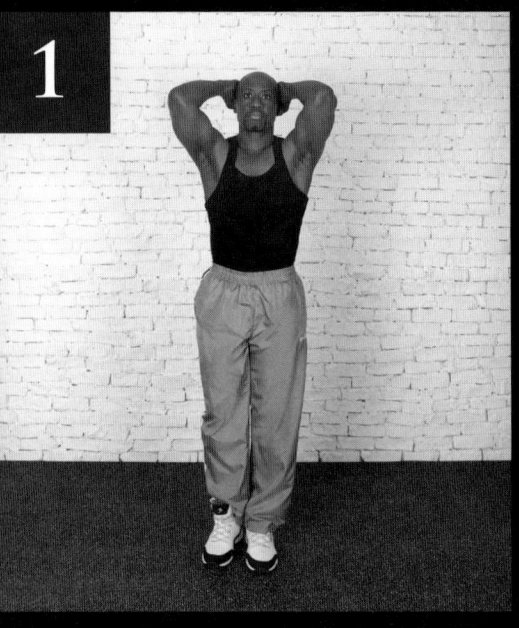

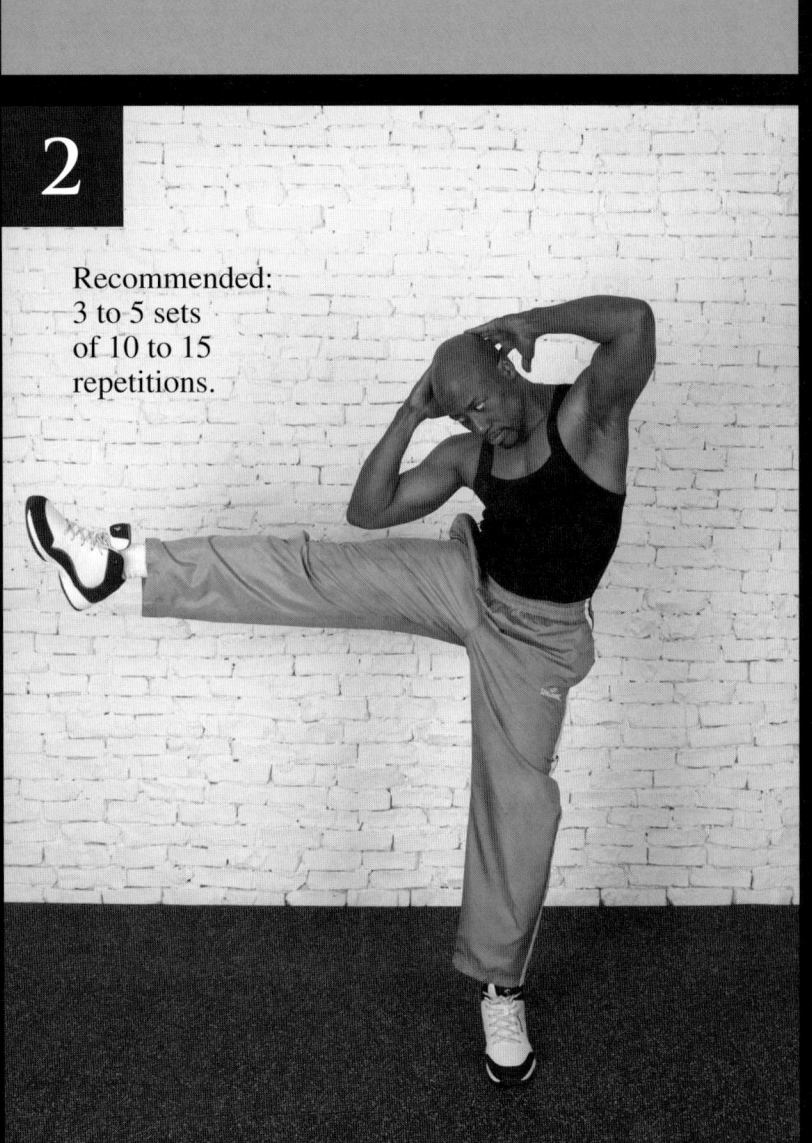

Recommended: 3 to 5 sets of 10 to 15 repetitions.

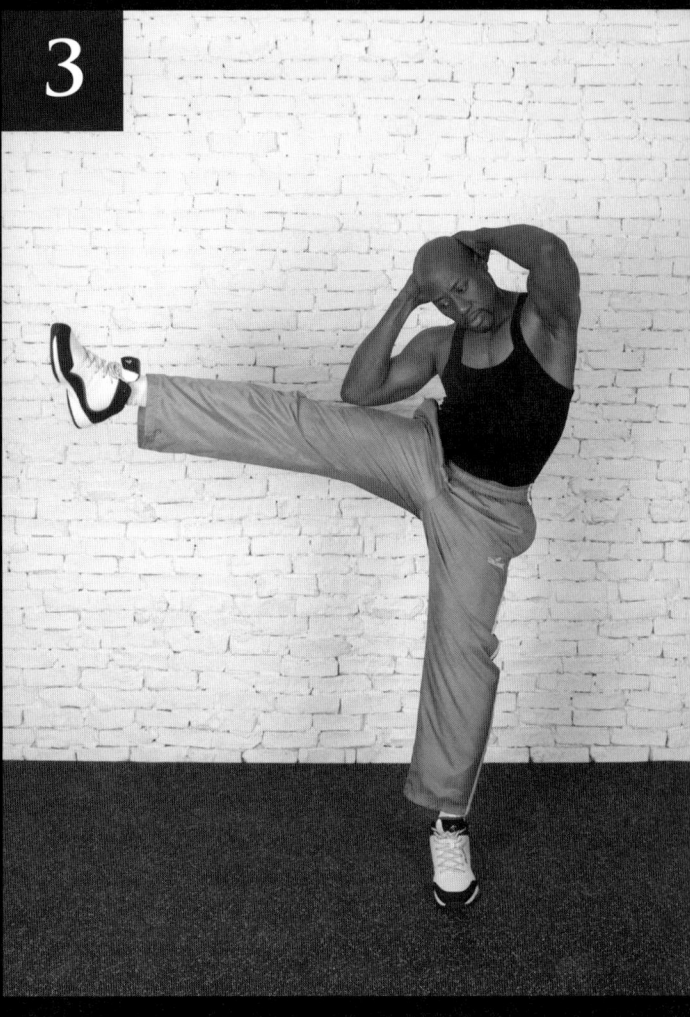

Start in the standard position. The leg is lifted laterally, and the elbow on that side is brought toward the thigh until the leg is perpendicular with the floor and the torso is laterally bent toward the thigh with the elbow flexed.

COMBINED ONE-ARM MILITARY SHOULDER PRESS AND ANTERIOR KNEE LIFT

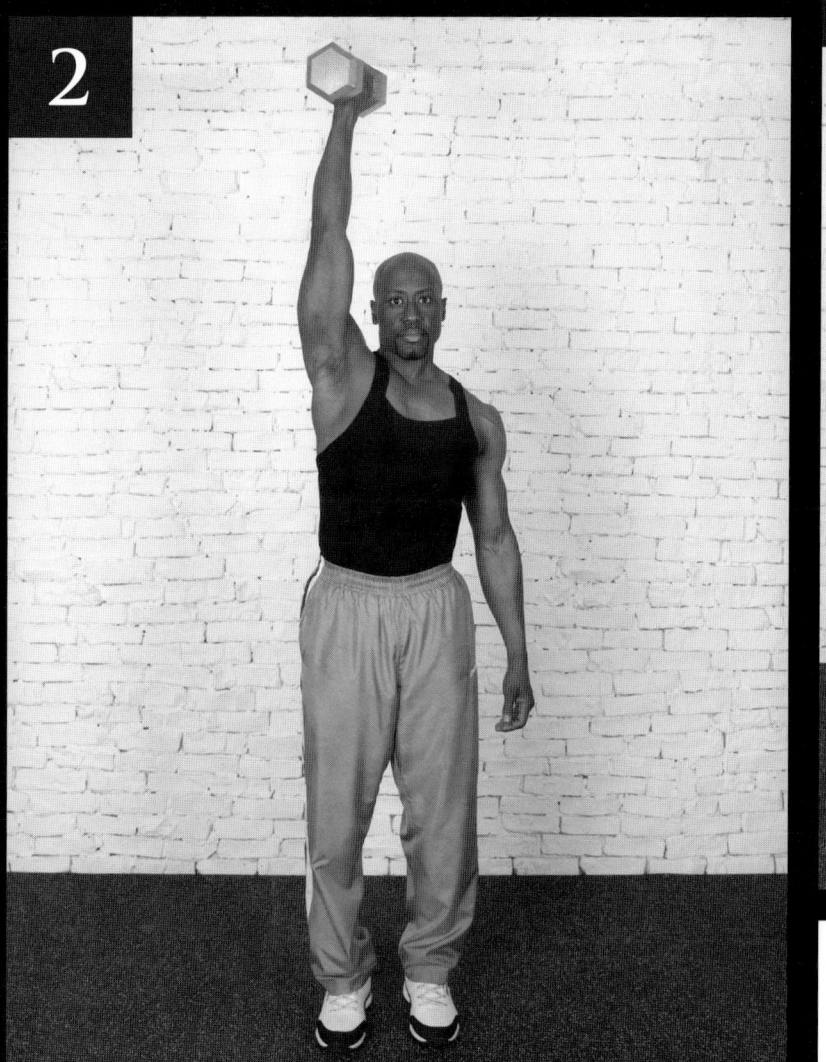
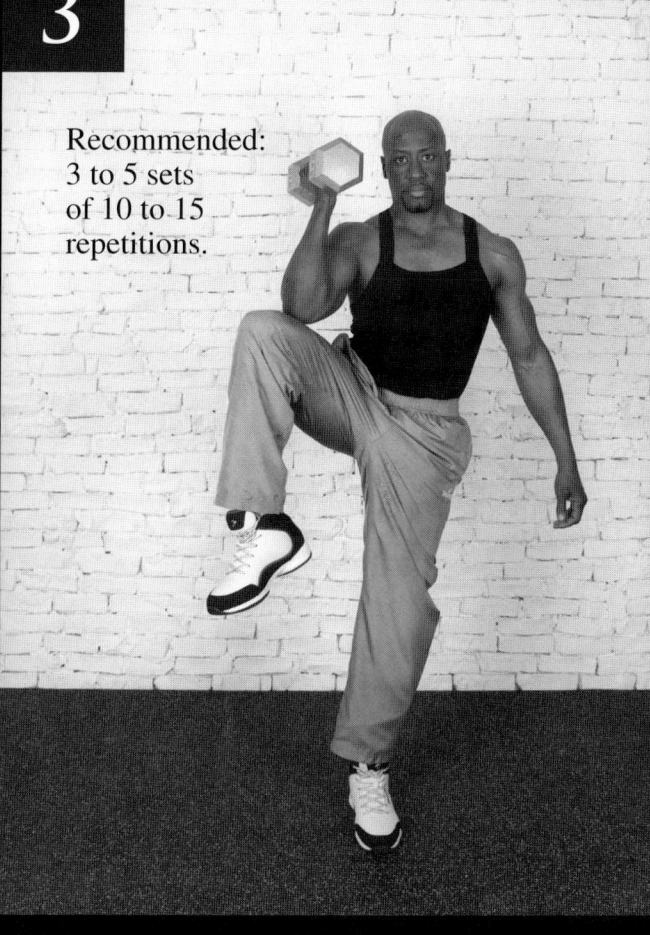

Recommended: 3 to 5 sets of 10 to 15 repetitions.

The exercise is done by starting in the standard position with a weight. Starting on the right side with the weight in the right hand and with the palm facing the thigh, lift the weight overhead. The knee is bent, and the elbow is brought down to the thigh, and then pressed again overhead.

Combined One-Arm Military Shoulder Press and Lateral Knee Lift

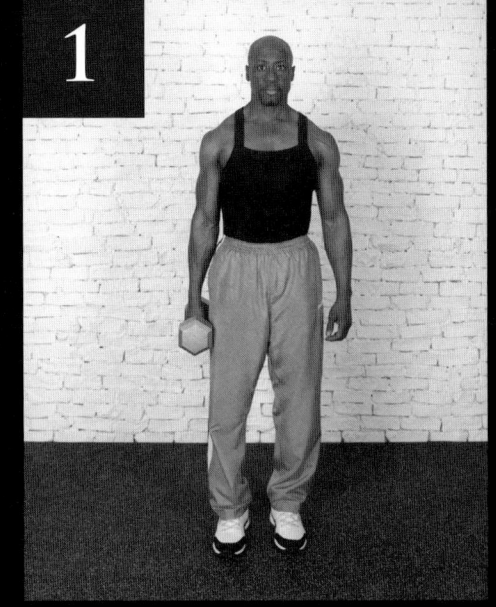

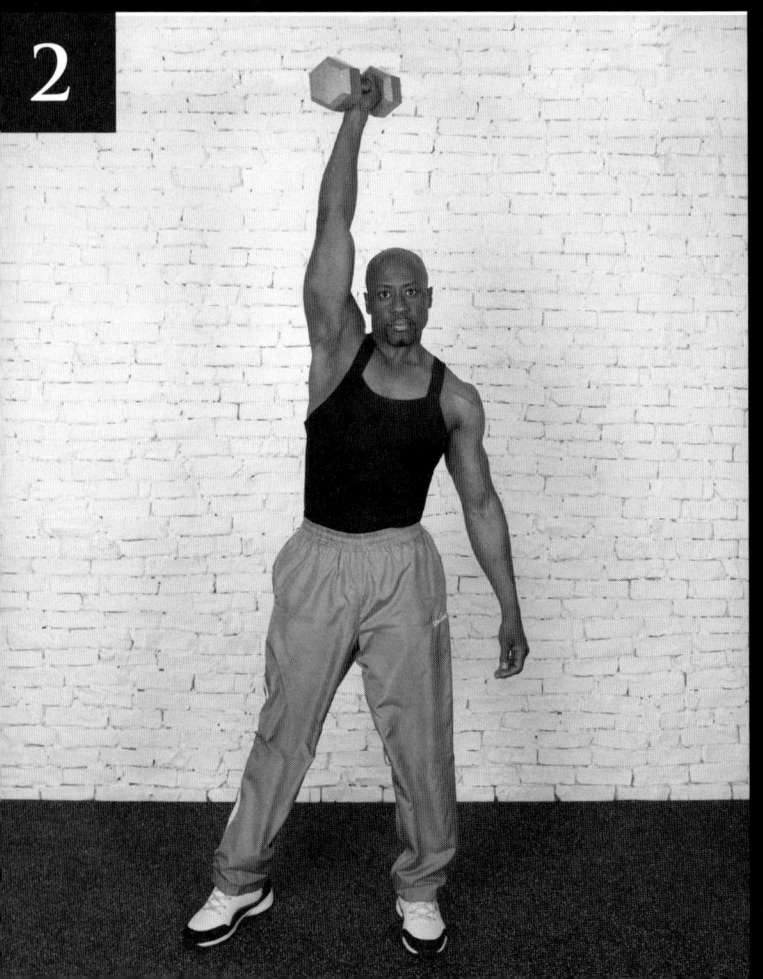

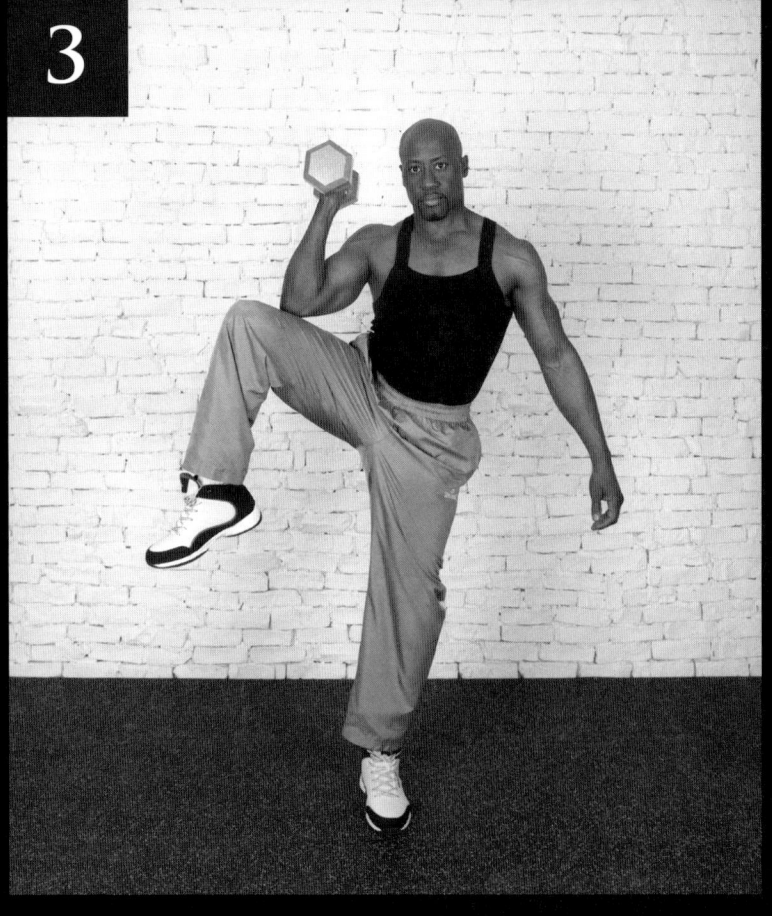

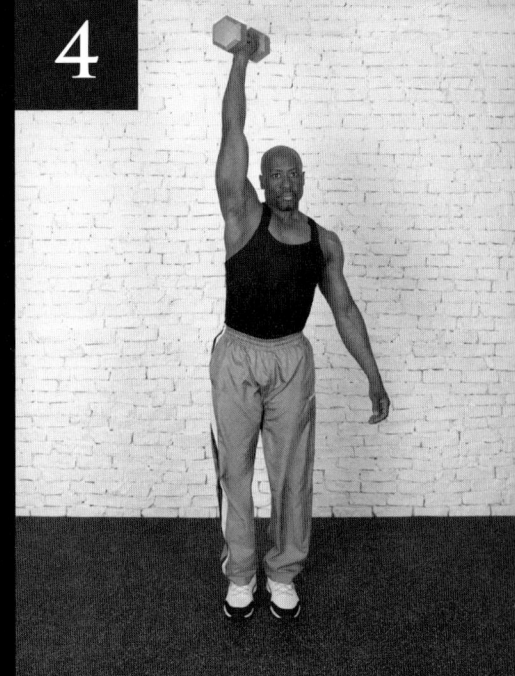

FIT TIP:
Bring the knee and elbow outward and lateral.

The starting position is with weight next to the body with the palm toward the thigh. The weight is then pressed overhead. The knee is lifted and then the elbow is brought to the knee and the weight is pressed above the head again.

Jumping Rope

This should be done the way you did it as a kid, often and happily.

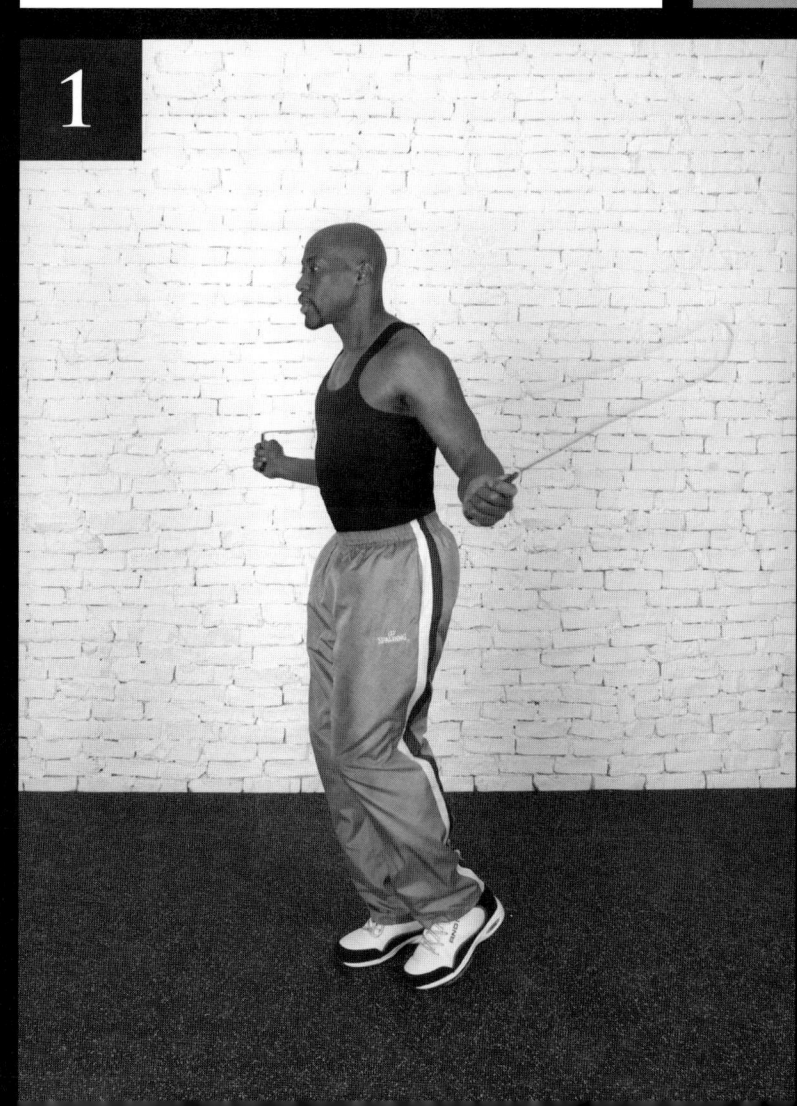

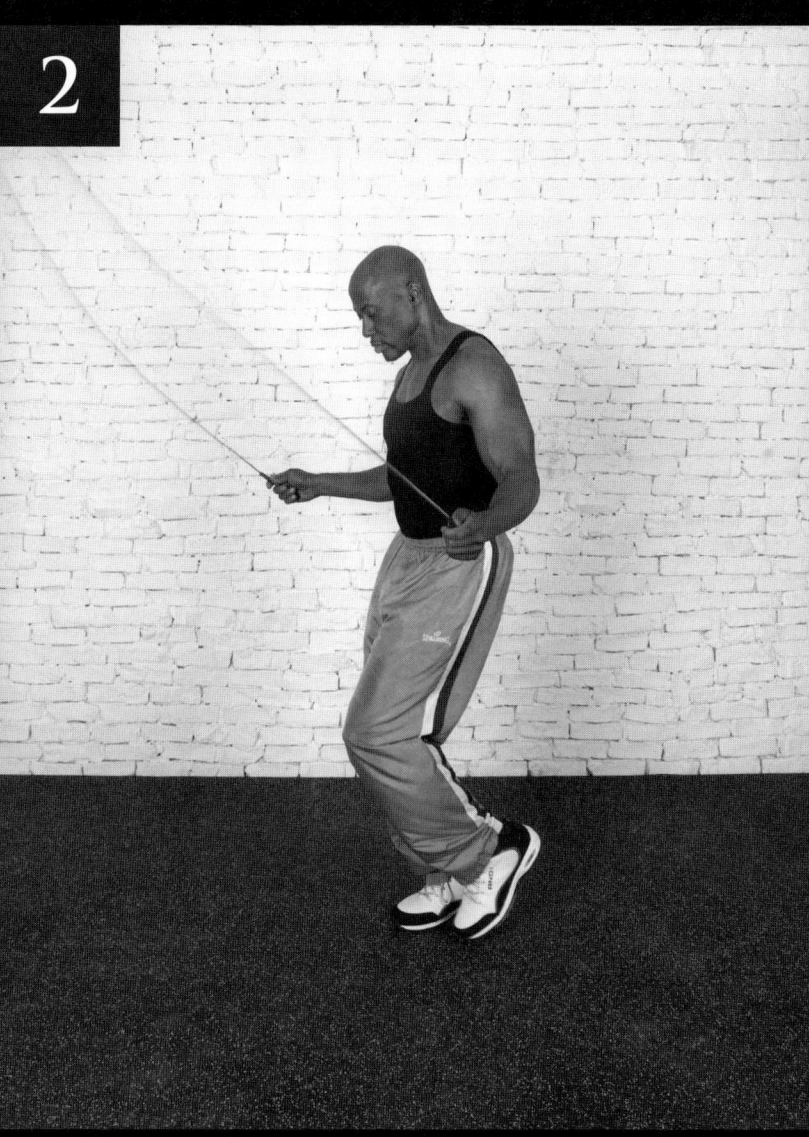

Recommended: 10 to 30 minutes, 3 to 5 times per week. Start with 5 to 10 minutes and build up. Change your speed to add variety.

Single Leg Jumping Rope

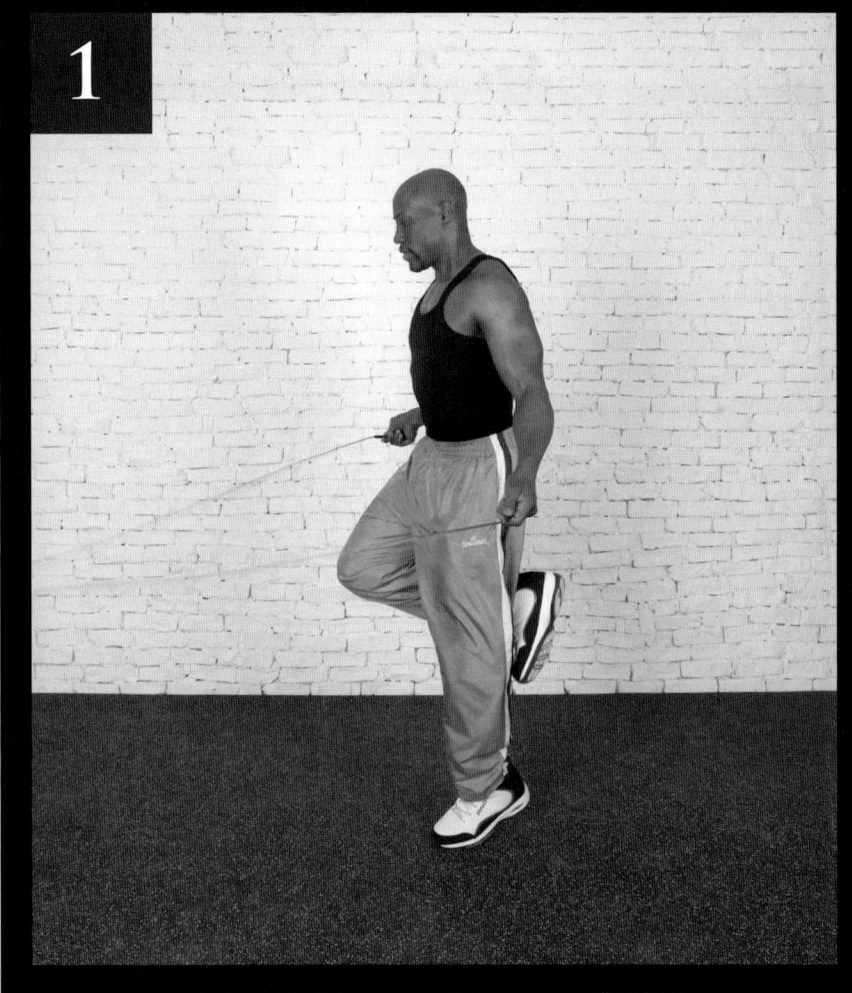

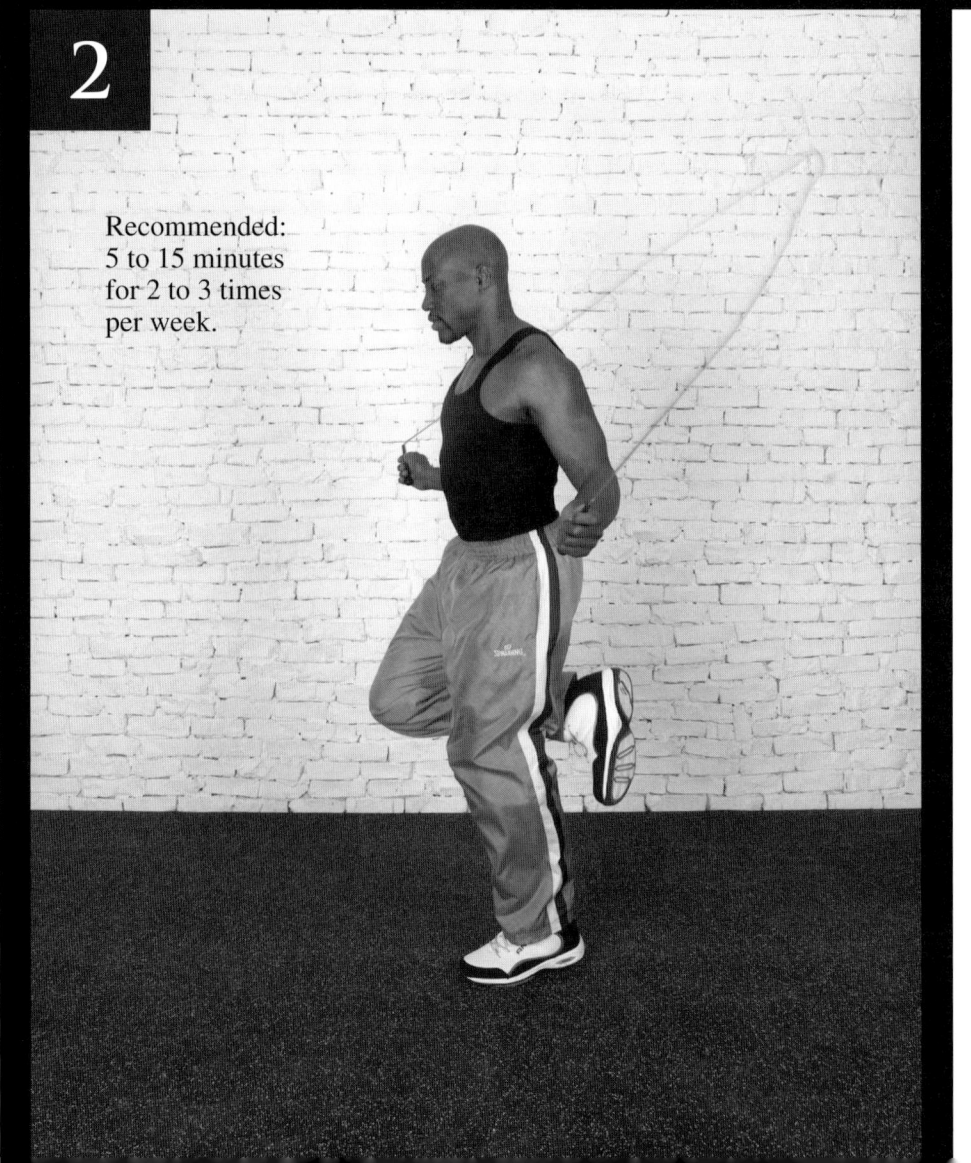

Recommended: 5 to 15 minutes for 2 to 3 times per week.

Single leg skipping is great when you want to intensify the workout and increase your balance.

The Jab

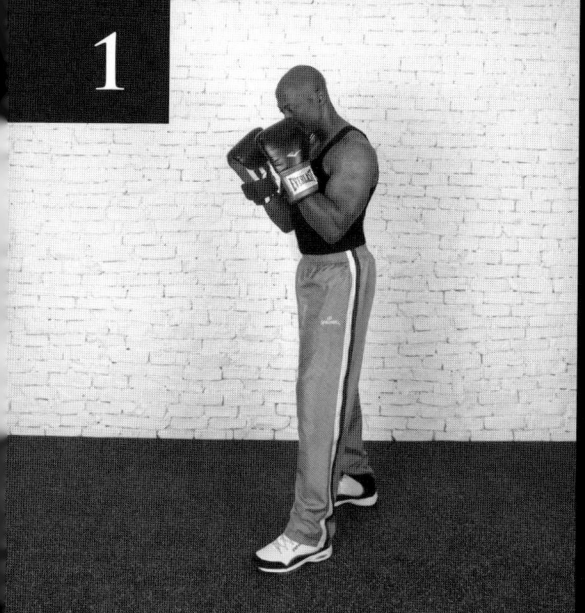

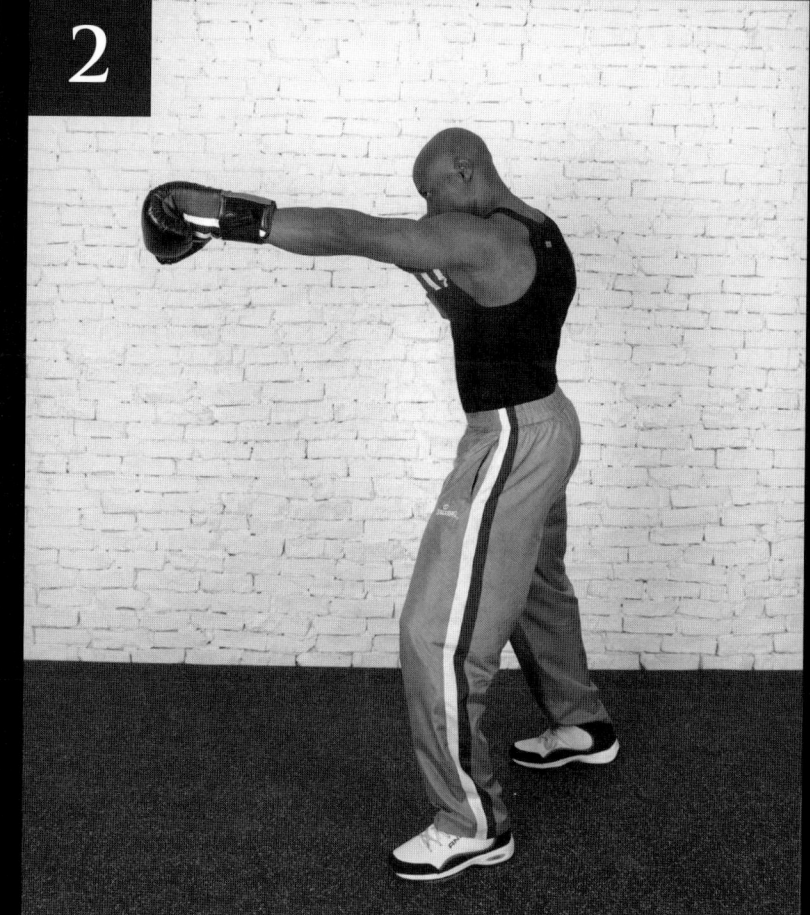

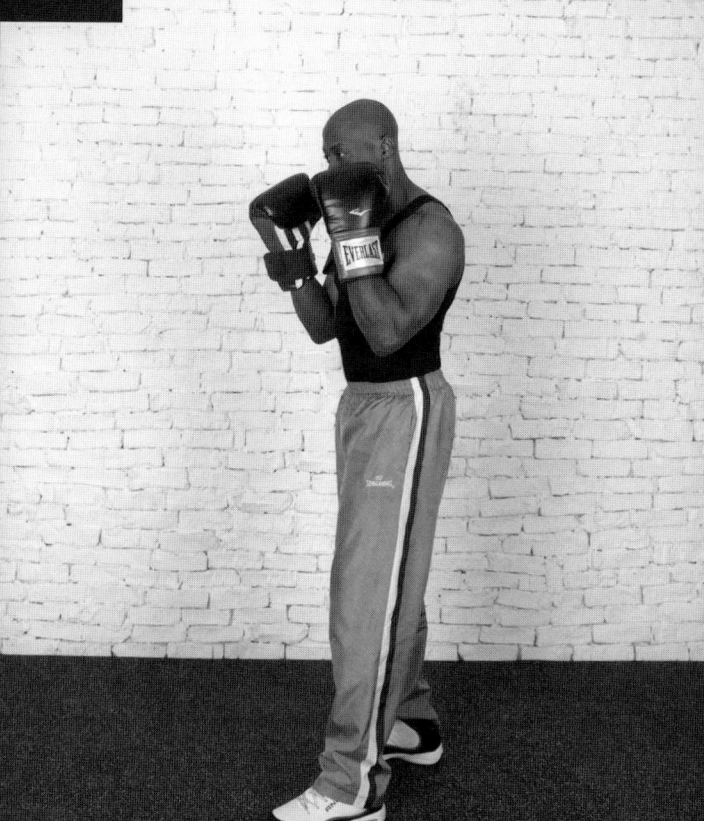

The Jab is executed by initially standing in the neutral boxer's stance with the feet slightly more than shoulder-width apart. The left foot is forward and the right foot is slightly turned out. The gloved hands should be at the level of the jaw. This punch is done by stepping forward on the left leg and twisting the left hand forward. The punch is completed by bringing the left hand back toward the face. The right hand should remain at the right jaw as cover protection.

The Cross

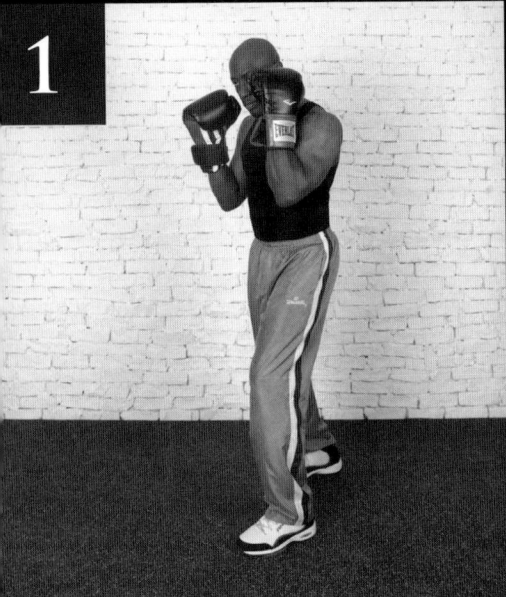

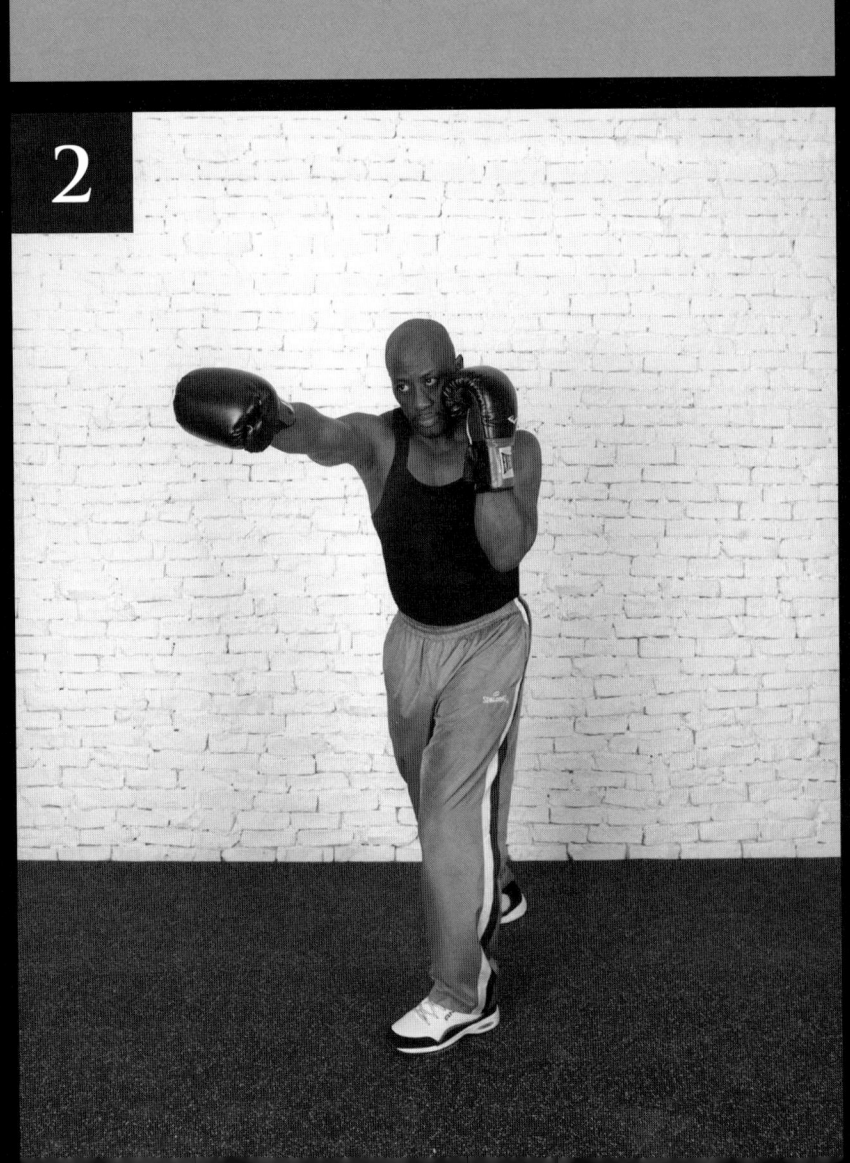

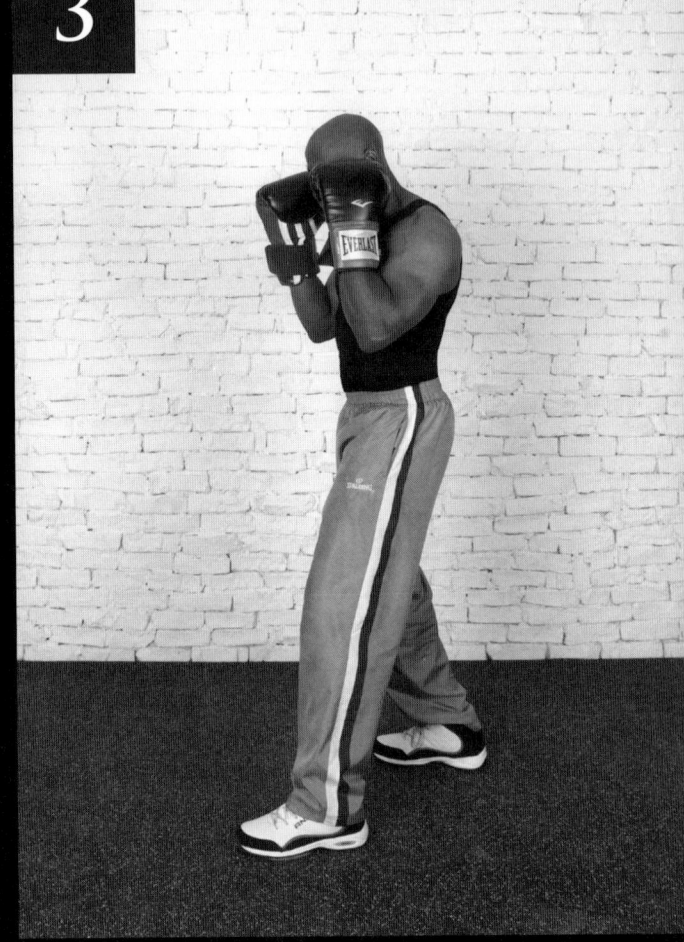

FIT TIP: Combine the Cross, Uppercut, Jab and Hook when shadow boxing or when using the heavy bag.

The exercise is done by standing in a neutral boxer's position as previously explained with both hands up toward the jaw line. The right hand is extended as it is rotated and twisted forward and a small step with the right leg is done. The exercise is ended by returning the right hand back to the face and going back to the neutral standing position.

The Uppercut

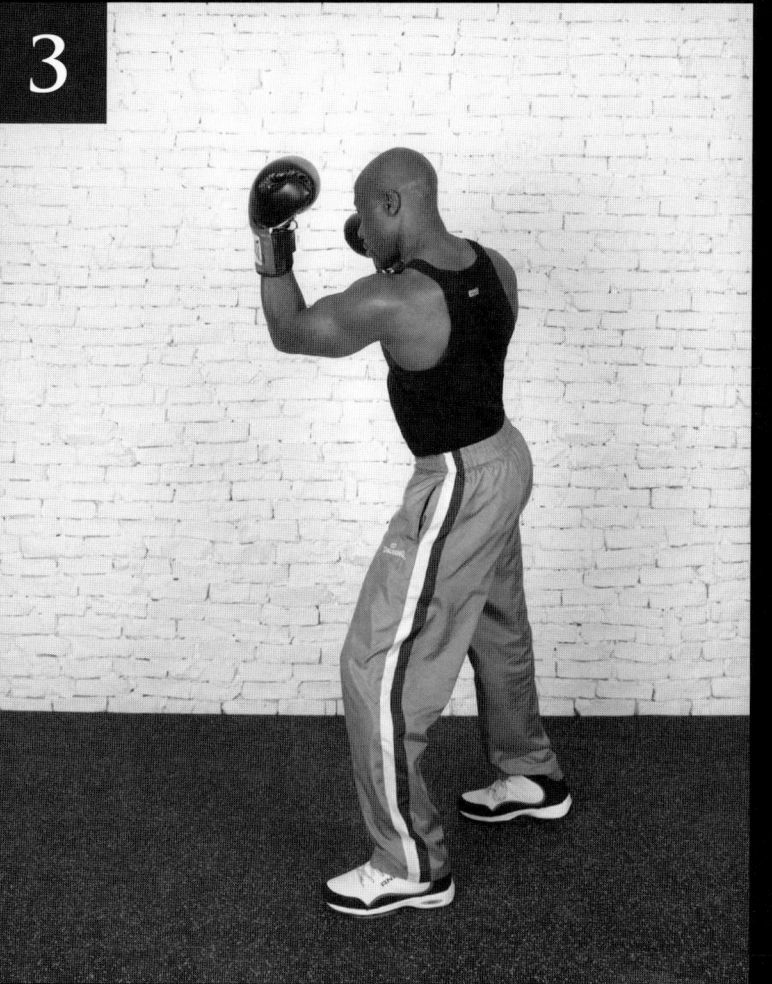

The neutral position is the starting point. Next, the left hand and body are dipped slightly down and forward. The left hand is turned with the palm toward the face with the hand going straight up from the shoulder. The elbow should stay close to the body in executing the punch and return back to the starting position.

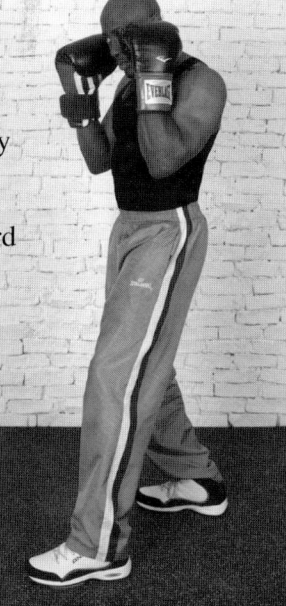

The exercise is actually called The Uppercut and Weave. The Weave is done by moving the body across to the left and downward in response to a punch coming toward the left side of the body which is dodged appropriately.

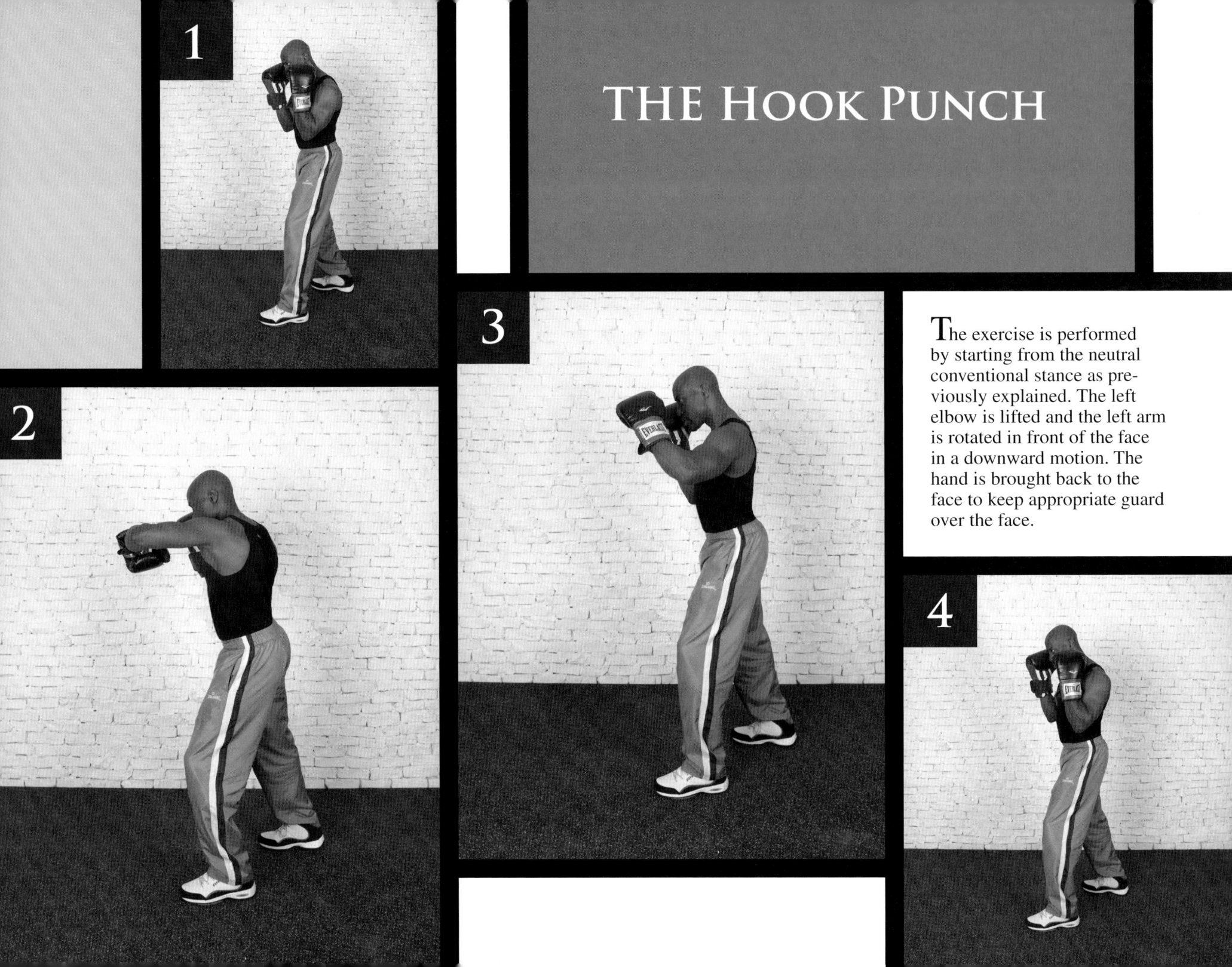

THE HOOK PUNCH

The exercise is performed by starting from the neutral conventional stance as previously explained. The left elbow is lifted and the left arm is rotated in front of the face in a downward motion. The hand is brought back to the face to keep appropriate guard over the face.

Chapter 4 • Diet

"Diet is the cornerstone for building a healthy, vibrant you!"

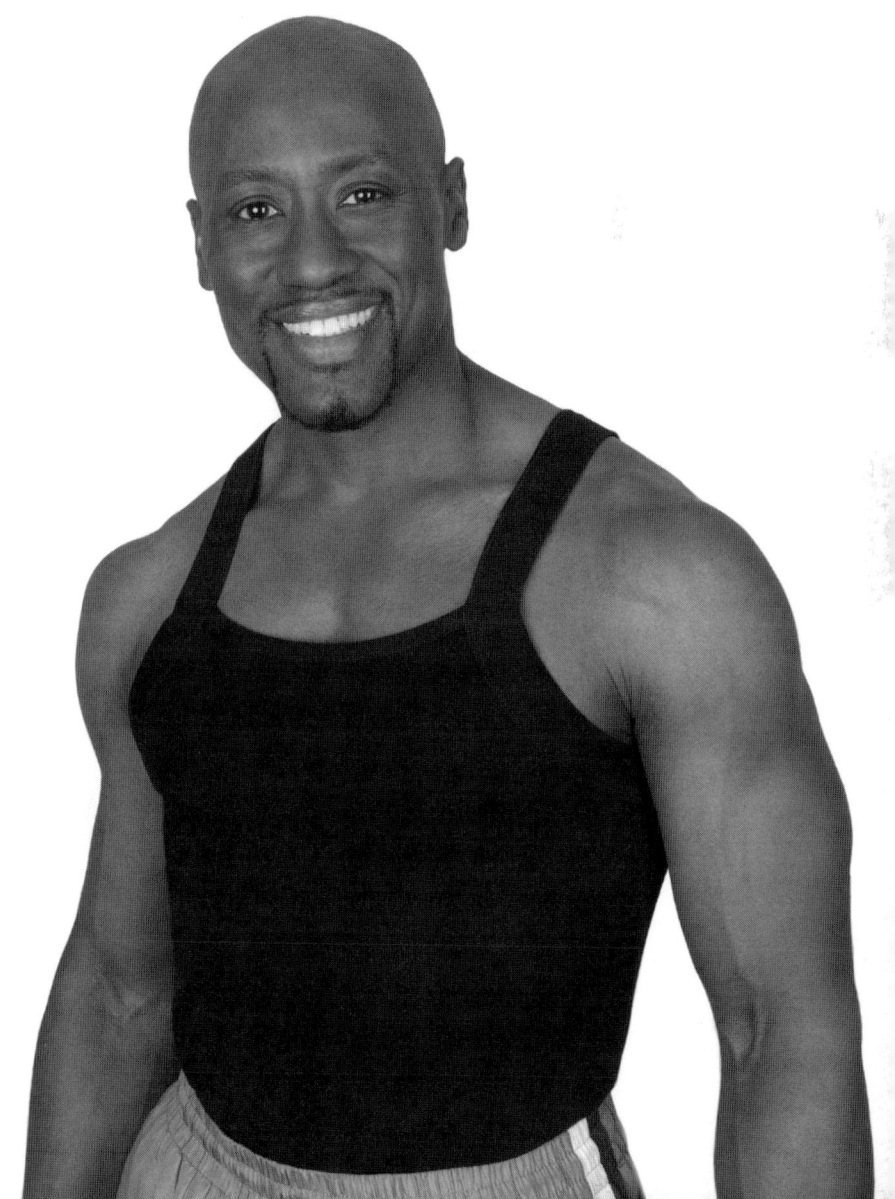

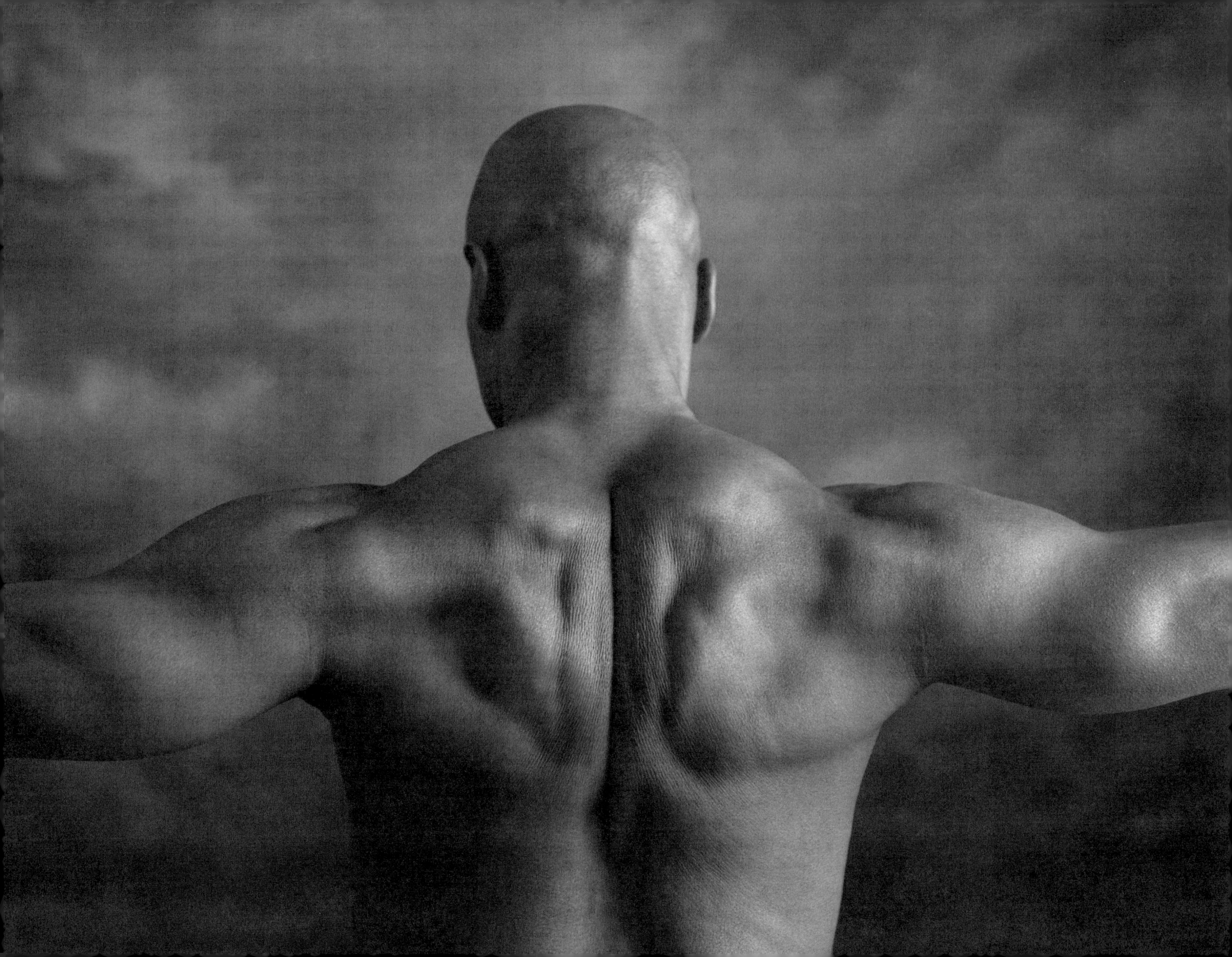

DIET

In addition to regular exercise, proper nutrition is another essential part of a healthy lifestyle. In this chapter, we will define diet and discuss how it impacts your life.

When I use the word "diet" I am not talking about depriving yourself or drastically restricting your food intake for a set period of time to help you lose weight. When I refer to diet, I mean providing your body with all the nutrients it needs to function optimally while, at the same time, providing the right amount of energy needed to achieve or maintain a healthy weight. A healthy diet, like good exercise habits, should be a way of life. In fact, without proper diet you will limit your body's ability to turn exercise into the health benefits and physique you desire. Think about it—a high performance engine cannot run well on low quality fuel!

Developing good eating habits does require time and effort, but it can also be fun and stress reducing if done properly. The types, frequency, and quantities of the foods you eat have powerful implications for your physical and emotional health as well as your mental capabilities. On the other hand, a poor diet can increase your potential for developing chronic diseases such as diabetes or heart disease, especially if they run in your family.

There is a lot to know and learn about diet, much more than I can share with you in this brief chapter. Similar to good exercise habits, creating healthier eating habits begins with accepting yourself just as you are, and being willing to take small, doable, sustainable steps in the direction you want to go. In this chapter, I will provide you with some very basic knowledge on eating a balanced, healthy diet. Hopefully, you will be able to recognize some small steps that you can take right away to improve your eating habits. I will also provide some basic information on what a healthy body weight is, and where to start if you need to lose weight. Finally, I'll share some tips I find especially helpful when it comes to food and fitness.

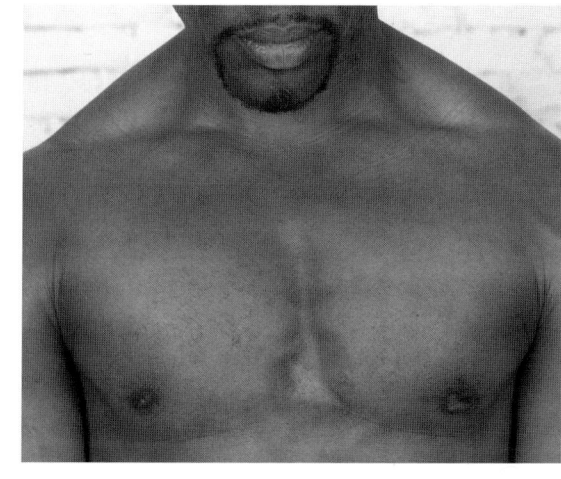

Eating healthy is about moderation; there should be no food that is off limits, unless you have food allergies or are instructed otherwise by your doctor. It's all about eating healthier foods most of the time and choosing less healthy foods much less often. Choose foods that are high in nutrients and low in calories, such as fruits, vegetables, whole grains, beans, and low-fat dairy. Minimize choosing high-calorie, low nutrient foods such as candy, cookies, pastries, chips, and processed foods. You can make big improvements in your diet, your overall health, your appearance, and your performance by making wise choices. Again, the key is moderation—and we will talk about that until the cows, the chickens, and the sardines come flying home!

Unless you are a high-performance athlete or have special dietary restrictions, everyone should be following the same basic plan when it comes to what foods to eat. Exactly how much to eat depends on your height, gender, activity level, and weight goals.

What and How Much to Eat

The FDA has just released new guidelines that make it easy to get started with eating healthier meals. According to the guidelines you should eat three meals per day. Each meal should contain the following main food groups: fruits and vegetables, grains, protein, and dairy. The FDA also recommends that one-half of your grains be whole grains, and that your dairy choices be non-fat or low-fat.

Imagine that you have a nine-inch dinner plate to fill for dinner, not the platter-sized plates that most restaurants use! One half of your plate should be fruits and vegetables. Now split the remaining half of your plate into two equal parts, one of those is for grains and the other for protein. In addition to your plate of food, you should also have some dairy, such as a medium glass of 1% or non-fat milk, some low-fat yogurt, or a small amount of low-fat cheese.

Just making these simple changes to daily meals would make a big improvement to the typical American diet! After you get comfortable with these portions and basic food groups you learn to make better choices within each food group.

All this information and more is available to you on www.choosemyplate.gov. There you can learn, for example, how to tell the difference between regular grains and whole grains, and how to get high-quality protein on your plate without a lot of the "bad" fats. You will also learn to figure out how much to eat each day in order to achieve or maintain a healthy weight. An adolescent male who is still growing and is very active in sports will need more food to fuel their body than a middle-age female who is moderately active. 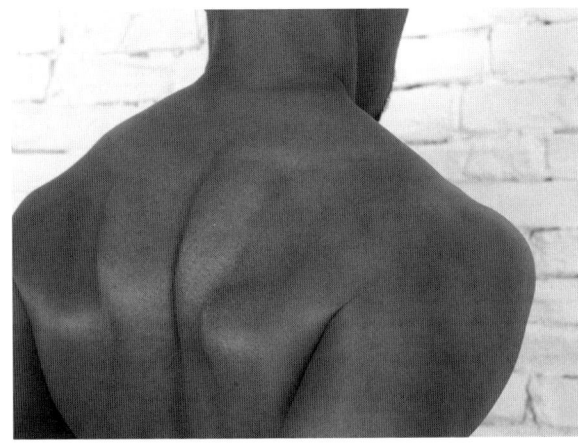 The one thing they have in common is that they both need healthy nutrition, and the plate method described above is a great place to start.

What Is a Healthy Weight?

That depends on how tall you are. A six foot man that weighs 170 pounds has a healthy, or normal, body weight. A six foot man that weighs 200 pounds will likely not. Body Mass Index, or BMI, is a measure that uses a person's height and weight in calculating his or her weight category: underweight, normal weight, overweight, or obese. Before we continue, let me remind you that it's important not to judge yourself, stress yourself, or worry about your current weight or BMI status. However, it is important to know your BMI and weight classification now so you can choose a realistic goal and create a doable plan should you need to lose weight. Most adults in this country fall outside of their normal weight range.

BMI	CATEGORY
Less than 18.5	Underweight
18.5 to 24.9	Normal weight
25 to 29.9	Overweight
30 and over	Obese

BMI is calculated by multiplying your weight measured in pounds times 703, and dividing that number by your height in inches squared. Below is an example of a BMI calculation.

If a man weighs 175 lbs and is 6 feet (72 inches) tall, his BMI would be calculated as follows:

$175 \times 703/(72 \times 72) = 23.73$

Therefore, we know that the BMI for this person is 23.73, which is considered to be in the "normal" weight category.

As you calculate your BMI, be aware that the weight category indicated may not be accurate for you. For example, a body builder will carry a lot more weight on his frame due to added muscle, not added fat. While his BMI may indicate that he is overweight, he may actually have a lower than normal amount of body fat. More of us should have that problem! What is important about the BMI is that for most people it is an accurate estimate of overall body fat content, which is a very good indicator of future health. The evidence is quite clear that elevated BMIs are associated with diabetes mellitus type 2, high blood pressure (hypertension), elevated blood cholesterol and triglyceride levels, cardiovascular disease, obstructive sleep apnea, osteoarthritis, as well as certain forms of cancer.

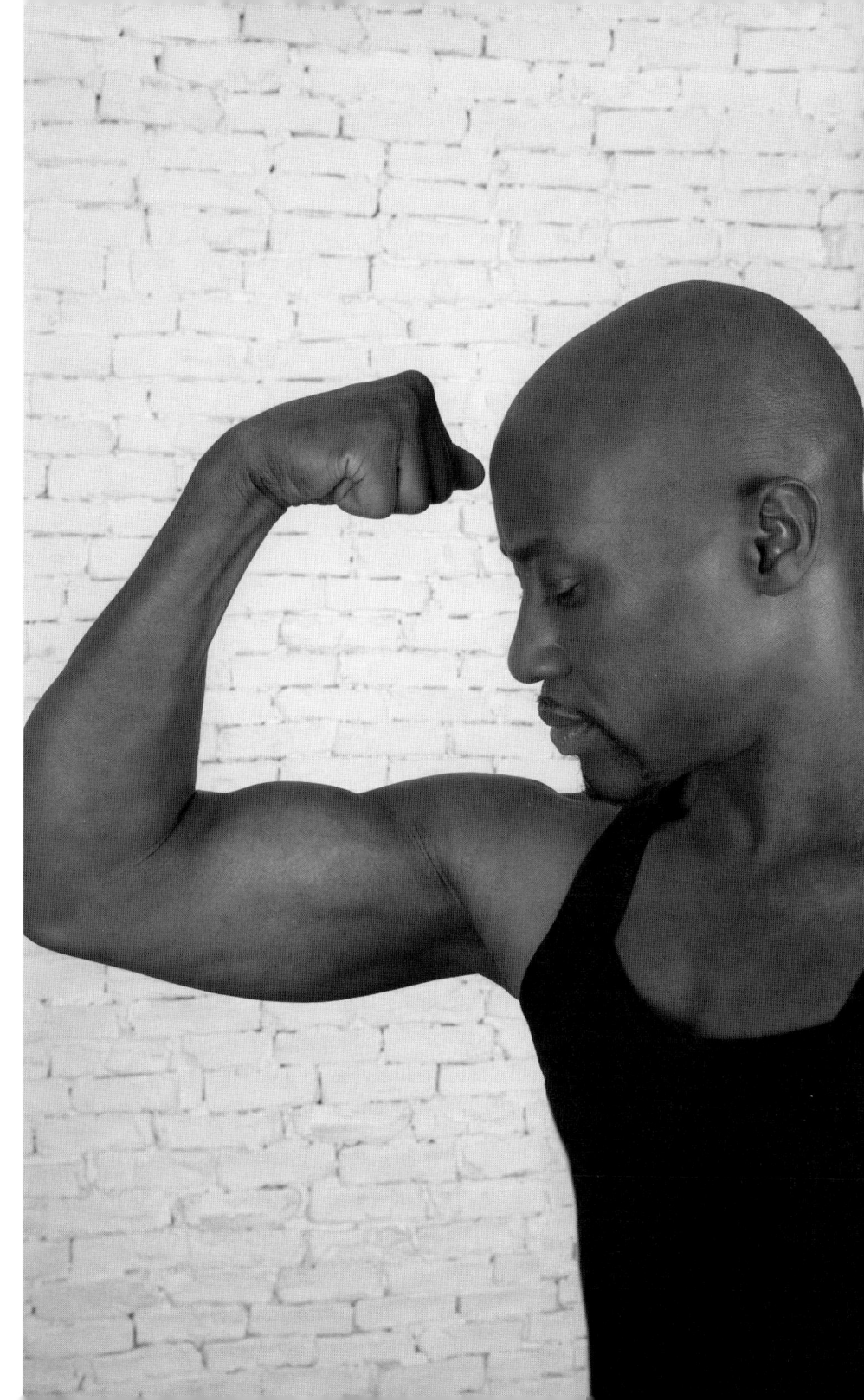

As you can see, the list of chronic diseases associated with elevated BMI levels are extensive. The bad news is that this is just the "short list." The good news is that with a healthy diet and regular physical activity, you can reduce your weight and BMI along with your risk of chronic health conditions.

About Losing Weight

Overweight and obesity are caused by both biological and behavioral factors. Research studies demonstrate that biology plays a role. For example, in one controlled study, people of the same age, sex, height and weight lost weight at very different rates even though they ate the same number of calories and did the same amount of physical activity each day. You will lose weight at a different rate than others. Don't judge or compare yourself to anyone else.

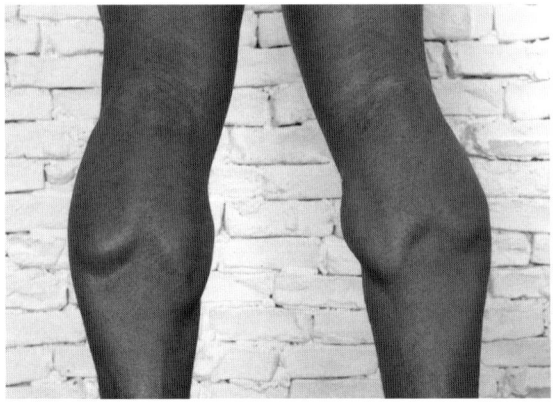

Focus your energy instead on tracking what you are doing and what results you achieve.

Take charge of your eating behavior patterns. Make slow, purposeful changes that will be easier to maintain. These adjustments to your eating plan (calorie intake) and your activity level (energy expenditure) will help you reach your weight loss goal. About 1 to 2 lbs per week is considered a healthy, sustainable weight loss.

This brings us to another important point: Obesity is not caused by very occasional episodes of overeating, but rather by a long-term imbalance between the calories taken in and the energy used through physical activity. Simply put, any calories we take in on a daily basis that our body doesn't burn get stored as fat. Over time, consuming even a few extra calories on a regular basis will result in extra inches on your waist and hips. This is why short-term or fad diets don't work. To achieve results that last, you will have to make lasting changes to your eating and exercise habits. Create a new healthier lifestyle to reveal a new you.

We all know this won't be easy for people who are overweight in this culture of "thin-is-in." Often people who carry excessive weight also carry the burden of being stigmatized and this can be traumatic. Even though overweight, where you are today is okay. What really matters is that you are making an effort to change your eating and activity habits and to enhance your health and life.

As you begin to make healthy changes to your diet, you will discover your own talent for eating and appreciating food. Avoid the detours of fad diets and weight loss supplements. Fad diets are not effective. Diets that suggest the amount of calories you consume doesn't matter as long as you keep your carbohydrate intake low enough are ineffective. Beware of diet supplement makers who make outrageous and unrealistic claims such as, "take our product and you'll lose inches while you sleep." You could imagine that if any of those products really worked there would be hardly any overweight adults left in this country! Remember, your goal is not simply to lose weight now but to maintain a healthier weight for life.

Starvation diets also are not effective because of the metabolic changes they cause. Maintaining a consistent, healthy insulin level is important to your weight and your health. This requires that you eat properly throughout the day. Start with a healthy breakfast and avoid going

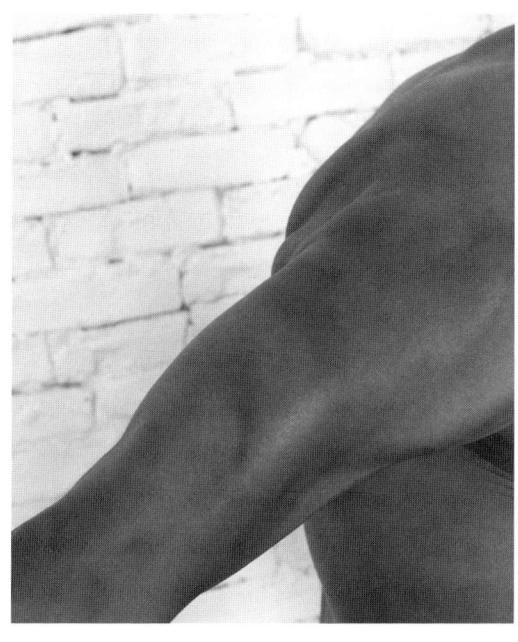

more than 4 to 5 hours between meals and snacks. A healthy diet has to be tempered with my favorite word, moderation. When you think about making changes to your diet, think about your diet as a fun way of living and a rewarding way of improving your health and enhancing your life.

As you gradually build healthier eating habits it will be helpful to plan ways to manage things that could trigger you to overeat. For example, feeling stressed, guilty, depressed, lonely, sad, bored, or excited can end up in an unplanned, excessive eating episode. Cues in your environment can also trigger what I refer to as situational overeating. Are you eating because the food is available or because you are actually hungry? For example, if you are at a party and there is a lot of food and everyone is eating, you may have a tendency to eat simply to be social. You want to participate by sharing food and drinks. Someone else at that same gathering may overeat because they feel awkward or uncomfortable in social gatherings and eating and drinking gives them something to do. Others may overeat in social situations simply because it is part of their family or native culture.

Triggers for situational overeating go beyond social situations. For example, it may be hard to stop thinking about having another piece of lemon cake when it is left sitting out on the kitchen counter. Have a slice and put the rest away. Drink some water flavoured with a slice of lemon instead of second helpings. Minimize purchasing snacks of low nutritional value and high caloric content. Always keep plenty of healthy snacks around and limit your access to less healthy ones. Reach for a small apple with some low-fat cottage cheese or whole grain crackers when you need some extra energy between meals. Do not deprive yourself. A practice of eating heavy meals and snacks loaded with saturated fats and carbohydrates and low in soluble fiber will not assist you in losing or maintaining a healthy weight.

To summarize, the biology of obesity is very complex and we still have a lot to learn. It appears that our genes do play a role, but they don't by themselves destine us to be overweight. What we understand much better are the behaviors that drive us to be overweight and obese. Your eating and activity habits are behaviors that you can take control of right now!

My Favorite "Food for Fitness" Tips

Fruits, vegetables, fiber rich foods such as whole grains and beans, and Omega-3 rich foods such as wild salmon, sardines, and flaxseeds should be a daily part of your diet. Note that foods that have a substantially high fiber content, especially when consumed with lots of water, are particularly good for promoting a feeling of satiety (fullness). Making high fiber foods a part of your daily diet can help control overeating.

There is a lot of information, and misinformation, about the benefits of taking vitamins and other nutritional supplements. In addition to a nutritionally balanced diet, I recommend adding a multivitamin and an Omega-3 supplement (EPA and DHA fatty acids). I am proactive about these supplements because clinical research has shown that Omega-3 fatty acids decrease inflammation in the body, which in turn reduces plaque formation in blood vessels, thus decreasing the risk for stroke and coronary artery disease.

Food can be like medicine or poison. Enjoy foods that are rich in vitamins, minerals and other nutrients that help your body to grow and renew itself, and to function at peak performance. Some foods will not add to your healthy lifestyle goals. Have foods such as these only occasionally and in very small quantities:

- Doughnuts
- Candy
- Fried foods
- Potato chips
- Pastries, cheesecake, cream pies, and cookies
- Regular ice cream
- White (non-whole grain) breads and pastas
- Highly refined and processed foods
- Sodas and sugary beverages

Diet and weight loss plans should be realistic. Safe weight loss is approximately two pounds per week. Do not stress if you only lose a pound each week in the beginning. Adjust your food intake and exercise level accordingly and be comforted in knowing that you are going in the right direction. Also know that you may not be able to lose all of the weight that you wish; very few people actually do. Keep in mind that weight loss of 5% to 10% may not seem like a lot. However, if you can lose that amount and keep it off, you can dramatically decrease your risk for type 2 diabetes as well as other chronic conditions while improving your health.

Finally, to eat well and manage a healthy, active lifestyle need not be complicated. You can make it fun by including others. Enrich your life; make it less stressful, simpler, and more enjoyable. *Eat well*.

Chapter 5 • Rest and Recovery

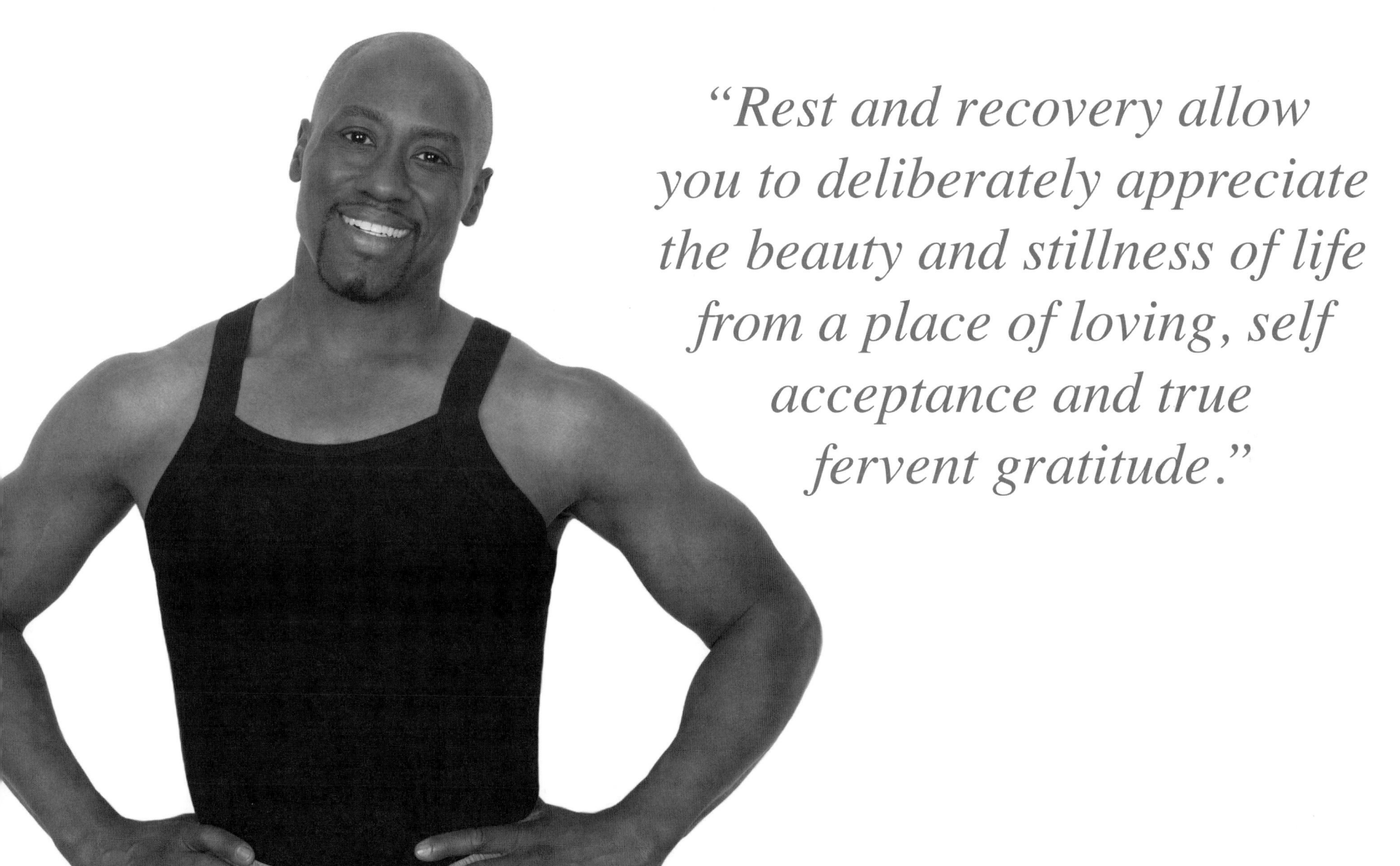

"Rest and recovery allow you to deliberately appreciate the beauty and stillness of life from a place of loving, self acceptance and true fervent gratitude."

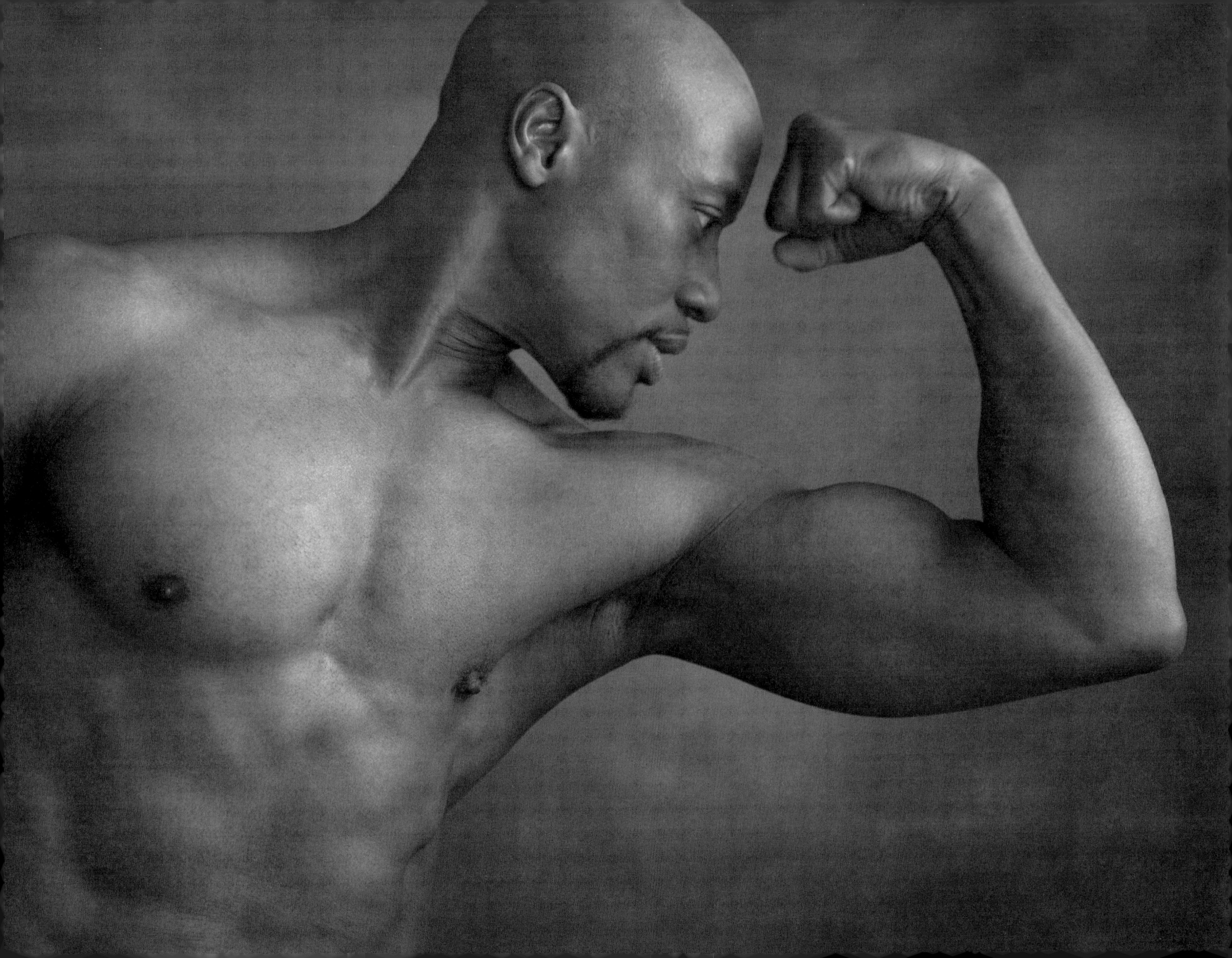

REST AND RECOVERY

A healthy lifestyle is a balanced lifestyle. Just as we need to balance the energy we take in with the energy we expend to maintain a healthy weight, it is also important to balance periods of exercise with periods of rest and relaxation. Rest is an integral part of your exercise and fitness program. It is important to let your body, mind, and spirit rejuvenate and recuperate. Rest is a vital part of the equation for attaining and maintaining good health.

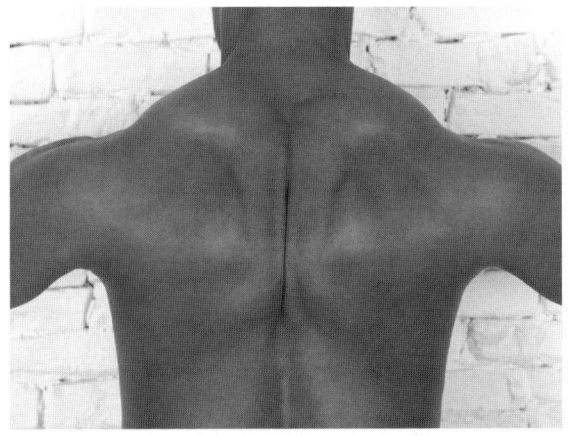

There are many different ways to allow our bodies to rest. Here are some of my favorite ways to relax:

Take 15-20 minutes a day to simply sit still and breathe. Sit in a quiet place in a chair with your back straight, shoulders relaxed, and feet flat on the floor. Begin to take long, slow deep breaths in and out at a pace that is comfortable to you. Focus on releasing the tension in your body with each exhalation. Notice how focusing on the movement of your breath allows your mind and body to become still. Appreciate the ease and power of taking a few deep breaths.

Meditation is another of my favorite ways to relax. During my daily meditation, I thank God for all the goodness in my life and for giving me the opportunity to be a vehicle for change—for myself and for others. I use this quiet time to be grateful for my family, my health and my life. Allowing time to rejuvenate on a consistent basis is vital to physical, mental, emotional and spiritual health.

There are many ways to create deep states of relaxation. Some take special training and others require special equipment or environments. Here are some simple, everyday activities that may help you find a greater sense of peace and calmness: taking time to work in your garden or taking a walk with your children, your partner, or your pet. There is great enjoyment to be found walking and spending time with those we love. I also recommend taking time to read an inspiring book or volunteering at a charity or a service organization in your community. There are many ways to find rest and rejuvenation, from exploring peace within to being of service to others.

REWARDS

Having developed skills and techniques to improve your health and well-being, and having reached your weekly goals, rewards are in order! Reward yourself as you become more fit. Be careful to select a reward that will not derail your progress or undo your hard-earned success. Here are some examples of some not-so-good rewards:

Patient: Dr. Harrison, I treated myself this weekend because I lost two pounds last week.

Dr. Harrison: What did you do?

Patient: Oh, Dr. Harrison, I had a super size hot fudge sundae. It was great. I feel good about treating myself.

Dr. Harrison: A hot fudge sundae or banana split is not a bad thing— as long as you remember the key: moderation. You can treat yourself once a week, but be careful with portions. A little bit of overeating can undo a lot of hard work. Think of splitting a regular sized dessert with your partner or a friend who would like to help you celebrate. And try not to get caught up in the habit of using food as a reward. Are there some non-food rewards you would enjoy? It's important to pay attention to how you reward yourself if you want to stay on track with your goals.

I had another patient who reported losing 50 pounds over an 8 month period. She and her husband celebrated with a bottle of champagne and chocolate-dipped strawberries.

This is a much better choice calorie-wise, and a much more appropriate reward for having lost 50 pounds as opposed to having just lost two. However, I will again take this opportunity to remind you of my favorite word — moderation. Be careful with alcohol. First, it is very high in calories. Second, it doesn't take much alcohol to begin dehydrating your system. And most importantly, alcohol can impair your judgment and reduce your resolve. This might result in an episode of overconsumption of food, alcohol, or both.

Broaden your perspective of what a good reward can be. Take some time off from work or your usual routines to participate in a charitable event or help the less fortunate in your community. The good feelings you get will last far longer than the good taste of a candy bar!

Consider buying some new clothes to enhance your improved physique, updating your hairstyle, or getting a professional massage as a reward. Treat yourself to some sessions with a personal fitness trainer or buy yourself some new workout gear. Consider joining a gym or fitness center as both a celebration and a continued commitment to a wellness lifestyle.

In this Chapter, we looked at the concept of rest, recovery and rewards in a new light. It's important to add periods of rest into your daily routines. Take a break, get some extra sleep, and enjoy quiet moments of reflection, meditation, or prayer.

I would also like to propose a new way to contemplate the concept of rest. Affirm the following:

- I will put to rest my habits and behavioral patterns that no longer serve me.

- I will put to rest things that I used to do which no longer benefit me.

- I will look at rest as releasing those things that no longer fit my vision of my future.

Redefine what rest, recovery and reward really mean in your life. Make these changes a part of your daily practice. *The Art of Fitness* can give greater depth to achieving this lifestyle in a safe and maintainable fashion.

Chapter 6 • Conclusions

"Exercise is an integral part of a healthy lifestyle. Embrace the new you!"

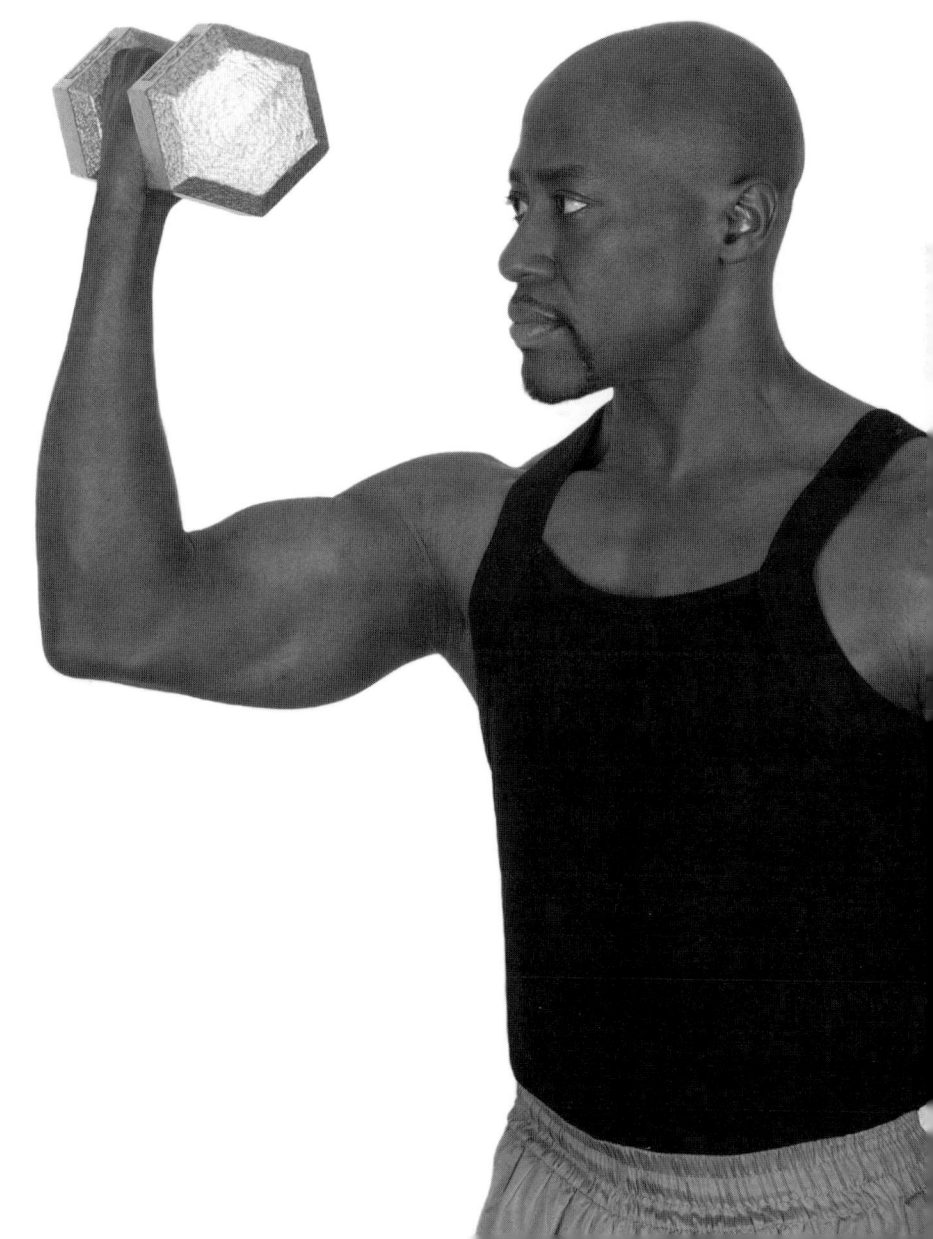

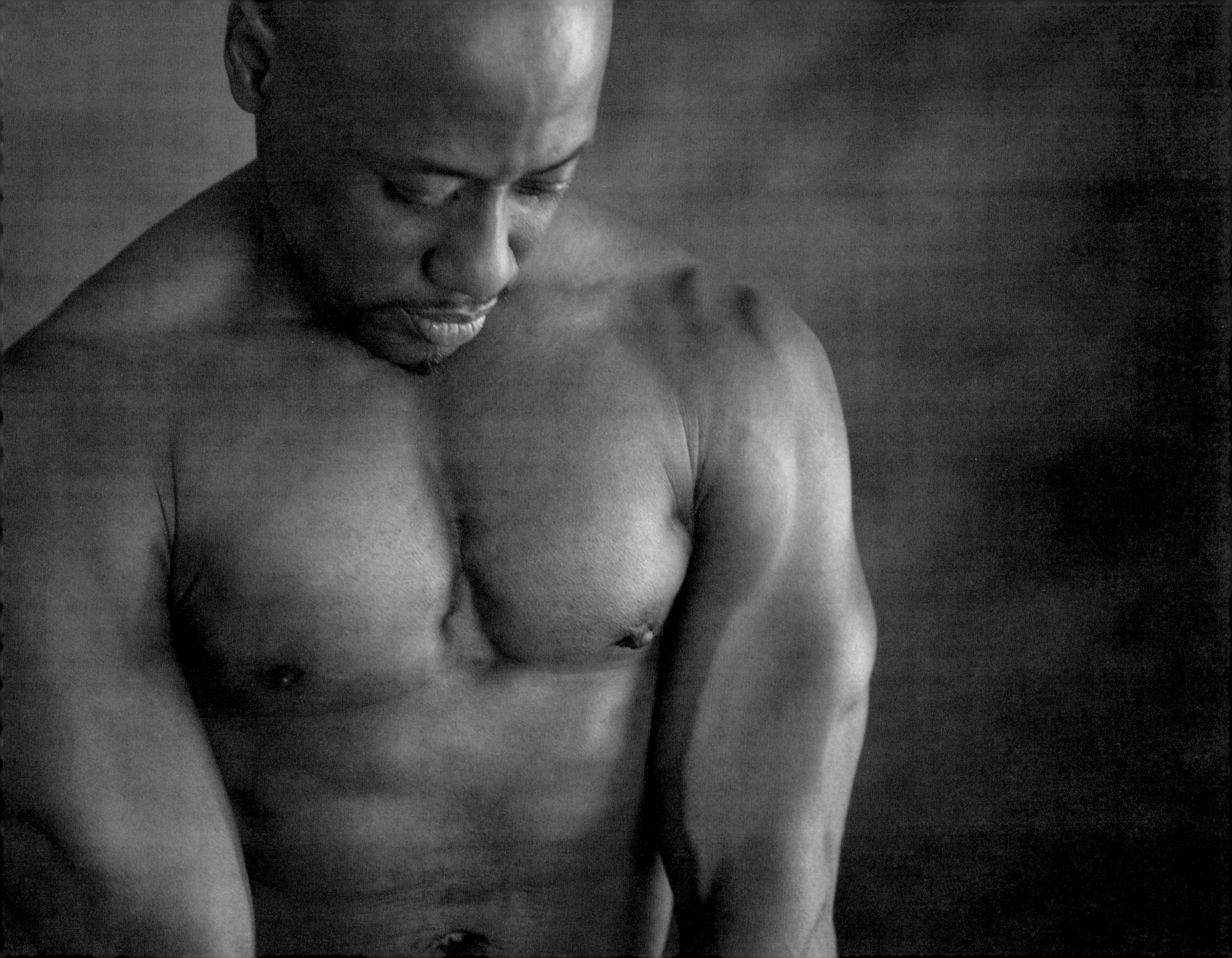

CONCLUSIONS

The *Art of Fitness* is a work of love and compassion. It was written with one goal in mind—to be of service to *you*.

This book was designed to help you start or advance your journey to physical fitness. The core principles of *The Art of Fitness*, along with the illustrated exercises, should lead you on your journey. Make *The Art of Fitness* your training companion.

We have stated that the journey to better fitness and a healthier lifestyle begins with commitment. Affirm that you will begin and continue your fitness program with a "no-matter-what" attitude. As you gain momentum, you will realize that it can be done. You have experienced greater motivation and inspiration through the techniques of this book.

Your commitment to fitness may decrease your chances of developing chronic illness, and has far reaching, positive effects on the quality of your personal, family, and work life. Your commitment to fitness can be contagious, inspiring those you love to join in on the journey to a healthier, happier life.

Learn that consistency is important in maintaining your commitment. Honor your plans to do something every day. Inevitably, from time to time, your plans will be interrupted. However, sticking with your exercise plan will aid you in reaching your goals.

Construct your program gradually by adding small steps to your exercise routine, easing into your new way of living and tracking your progress. Your new attitude of commitment and consistency will make exercise a regular part of your self-care program.

We have discussed how diet can assist you to improve your lifestyle. It's important to provide your body with the fuel it needs to convert exercise into strong bones, healthy joints, and functional, pliable muscles. Strike the right balance between total energy intake (calories you eat) with energy output (calories you burn). This is necessary to achieve and maintain a healthy body weight and contour. Moderation will be key as you fortify your body with whole grains, vegetables, fruits, lean protein, and low-fat dairy.

As you become a conscious, purposeful eater, take the time to eat slowly and enjoy the taste, texture, color, and presentation of your meals. We truly are what we eat. Choose foods that heal, restore, and fortify your body.

Exercise is another principle of healthy living, and is the central focus of *The Art of Fitness*. Exercise is something that I love to do and my hope is that you will come to share this love. Whether you are exercising alone or with others, indoors or outside, at home or at a gym, variety keeps you interested and motivated.

I am a dedicated advocate of Dynamic Core Cross-training. Cross-training adds substantial diversity to your routine. It also accelerates the development of your muscles and helps you prevent overuse injuries.

Finally, rest and recovery are just as important as the other core principles presented in *The Art of Fitness*. Take time to let your mind and body rest. Congratulate yourself on taking purposeful steps on your journey to better health. Feel good about you. Stillness does the body good on so many levels. You will learn to appreciate the stillness of meditation, prayer, or simple quietness as it energizes your mind, replenishes your body and lifts your spirits.

Life is neither good nor bad—it's only in your perception. Focus on the good and you will experience more of the good. Create a good life!

Utilize the core principles in *The Art of Fitness* to achieve new heights of health and well-being. Be grateful everyday and stay hopeful that the best is yet to come. Know that your body is beautiful as it is, you are simply enhancing your current perfection. I believe in you. Now it's your turn to believe in yourself. I wish you the greatest peace and joy on your journey. You are a winner!

Appreciate and acknowledge every step you take to enhance your life through *The Art of Fitness. Get moving!*

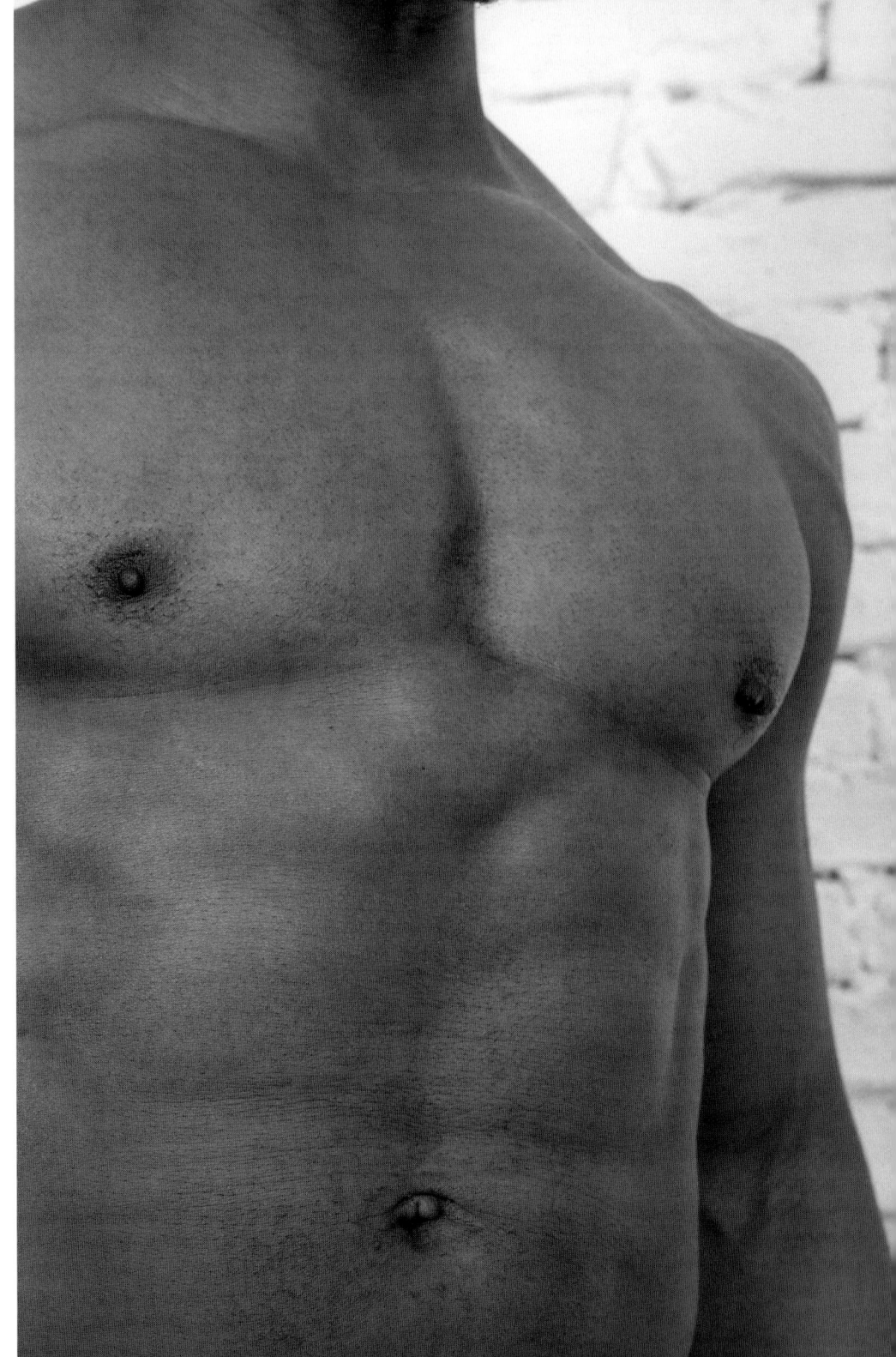

Gym Basics

Here is a list of items, which are truly investments in your life–

- A pair of well made, comfortable running or walking shoes.

- A pair of fitness or workout gloves.

- A well-marked water bottle.

- A dedicated workout towel for your gym use.

- Several pairs of hand-held weights: 2, 5, 10 and even 20 lbs.

- A pulley system, which may have resistance of 10, 15, 20 or 30 lbs.

- A fitness journal to log your progress.

- A medicine ball of 8, 10 or 20 lbs.

- A BOSU ball.

- An exercise mat.

Please note that these gym basics are simply tools that will help you use *The Art of Fitness* to enhance your life.

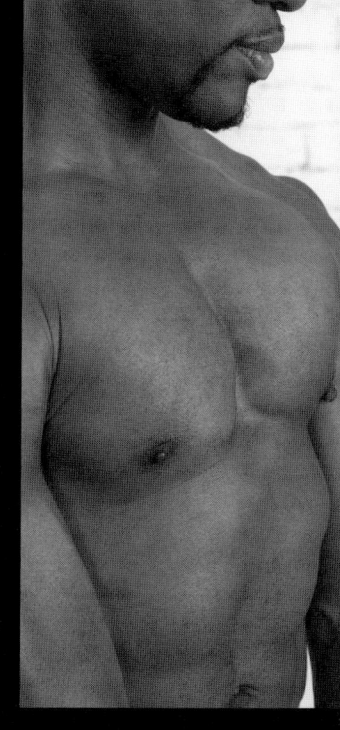

Master Exercise Guide • Part 1

Exercise	Muscle Group Affected	Level of Exercise Participant
Lateral Neck Side Bends	This allows one to stretch the muscles in the cervical area of the neck and the trapezius.	I – IV
Shoulder and Arm Overhead Stretch	This allows one to stretch the arms, shoulder, trapezius and latissimus dorsi.	I – IV
Lateral Neck Stretches	This allows one to stretch the muscles around the cervical spine and the trapezius.	I – IV
Shoulder Shrugs	This allows one to stretch the muscles around the cervical spine and the trapezius.	I – IV
Posterior Shoulder Rolls	This allows one to warm up the trapezius, cervical muscles and the latissimus dorsi.	I – IV
Shoulder and Back Stretch	This allows one to stretch the upper and midback.	I – IV
Right and Left Side Bends	This allows one to stretch the latissimus dorsi, obliques and serratus and back.	I – IV
Triceps and Torso Stretch	This allows one to stretch the triceps, latissimus, serratus, and obliques.	I – IV
Right and Left Side Bends and Torso Stretch	This allows one to stretch the back, obliques, latissimus dorsi and serratus.	II – IV
Deep Lateral Side Bends and Torso Stretch	This allows one to stretch deeply the latissimus, serratus, obliques, quadriceps and hamstrings.	II – IV
Trapezius and Neck (Cervical) Stretch	This allows one to stretch the trapezius and cervical muscles.	I – IV
Quadriceps, Hamstring and Calf Stretch Combined	This allows one to stretch the quadriceps, hamstrings, calves and the latissimus dorsi.	II – IV
Torso and Oblique Stretch	This allows one to stretch the serratus, as well as the obliques as well as the muscles of the back.	I – IV
Squats and Seated Calf Raises	This exercise allows one to stretch the calves, muscles of the lower leg as well as quadriceps and hamstrings.	II – IV
Hamstring and Quadriceps Stretch and Balance	This exercise allows one to stretch the quadriceps and hamstrings as well as providing appropriate balance technique.	III and IV

Exercise	Muscle Group Affected	Level of Exercise Participant
Toe Tap, Buttocks Tone, and Balance Exercise	This exercise allows one to tone and stretch the gluteal muscles as well as hamstrings and quadriceps.	III and IV
Calf Stretch, Hamstring Stretch and Balance Exercise	This allows one to stretch the calf muscles, hamstrings, latissimus and tibialis anterior.	I – IV
Hamstring Stretch	This allows one to stretch the hamstrings.	I – IV
Super Hamstring Stretch and Balance	This allows one to extensively stretch the hamstrings.	III – IV
Lateral Super Hamstring Stretch and Balance	This allows one to stretch the hamstrings as well as the calf muscles because the toes are flexed toward you.	IV
Back Stretch	This allows one to stretch the muscles of the back as well as the calves because the toes pointed toward you.	I – IV
Seated Hamstring and Calf Stretch	This allows one to stretch the hamstrings, calf muscles and the back.	I – IV
Standing Pulley Squats and Shoulder Press (Military Style)	This allows one to work the quadriceps, hamstrings, shoulders and triceps.	I – IV
Anterior Deltoid Raises	This allows one to work the anterior shoulder muscles and the latissimus dorsi.	I – IV
Posterior Deltoid Raises	This works the posterior shoulder muscles and the latissimus dorsi.	II- IV
Seated Biceps Hammer Curls	This allows one to work the biceps of the upper extremity.	I – IV
Combination Biceps Curl and Shoulder Press	This allows one to work the biceps, shoulders and forearms.	II – IV
Seated Inner Leg Biceps Curls	This works the biceps and forearms.	II – IV
Chair Triceps Dips	This works the chest pectoral muscles, triceps and forearms.	I – IV
Rotator Cuff Stabilizing Side Raises (External Rotation)	This exercise allows one to strengthen the muscles of the rotator cuff and forearms. Target Muscle: Infraspinatus*	I – IV
Rotator Cuff Stabilizing Side Raises (Internal Rotation)	This exercise allows one to strengthen the muscles of the rotator cuff and forearms. Target Muscle: Subscapularis*	I – IV

*Very Important Exercise to maintain shoulder stability and to prevent injury to the shoulder

Exercise	Muscle Group Affected	Level of Exercise Participant
Triceps Kickbacks	This allows strengthening of the triceps and forearms.	I – IV
Overhead Triceps Extensions	This allows strengthening the triceps and forearms.	II – IV
Combined Front Deltoid Rows and Lateral Triceps Extensions	This allows one to strengthen the deltoids, triceps and forearms.	II – IV
Front Dumbbell Deltoid Rows	This allows one to work the deltoids (Specifically the anterior deltoids.) and the trapezius.	I – IV
Combined Rhomboid Rows Tricep Kickbacks	This strengthens the rhomboids, triceps and forearms.	II – IV
Front Lateral One Arm Dumbbell Lat Rows	This exercise strengthens the latissimus, obliques and serratus.	II – IV
Variation of a Lower Triceps Kickback	Strengthens the triceps and the forearms.	I – IV
Posterior Wrist Curls of the Forearm (Wrist Extension)	Strengthens the extensors of the forearm and wrist.	I – IV
Anterior Wrist Curls (Wrist Flexion)	Strengthens the flexors of the wrist and forearm.	I – IV
Leg Extensions	This exercise strengthens the quadriceps.	I – IV
Hamstring Curls	This strengthens the hamstring muscles of the posterior thigh.	I – IV
Short Curl Bar Upright Rolls	This exercise strengthens the trapezius and forearm muscles.	II – IV
Combined Upright Rows and Squats	This exercise strengthens the quadriceps, hamstrings, trapezius and back.	II – IV
Bench Assisted Lunge	This strengthens the gluteal muscles, quadriceps and hamstrings.	III – IV
Bench Squats with Weights	This strengthens the quadriceps, gluteal muscles, hamstrings and forearms.	II – IV
Wide Squat with Anterior Deltoid Raises	This strengthens the deltoids, latissimus and forearms.	II – IV

Exercise	Muscle Group Affected	Level of Exercise Participant
Wide Squat with Weight	This strengthens the quadriceps, hamstrings and back.	II – IV
Forward Standard Calf Raises	This strengthens the calf muscles, the gastroc-soleus complex and tibialis anterior.	I – IV
External Calf Raises	This works the outer aspect of the calf muscles.	I – IV
Internal Calf Raises	This works the inner aspect of the calf muscles.	I – IV
Lateral View of Calf Stretch	This allows stretching of the gastroc-soleus complex and tibialis anterior muscles.	I – IV
Lateral Rhomboid Raises	This allows strengthening of the rhomboids and posterior deltoids.	I – IV
Posterior Pulley Raises	This strengthens the posterior deltoids and the latissimus dorsi.	II – IV
Declined Bench Press	This works the lower pectoral muscles of the chest, triceps and the forearms.	I – IV
Inclined Bench Press	This works the upper pectoral muscle of the chest, triceps and forearms.	I – IV
Inclined Pectoral Flys	This works the pectoral muscles of the chest, latissimus, arms and the forearms.	II – IV
Declined Bench Press Flys	This exercise works the pectoral muscles lower chest, latissimus, arms and the forearms.	II – IV
Standard Bench Press	This works the pectoral muscles, triceps, arms and forearms.	I – IV
Seated Safe Shoulder Shrugs	This allows strengthening of the trapezius and forearms. (Keep the back straight during this exercise.)	I – IV
Medicine Ball Side Twist	This is for stretching and strengthening the obliques, serratus and back.	II – IV
Short Medicine Ball Twist	This strengthens and stretches the obliques and serratus.	I – IV
Standard Bosu Ball Plank and Push Up	This exercise works the triceps and core muscles.	II – IV

Exercise	Muscle Group Affected	Level of Exercise Participant
BOSU Ball Flying Push Ups (also called Superman Push Ups)	This exercise strengthens the chest, triceps and core muscles.	IV
Advanced Superman BOSU Push Up	This allows strengthening of the triceps, chest and core muscles.	IV
Triangle BOSU Push-Up	This strengthens the chest pectoral muscles, triceps, arms and core muscles.	II – IV
Modified Triangle BOSU Push- Up	This exercise allows strengthening of the chest pectoral muscles, triceps, arms and core muscles.	II – IV
Oblique Mountain Climbers	This allows strengthening of the core muscles, obliques, serratus and latissimus.	III – IV
Wide-based Spider Push Up	This allows strengthening of the chest pectoral muscles, core muscles, arms, triceps and forearms.	III – IV
Mountain Climbers	This strengthens the quadriceps, hamstrings, forearms and core muscles.	II – IV
Exchange Medicine Ball Push- Ups	This strengthens the core muscles, chest pectoral muscles, triceps and forearms.	III – IV
Medicine Ball Modified Push- Up with Extension	This strengthens the core and pectoral muscles, triceps, forearms and back.	III- IV
Side Perspective Triangle Push Ups	This strengthens core muscles, chest pectoral muscles, triceps, arms and forearms.	II – IV
Modified Triangle Push Ups	This strengthens core and pectoral muscles, triceps, arms and forearms.	II – IV
Front/Anterior Perspective Standard Triceps Push Up	This strengthens the core and pectoral muscles, arms, triceps and forearms.	II – IV
Same Side Plank and Knee Lift	This strengthens core muscles, quadriceps and hamstrings.	III – IV
Half-ups	This strengthens abdominal core muscles.	II – IV
Knee Raises from the 6-inch Position	This strengthens the abdominal muscles. (Hand should be under the buttocks to protect the back.)	IV
Balance Plank	This strengthens core muscles.	III – IV

Exercise	Muscle Group Affected	Level of Exercise Participant
BOSU Ball Plank	This strengthens core muscles as well as forearm and chest pectoral muscles.	II – IV
BOSU Ball Hyperextension Balance Plank.	This strengthens the core muscles and lower back muscles also increases overall spatial balance of muscles.	III – IV
One Arm Side Plank	This strengthens all core muscles.	III – IV
Double Balance Elbow Plank	Strengthens core muscles.	III – IV
Regular and Abdominal Crunch	Abdominal muscles.	I – IV
Elevated Leg Crunches	The abdominal muscles.	II – IV
Extended Leg Crunches	Abdominal muscles.	II – IV
Seated Leg Lifts	Core, quadriceps, hamstrings, abdominals and hip flexors.	III – IV

Master Exercise Guide • Part 2

Exercise	Muscle Group Affected	Level of Exercise Participant
Combined V-ups and Leg Lifts	This exercise strengthens the hip flexors, abdominals and core muscles.	III – IV
Overhead Leg Lifts	This strengthens the core abdominal muscles as well as hip flexors.	III – IV
Superman Rocky Overhead Leg Lifts	This strengthens the abdominal core muscles and hip flexors.	IV
The Plank Exercise also called the Elbow Bridge Plank Exercise	This strengthens core muscles.	II – IV
The Captain's Chair Core Position	This strengthens the core muscles as well as the forearms. (Avoid swinging during this exercise.)	II – IV
Triceps Dips (from the Captain's Chair)	This strengthens the triceps as well as the core muscle. The core muscles assist with stabilizing the torso and in preventing swinging during this exercise.	III – IV
Captain's Chair Knee Lifts	This strengthens the core abdominal muscles as well as the hip flexors.	II – IV
Captain's Chair Combined Knee Lifts and Leg Extensions	This strengthens the quadriceps, hamstrings, hip flexors, abdominals and core muscles.	III – IV
Wide Grip Pull-Ups	This strengthens the triceps, biceps, trapezius, latissimus dorsi, forearms and core muscles.	II – IV
The De-Rotation Straight Leg Lifts	This exercise strengthens the abdominal core muscles, hip flexors and muscles of the arms.	III – IV
Captain's Chair Oblique/Side Leg Lifts	This exercise strengthens the obliques, serratus anterior, abdominals and core muscles.	II – IV
Flying Triceps Dips or Superman Dips	This strengthens the triceps, forearms and pectoral chest muscles and the core muscles.	IV
Roman Chair Sit-ups	This strengthens the lower back as well as the abdominal core muscles and hip flexors.	II – IV
Lateral/Side Roman Chair Sit-Ups	This strengthens the obliques, serratus anterior, rectus abdominis, and core muscles.	III – IV
Roman Chair Back Extensions	This strengthens the lower back, abdominals and core muscles.	II – IV

Exercise	Muscle Group Affected	Level of Exercise Participant
Captain's Chair Straight Leg Raises	This strengthens the abdominals, core muscles and the hip flexors.	II – IV
6-inch Crunches	This strengthens the abdominals and core muscles.	IV
Bicycle Crunches	This strengthens the abdominal core muscles and the hip flexors.	II – IV
Straight Leg V-up Crunches	This strengthens the abdominal core muscles and the hip flexors.	III – IV
Lateral Side Crunches (with Elevated Knees)	This strengthens the core abdominal muscles, serratus anterior, and the obliques.	III – IV
Standing Front Abdominal Curl and Knee Lift	This strengthens the core abdominal muscles, back muscles and the hip flexors.	III – IV
Standing Lateral Side Crunches and Knee Lift	This strengthens the hip flexors, hamstrings, obliques and the core muscles.	III – IV
Standard Forward Abdominal Crunch (with the Straight Leg Elevated)	This strengthens the abdominal core, gluteal muscles and the hip flexors.	III – IV
Lateral Side Crunch (with Lateral Straight Leg Raise)	This strengthens the core abdominal muscles, obliques, serratus and gluteal muscles.	III – IV
Combined One Arm Military Shoulder Press and Knee Lift	This strengthens the hip flexors, abdominal core muscles, the deltoids, obliques and the serratus.	II – IV
Combined One Arm Military Shoulder Press and Lateral Knee Lift.	This strengthens the deltoids, abdominal core muscles, back and gluteal muscles.	III – IV
Jumping Rope	This is aerobics training.	I – IV
Single Leg Jumping	This is aerobic training.	II – IV
Shadow Boxing: The Jab, The Cross, The Upper Cut, and The Hook	Arms, forearms, latissimus dorsi and the core muscles.	I – IV

INDEX

abs and core strengthening, 113
advanced "Superman" BOSU ball push-up, 118
aerobic equipment, 4
aerobics, 4, 17, 25
anterior deltoid raises, 56
anterior wrist curl, 80

back stretch, 49
balance plank, 138
bench assisted lunge, 88
bench squat with weights, 90
bicycle crunch, 178
blogging about exercise goals, 3
blood glucose level, 3
blood pressure, 3–5
blood sugar levels, 3
body mass index (BMI), 196–197
BOSU ball flying push-up, 117
BOSU ball hyperextension balance plank, 140
BOSU ball modified triangle push-up, 121
BOSU ball plank, 139
BOSU ball triangle push-up, 120

calf and hamstrings stretch and balance exercise, 45
calories, 5
Captain's Chair core position, 155
cardiovascular health, 4
chair triceps dip, 64
challenges to committing to exercise, 4–5
cholesterol level, 3
combination biceps curls and shoulder press, 60
combined front deltoid rows and lateral triceps extensions, 72
combined knee lifts and leg extensions, 160
combined one-arm military shoulder press and anterior knee lift, 185
combined one-arm military shoulder press and lateral knee lift, 186
combined rhomboid rows and triceps kickbacks, 74
combined upright row and squats, 83
combined V-ups and leg lifts, 148
commitment to exercise, 1, 3–5, 207
conclusions, 205–207
consistency, 11, 13, 207
core strengthening, 18–19, 25, 113, 155, 208
cross, (boxing), 190
crunch exercises, 143–145, 177–180, 182–184

declined bench press, 104
declined bench press flys, 110
deep lateral side bends and torso stretch, 37
depression as commitment challenge, 5, 8
derotation straight leg lifts, 164
diet, 193, 195, 207
double balance elbow plank, 142
dynamic core cross-training, 13, 18–19, 25, 208

elevated leg crunch, 144
exercise
  basics of, 15, 17
  commitment and challenges to, 3, 6, 9
  consistency of, 13
  importance of, 207
extended leg crunch, 145
external calf raises, 95

family commitments, 7
fitness levels, 4, 13, 20–25
flying triceps dip or "Superman" dip, 168
food groups, 4
forward standard calf raises (Captain's Chair), 94

front and lateral one-arm dumbbell lat (latissimus dorsi) rolls, 76
front dumbbell deltoid rows, 73
front perspective standard triceps push-up, 134

glucose, 3
goals, 3–4
guilt, 4
gym membership, 3, 6, 8
gym basics, 209

half-up exercise, 136
hamstring and quadriceps stretch and balance, 42
hamstring curls, 87
hamstring stretch, 46
hamstring super stretch and balance, 47
hook punch, (boxing), 192

illness and effects on exercise, 7–8
incline bench press, 106
incline pectoral fly, 108
internal calf raises, 96

jab, (boxing), 189
journal for tracking goals, 3
jumping rope, 187

kinetic stretching, 18
knee lifts (Captain's Chair), 158
knee raises from the 6-inch position, 137

lateral hamstring super stretch and balance, 48
lateral neck side bends, 28
lateral neck stretch, 30
lateral rhomboid raises, 100
lateral side crunch with elevated knees, 180

lateral side crunch with lateral straight leg raise, 184
lateral side profile of wide squat with anterior deltoid (shoulder), 93
lateral view of calf stretch, 98
laziness as commitment challenge, 5, 8
leg extension exercise, 86

Master Exercise Guide: Part 1, 210–215
Master Exercise Guide: Part 2, 216–217
medicine ball exchanged push-ups, 126
medicine ball modified push-up with extension, 128
medicine ball side twist, 114
moderation, 195–196, 207
modified triangle push-up, 132
money, lack of, 5
motivation, 207
mountain climber exercise, 125

nutrition, 200

obesity, causes of, 198
oblique exercises, 40, 122
oblique mountain climber exercise, 122
omega-3, 200
one-arm side plank, 141
overhead leg lift, 150
overhead triceps extension, 70
overweight, 198

pain, as commitment challenge, 5, 7
physical baseline, 3, 19
plank exercise, 154
posterior deltoid raises, 58
posterior deltoid row, 84
posterior pulley raises, 101
posterior shoulder rolls, 32
posterior wrist curls of the forearm, 79
preservatives and food choices, 4

quadriceps, hamstring and calf stretch combined, 39

regular abdominal crunch, 143
regular bench press, 102
relaxation, 203
rest and recovery, 201, 203, 208
rewarding yourself, 4, 203–204
right and left side bends, 34
right and left side bends and torso stretch, 36
Roman chair back extension exercises, 174
Roman chair sit-up, 170
rotator cuff stabilizing side raises, external rotation, 66
rotator cuff stabilizing side raises, internal rotation, 67
running, 4

salt-free food, 4
same side plank and knee lift, 135
seated biceps hammer curl, 59
seated hamstring and calf stretch, 50
seated inner leg biceps curl, 62
seated leg lift, 146
seated safe shoulder shrug, 112
short curl bar upright row, 82
short medicine ball twist, 115
shoulder and arm overhead stretch, 29
shoulder and back stretch, 33
shoulder shrug, 31
side bend, right and left, torso stretch, 24, 26
side leg lifts, 166
side perspective triangle push-up, 130
side Roman chair sit-up, 172
side views of the declined bench press, 105
side views of the declined bench press flys, 111
single leg jumping rope, 188
six-inch crunches, 177
spouse as supporter, 3
squats and seated calf raises, 41
standard BOSU ball plank and push-up, 116
standing forward abdominal crunch, 183

standing forward flexion lateral deltoid raises, 55
standing front abdominal curl and knee lift, 181
standing lateral side crunch and knee lift, 182
standing pulley biceps curl, 54
standing pulley squat and shoulder press, 52
starvation diets, 199
straight leg raises, 176
straight leg V-up crunch, 179
strength training, 17
stress as commitment challenge, 5, 7
stretching, 17, 26–27
sugar-free food, 4
"Superman" overhead leg lifts, 152
support system, 3
swimming, 4

television as commitment challenge, 5, 9
time as commitment challenge, 5
toe tap, buttocks tone and balance exercise, 44
torso and obliques stretch, 40
trapezius and neck (cervical) stretch, 38
triceps and torso stretch, 35
triceps dip, 156
triceps kickbacks, 68
triggers for overeating, 199
triglycerides, 3

uppercut, (boxing), 191

variation of a lower triceps kickback, 78

walking, 3, 4
water aerobics, 4
weight baseline, 3
wide based spider push-up, 124
wide grip pull-up, 162
wide squat with anterior deltoid (shoulder) raises, 92
wide squat with weight, 91
workout partner, 3, 13